Grandma Miller
we ♡ you!
♡Andrew
+
Abby

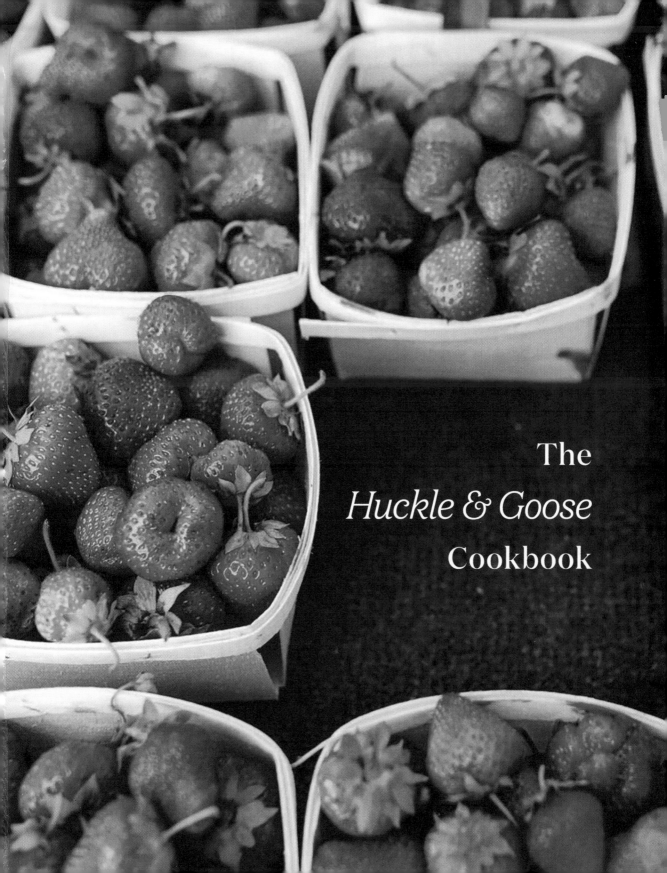

The
Huckle & Goose
Cookbook

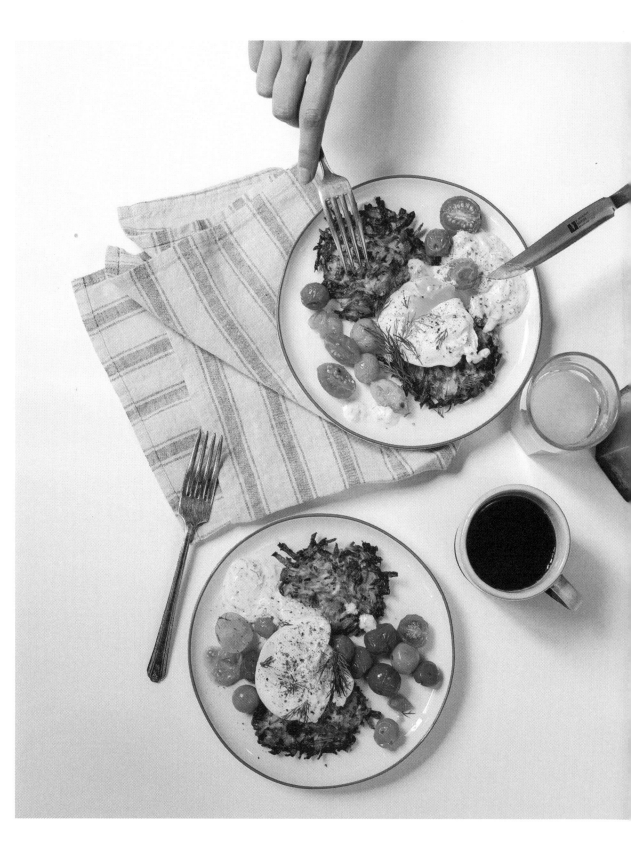

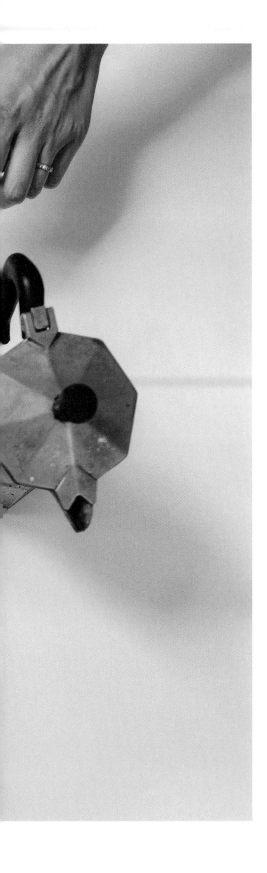

THE
Huckle
& Goose
COOKBOOK

---

152 Recipes & Habits

to Cook More, Stress Less,

and Bring the Outside In

ANCA TODERIC & CHRISTINE LUCACIU

PHOTOGRAPHS BY
MANDALYN RENICKER

HARPER WAVE
An Imprint of HarperCollins*Publishers*

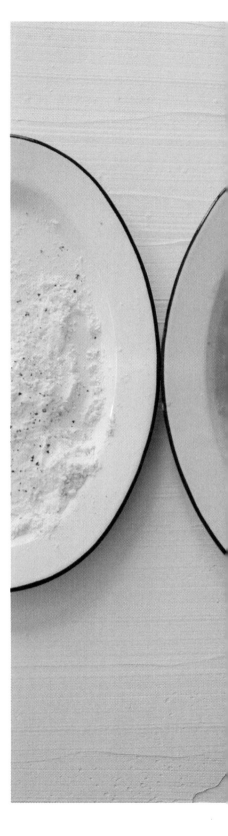

HarperCollins books may be purchased for educational, business, or sales promotional use. For information, please email the Special Markets Department at SPsales@harpercollins.com.

FIRST EDITION

Designed by Leah Carlson-Stanisic
All photographs © Mandalyn Renicker
Cover photograph © Christine Lucaciu
Cover designed by Cast Iron Design

Library of Congress Cataloging-in-Publication Data has been applied for.

ISBN 978-0-06-283968-8

19 20 21 22 23   LSC   10 9 8 7 6 5 4 3 2 1

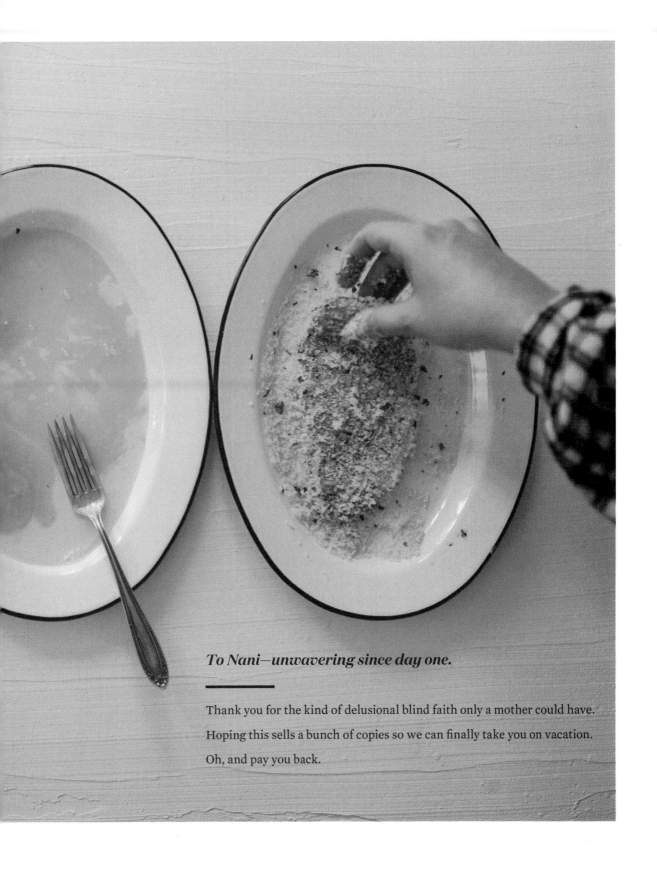

To Nani—unwavering since day one.

Thank you for the kind of delusional blind faith only a mother could have.

Hoping this sells a bunch of copies so we can finally take you on vacation.

Oh, and pay you back.

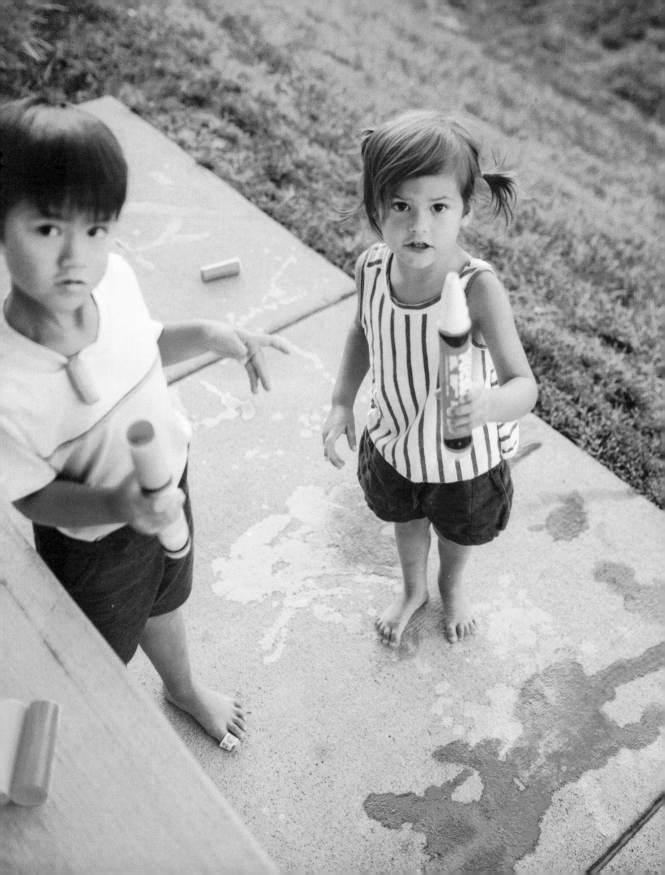

HUMAN *(hyu mən)* NOUN: person that needs to eat daily and figure out why they exist.

———————

Feels a little weighty for a cookbook, huh?

But how well we accomplish the big life stuff is directly dependent on how well we eat.

We've just gotta plan it out a little.

Welcome to *Huckle & Goose*. Where good food, life habits, and nature all connect.

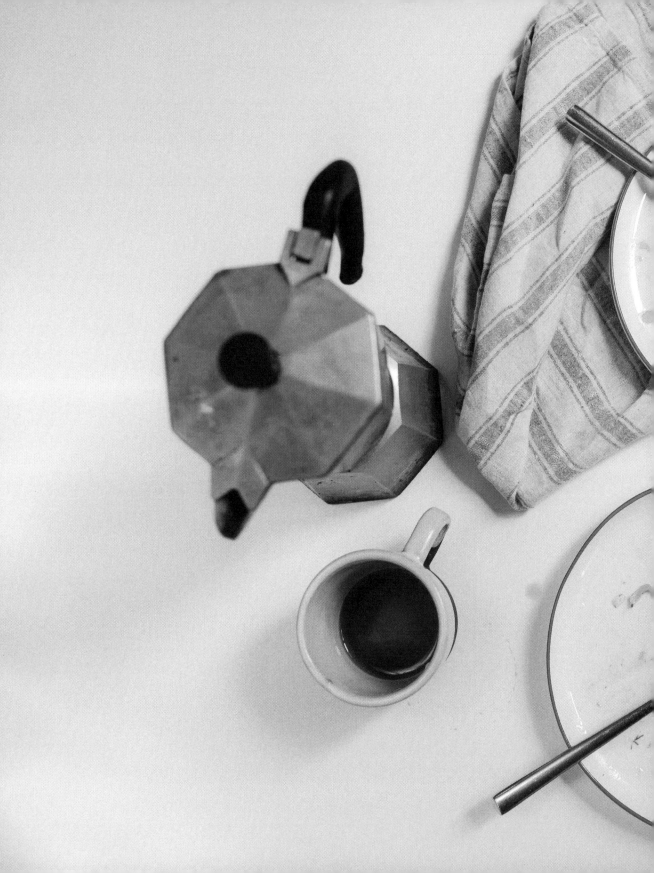

Contents

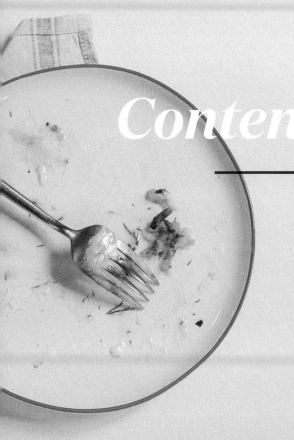

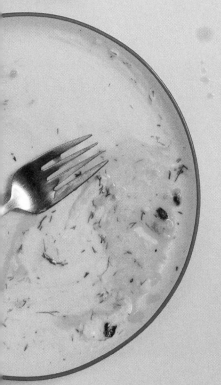

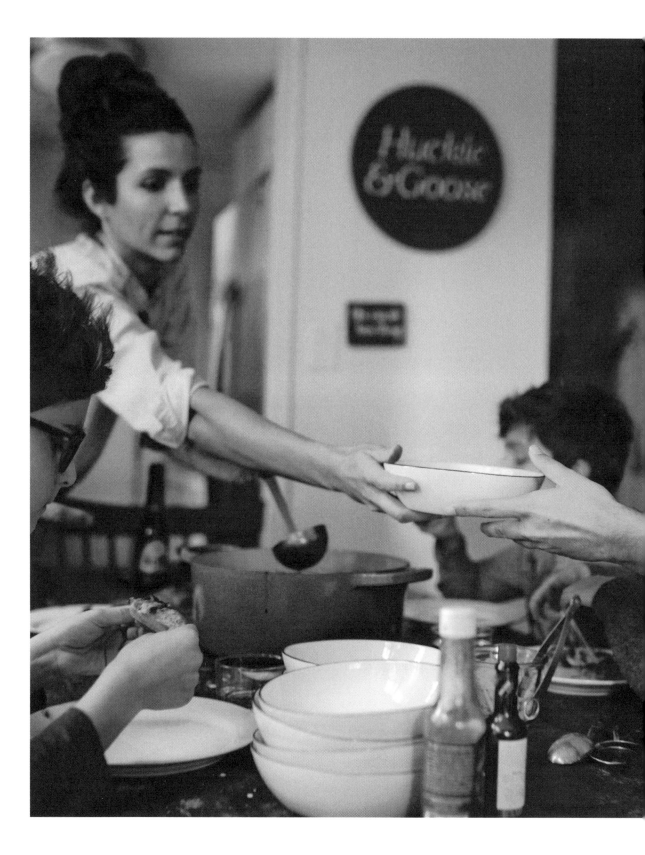

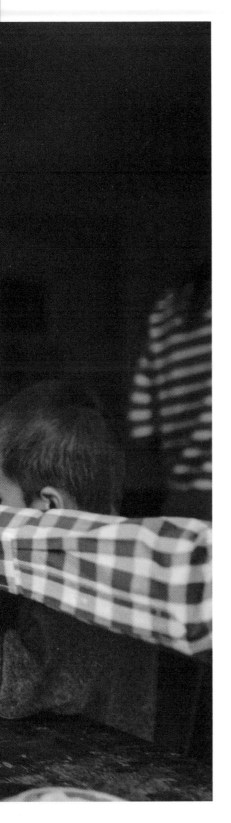

This Book Is for You

―――――

Let's be honest. We've all complained about keeping ourselves alive at some point.

You: "I should probably cook more."

Also you: "I hate cooking. It really is a waste of time."

Sound familiar?

Maybe you used to like cooking, but now you kinda don't. You're burned out.

Maybe it's always felt like going to the dentist . . . but in a more plaguing, eternal, unrelenting way. You dread it.

Maybe you try to like it but you're convinced you don't have the requisite cooking gene. You're unsure where to even start.

Or inevitably you find yourself panic-staring into an empty fridge at the end of each day, despite your best efforts. You're stressed and stuck.

We get it.

"What am I going to eat?" is playing on a near-constant loop in our brains. Day in, day out. We're human; we need that internal nag to not die. But pile on extra stuff like kids asking what's for dinner in their best whiny voice, feeling like we don't have the necessary skills, trying not to spend a fortune on food, and too many recipes to choose from, and it's no wonder we complain about the never-ending-ness of cooking.

But the truth is, we'd all like to have more of *this*:

Laughing way past sunset under the twinkle lights, eating an incredible grilled feast, sipping sangria. Planning a week's worth of meals and sticking to an actual budget. Having friends over for taco nights or impromptu brunch and coffee. Packing a killer sandwich on a workday and eating it on a park bench while the leaves fall. Kids sharing something vulnerable about school around the dinner table *and* eating a vegetable, not necessarily both in the same night. Having a simple and organized kitchen that practically begs you to cook. Being able to make someone's favorite pancakes for a big day. Having vegetables in the fridge, actually cooking with them, and discovering you don't have to force yourself to eat them. Surprising yourself, mid-recipe, and switching up the ingredients—you know how to cook by instinct.

Before the last page of this book, you'll get there. We promise.

Even if right now you can't possibly imagine yourself cooking most nights or your blood pressure rises at the mere thought of inviting people over. We will show you not only how to cook some of the best food you've ever eaten but also how to figure out why you've been feeling kinda burned out and generally annoyed by cooking. And how to fix it.

As we've learned on our own journey with cooking, the best kinds of changes, the ones that stick, begin with noticing. Noticing those tiny details about our internal thoughts and external circumstances and surroundings, then acting with consistency, over and over again. The results are rarely instantaneous. Choose the easiest, most organic place to start, and let that carry you forward. Little by little, in almost undetectable increments. The success of the Huckle & Goose Method hinges on this mindset. Here's the method:

NOTICE WHAT'S HAPPENING OUTSIDE (NATURE) + INSIDE (HUMAN NATURE).

COOK 3X A WEEK.

The magic here is that food and nature are so foundational for us that, when we choose to engage consistently, these elements have the power to carry us forward with a quiet, steady force unlike anything else. You'll look back in a year, surprised—but not—to see how far you've come.

That's how Huckle & Goose was born, by noticing, kind of by accident. During a trip to the farmers' market on a sunny June morning, there were pints of gooseberries. And those little striped berries sparked a bunch of questions: *Why haven't we seen these before? Why can't we buy them at the store? How many other fruits and vegetables are there that we don't know about?* Turns out there's purple asparagus, dozens of pepper varieties, pattypan squash, golden raspberries, a million different lettuces, husk cherries, new-to-us herbs, kohlrabis, and a ton more. But what the heck do you do with them?

So we set out to create a meal-planning company that would help people be in nature, cook from nature, and learn the rhythm of seasonal, healthful cooking—with craveable, non-diet-focused food. This has the power to shift your mindset from what you shouldn't eat to the abundance and inspiration Mother Nature provides.

Huckle & Goose is a sure place to start if you want to get out of survival mode and learn to make cooking a habit you actually like, with a plan that doesn't feel like a plan.

The book starts with 7 Elements—general areas that affect our well-being and contribute to our attitudes about cooking. Because it's not just about the cooking and the eating. It's about pairing that with good-for-you habits, too. The wrong details clutter the process (you don't need the right pots or amazing knife skills). The right details transform cooking (or anything else you're hoping to improve) into everyday second nature.

Then the recipes are planned out for you every single season.

As you follow along, little by little, you'll notice more sparks and lightbulb moments—those tiny electric currents in our minds—that can give us brighter ideas, help new habits click, and change the trajectories of our lives if we let them. Cook 3x a week, and wherever those little sparks lead, you follow. It won't be long before you'll feel fully at home in your kitchen.

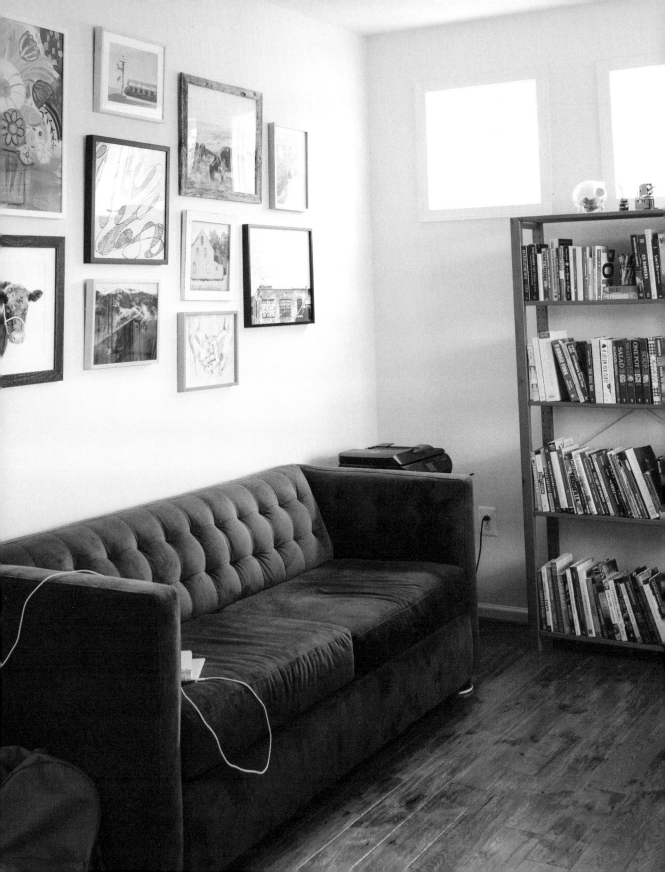

Part I

The 7 Elements

———

(AND THE HABITS THAT SUPPORT THEM)

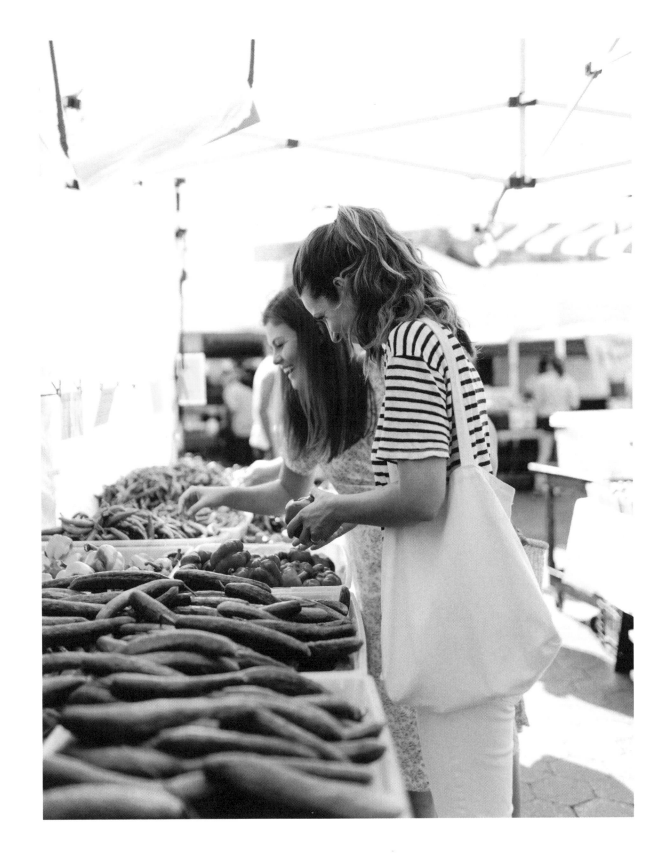

Mindset Creates Momentum

OVERRIDE HUMAN NATURE TO ENJOY COOKING
(AND ACCOMPLISH OTHER LIFE STUFF).

Oh, the mother element of them all, changing your mind about cooking (and everything else you might be telling yourself you can't do, won't do, don't like, won't try, or won't try again).

And it's really not just about the cooking; it's the planning, shopping, prep, the mess afterward, recipes turning into *meh*, picky eaters, lack of appreciation . . . you know, just to name a few.

All right, so you don't like cooking. That's a good place to start, and here's why. When you don't like something, you build an internal resistance. Every time you utter "Ugh, I hate cooking" or "I'm so tired of cooking dinner all the time," you're adding a brick and then another brick. The resistance is getting stronger and turning into a wall. You've labeled yourself as the non-cooking type. Why fight the truth? What do you do now?

First, let's talk about the reasons you loathe it. Take a good look at that brick wall. Name every brick in it. Write it all down if you have to.

If you're drawing a blank as to why you kinda hate cooking, here are some universal *ughs*. No one is immune to these—we've encountered them, still do sometimes. Here's how to overcome them:

1. IT'S NEVER ENDING, HAVING TO EAT. Yes, it is, and it won't end until you die. That's like complaining that you're getting old. It's a fact of life: you can complain about aging, but it sure isn't going to stop it.

2. BECAUSE NOTHING I MAKE EVER TURNS OUT. It could be the recipes you've tried to cook (that's where we've got you covered). It could be the technique. Overcooking and

underseasoning are often the main culprits of food not tasting good. Start simple and be consistent. Try cooking three times a week; don't pressure yourself to cook every day.

3. BECAUSE PLANNING MEALS AND MAKING GROCERY LISTS ARE THE WORST THINGS EVER. They are. That's why we wrote this book. Tools to make this task less awful.

4. BECAUSE MY KIDS ALWAYS COMPLAIN ABOUT PRETTY MUCH ANYTHING I MAKE. For now they do. Their palates are still forming, and if they've been used to processed food and excessive snacking before dinner, you'll have a bit of a battle on your hands. You're going to slowly change their taste buds. Some things they may never like, and that's okay. The first twenty times they may "hate" broccoli, but the trick is to cook it in different ways. Don't hide, don't sneak, don't pretend it's not there. If vegetables are making a consistent appearance at dinner and you're nonchalant about it, they will at least be more willing to try them.

5. BECAUSE EATING HEALTHY IS EXPENSIVE. Yes, it costs money to buy food, but it costs more money to buy takeout and go to restaurants. You can eat healthy and not break the bank. The problem is that we buy too much produce on a whim, with no real plan, then forget to cook it and toss it out.

6. IT'S TOO MUCH WORK TO CHOP. Get a good knife and make sure to sharpen it regularly. It'll change your life. It gets the job done in half the time and keeps your fingers safe (dull knives can do damage).

7. IT'S ALWAYS A MESS DURING AND AFTER. Chefs keep immaculate work spaces. If we follow their lead and clean as we go, it's not quite as daunting.

Okay, now that we've thoroughly re-annoyed you about cooking, we can begin. You specifically named your internal nag. What's next?

We're all wired to do the easiest thing rather than the better thing that might be harder. So accept this about yourself. You're difficult and almost impossible to change. Almost.

Tackle the easiest annoyances first, and little by little by little you'll notice the hate is kinda gone. Maybe you just don't like it now. Then you're okay with it. And then maybe you just might start to like it. Maybe. Our goal is to give you the tools to pluck yourself out of the negative-thinking phase as quickly as possible.

Habits

The Morning Minute

It's one of the most powerful ways to transform your entire day. And it can be a game changer for cooking.

When you wake up, before you check your phone, before your feet even hit the floor, before you brush your teeth, focus—with a meditation-like focus—for one entire minute. You're not transcending anything, there aren't sounds of trickling springs in the background. You're simply but routinely taking one full minute every morning to pause before the incoming flood of thoughts and to-dos. This pause is first and foremost to be grateful for being alive. It's focusing on a phrase, a morning mantra, or a single word that guides you through your day.

You want to stop making excuses to avoid cooking? Use your morning minute to reinforce your commitment to your routine. You could even write down your phrase or word and stick it on your kitchen cabinet. Keep the word in mind before and while you cook. It helps keep the negativity at bay and funnels your mental energy down the right path—so that you focus on what's important instead of on excuses and complaints.

One Day Off

Are you a Monday complainer or perpetually TGIF-ing? No one wants to be stuck in a just-get-through-the-week cycle.

Many factors play a role in creating optimal work-life balance, but in our experience, there is *one* habit that can make you feel surprisingly more at peace throughout the *entire* week, not just on Saturday and Sunday: taking a consecutive twenty-four-hour break every seven days. No excuses.

Here's how:

- CHOOSE A DAY THAT MAKES THE MOST SENSE FOR YOU. For us it's Sunday. It'll probably be a weekend day for most of you, too, but if you can set your own schedule, why not make it in the middle of the week, when everyone else is at work? Then repeat, on the same day, every single week. Guard this day from obligations and distractions like a mama bear.

- ZERO WORK. Zero. Don't put "just one load of laundry" in. Don't pull stuff like "But I just need to respond to this one email and that's it." That's always a slippery slope, and your brain needs to breathe from the burden of responsibility. Even the tiniest bit. The world will keep on spinning if you set boundaries with yourself and with your boss (especially if your boss is you). You don't want a life where you have to be working seven days a week. That's the very definition of a vicious cycle. Taking that one day off makes you more productive the other six days anyway.

- NO SOCIAL MEDIA. Your brain also needs a break from "the life you should be living." Don't let yourself be robbed of gratitude. Give your life the full attention it deserves for at least one full day.

- THAT COVERS ALL THE DON'TS. Now that you've decluttered your day off, fill it with things that feel good for you. For us, it's naps, reading, walks, time with family and friends, a day trip, time in nature. Any of your restful weekend ideas you've been saving for someday.

Once you do this regularly, you get to the point where you're actually, truly resting. Not semi-resting.

Wake with the Sunrise

For the past decade of my adult life, I (Christine) have tried desperately and failed miserably to be a morning person. I'd read those "Nine Things Highly Successful People Do Better Than You" or "How to Not Be a Crazy Mom Who Yells at Her Kids and Has It All Together" type articles and inevitably one of the bullet points was always, without fail, "Wake up before dawn." And there might as well be a *dot dot dot* "or your day will fall apart." I would nod along, acknowledging the logic; it made perfect sense. I'd have visions of opening my non-mascara-streaked eyelids and doing yoga, meditating, writing, drinking coffee while the sun's first rays stream through the window. There'd be stillness to prepare well for the day.

But there was a bigger problem. It turns out that functioning on a consistent less than eight hours of sleep per night (four in my case) is not very productive. Nor was it a good starting point for becoming a morning person.

Most of us know getting more sleep would solve about 90 percent of our problems, but for various, not very good reasons, we still don't do it. Instead we're on our tablets or phones until the very last possible second before closing our eyes. And it messes with our natural, inherent rhythm: *Wake up with the sun, get sleepy as the sun sets.* That blue-screen light tricks our brain into staying awake longer and longer, even if our body is actually asleep. We're in some limbo state, our mind unable to shut down.

One day, out of sheer necessity and against my workaholic will, I fell asleep at 9:30 P.M. (no screen before bed either because I misplaced my phone). Miraculously, I woke up at 5:30 the following morning. I got eight hours of Such. Good. Sleep. No blaring alarm, just calm. I stepped outside on the porch with a mug of ginger-lemon tea and watched the sun rise.

I am not the kind of person who watches the sun rise. I did not intend to become the kind of person who watches the sun rise. But I am now, and I'm wondering why more of those articles don't urge readers, in all caps, to WAKE UP AND WATCH THE SUN RISE.

Because here's what happens. You get to watch the day preparing for the day. There is something palpably energizing and perspective-shifting in the air that's not present at any other time of day. It's contagious. And somehow your problems seem to shrink. If you need inspiration, it's there. If you need direction, you'll probably find it there, too.

You will head back inside with a "battery sufficiently charged" message for your mind and spirit. Try it once a week, once every few weeks, whatever you find works well for you—aspire to become a sometimes morning person.

Notice Nature

At the very center of our brain, in the hypothalamus, we have a circadian clock. It pays attention to when the sun rises and sets and determines the daily rhythms and routines of our bodies. We're literally wired from the inside out to sync with nature.

After all, we're biological beings, right? Our bodies are made to move, to breathe in real air, not cranked-up-A/C office air. To feel sunshine on our faces, not fluorescent lighting. To sync up with the seasons and what's happening around us. In this modern age, we're neglecting what we actually need to thrive. Our meat and vegetables arrive for dinner on our doorsteps, pre-measured and plastic-wrapped in cardboard boxes. We connect with friends on screens while we eat lunch at our desks. We go from the gym to work to watching TV on the couch with takeout, rarely noticing that first day the spring blossoms finally appeared in the front yard. The consequences are, of course, a constant, subtle fog over the way we think, live, and eat. And ultimately, we start to feel bad—in mind and body. Which is usually when we start to care. Medicine, diets, and detoxes certainly have their place, but a lifestyle change that addresses the root of our symptoms is often what we need most.

The more you match your external environment (nature, your outdoor activities) with your internal environment (your home, your body), the more in tune you'll feel. And then, in turn, you'll appreciate cooking more, or at least the *idea* of cooking. When nature's everyday details overlap with the way you cook and you make it a habit, you discover the connection. For instance, you don't crave a hearty beef stew after a refreshing summer swim. Eating watermelon and corn on the cob after building a snowman would be odd. But seriously, stop and think about that for a moment. Everything is available for us everywhere now, year-round, yet it still goes against our natural instinct. The food that grows around us during each season is exactly what our bodies need and crave for that time of year. Always listen for that tug.

Habits

Go to the Market

It often feels like cooking is this isolated chore that millions of people around the world collectively grumble about at 8 A.M., 12 noon, and 6 P.M. each day. But cooking, ultimately, is a story. So let's click the zoom-out button a few times and give ourselves the chance and the perspective to see it unfold.

Someone, somewhere (with a story of their own) plants a seed in the ground. That seed grows into something we can eat. And that someone works really hard to water it, pull out weeds, weather storms and pests—so they can make a living feeding you and me. Then we bring that food home.

A great ending actually continues the story. You make yourself an amazing breakfast that prepares you for a challenging workday and helps you be a little more patient with all your co-workers. Or your family feels loved and noticed—and they go off to school and choose to be kinder to their classmates. Or you invite friends over for dinner and linger over flickering candles. Everyone goes home thinking life is good.

But if we're not *there*, present in some of these details that get our food from the ground to our fridge, there will always be a disconnect. It's one of the main reasons we view feeding ourselves as insignificant drudgery.

Outsourcing too many steps results in not really knowing what you're doing, why you're doing it, or where you're going. Convenience can steal our awareness. We miss the bigger picture: our own lives, the environment, our culture—they're all linked. We're the only ones who can help them function in harmony.

The most effective way to experience the full story is to grow our own food. Put a seed in the ground, water it, watch it grow, harvest it. You're part of the story from start to finish. But for most of us, the next best thing is local farmers' markets and CSA programs. The next best thing after that is a local co-op or grocery store that buys from local farmers.

The problem is that many of us have preconceived notions about the farmers' market. Take your pick: *Only snobby people eat this way; it's too expensive; I don't have time to shop there; I don't like vegetables.* We thought the same, yet here we are telling you it completely changed the way we cook.

We're asking you to just dip your toe in the water a little bit. Walk through the market. That's it. Just walk through. For three consecutive weeks. Find the best market near you, note the opening hours, and make it happen. Week 1, walk through. Week 2, walk through. Week 3, walk through. Don't stress about buying a thing. Just be a part of it.

This is an actual place you can go to remember you need nature and nature needs humans. The pull to eat green stuff and support the people who grow it is magnetic. We're willing to bet you'll be making it tradition before you know it. The whole cooking-is-a-story thing will make a lot more sense, and participating in it will inspire new ways of getting creative in your kitchen.

Eat Outside

Just as walking through the market can spark a deeper connection to nature, so can enjoying a meal alfresco. You know that feeling you get when you score a patio table at your favorite restaurant just as the sun is setting? For some reason, everything tastes extra-good. There's just something about it.

Sure, there's science behind it: Fresh oxygen shoots to your brain, giving you a boost of energy. Serotonin is activated by the sunshine, improving your mood and appetite. But doing almost anything outside, really, is going to help you feel good. All your senses are heightened in the presence of fresh air and natural light. So, adding good food to the mix will make your meal taste that much better. Eating a spring quiche at your dining room table will be really good, but if you pack that same quiche for a picnic, it's an experience you're going to want to bottle up for a long time.

You can re-create that eating-outside-at-a-café feeling way more often, but right at home. Even being next to a window can inspire a similar effect. Try it and see what it does for your cooking motivation.

Walk

You sleep in a box, travel in a box so you can go work in a box, leave work in a box to go buy food that's in a box, drive back home to your box and watch a box on the wall for entertainment until you repeat the process the next day. Sadly, that's life for most of us. The part spent in nature is about 10 percent, and usually that's just because we had to walk from one box to another. We're a bunch of box people. Confined, lethargic, unhappy, and anxious. While getting outside the box won't fix all our ailments, it could probably make a lot of stuff better.

No matter where you live, you can go for a walk. And, no, that doesn't have to be the same walk you take every morning on the way to work, or the lap around the block with your dog in the evening. Remember, the goal here is just to be outside, notice the small things, and reconnect with the natural world.

THE TAKING-THE-LONG-WAY-HOME WALK: Your usual route home with a spirit of adventure. New paths can stir new thoughts. Skip the shortcut and forget about the to-do list that's waiting for you at home.

THE YOU'RE-UPSET-AND-NEED-TO-WALK-IT-OFF WALK: You're fuming. Do not say another word. Grab your coat and headphones and get some air. You'll have less to apologize for later if you walk it off instead.

THE SUNRISE WALK: These are life altering. There's no overstating it. If you're in a rut or need a fresh start (again?) wake up just before the sun comes up and take a walk to meet it. Bring your journal. Because there's nothing like watching a new day emerge to stir up some philosophical ponderings.

THE AFTER-DINNER SUNSET WALK: Dinner with the family—check. Dishes washed (but not necessarily)—check. Adorable frog pj's on kids—check. Sneakers on—double check. Phones left on the counter—seriously. Look up. The sky is a muted blue with orange and purple streaks.

THE EARLY-AFTERNOON HIKE FOR PLOTTING: Have a list of things you need to sort out, plans you need to make? Get outside, walk through the woods, take in the colors of the autumn leaves, and clear your mind so you can actually get things done later.

THE ACTUALLY-LEAVE-THE-OFFICE-AND-HAVE-LUNCH-OUTSIDE WALK: Summer's almost over and you've eaten lunch outside once. Once. Pick the day this week and then stroll through the park and find the perfect bench with the perfect shade and actually take the full hour you're supposed to have. Bring that novel you keep meaning to finish.

THE QUIET-SNOWFALL-IN-THE-EVENING WALK: Yes, it's cold outside. But your lungs need a reminder that crisp air is good for them. So bundle up and go for a walk. Snow has a way of making everything it touches silent. Hopefully, it will even silence your mind.

THE ONE-ON-ONE-TIME WALK: No big explanation here—grab some hands (spouse, kid). Make someone feel special by taking a walk and giving them your undivided attention. None of this on-the-couch, half-looking-at-your-phone, half-listening nonsense. Go for a walk and simply say, "I want to hear all about your day," and then just listen, but really listen.

THE CHECK-YOURSELF WALK: Sometimes you just need an honest talk with yourself. You're not doing what you keep saying you'll do. And now it's just annoying. What things are unacceptable? Don't go home until you decide that one thing that can help you shift.

Home Is a Haven

If we don't feel rooted in our own homes, we'll always wander or want to be somewhere else—physically, emotionally, mentally. Deep down, we're always longing for home. We want to be tucked away inside a home with candlelight on a snowy day. A shelter from the cold and crowds. Somewhere with laughter and music inside. To know, without a doubt, that we have a place to go at the end of the day. A place where we belong. And there's always something really delicious simmering on the stove.

Think back to the things that made home feel like home. Maybe it was the worlds you visited in your childhood book nook, Christmas mornings, or Sunday game nights. But more often than not, we instantly think of Dad's mac-and-cheese or the famous Thursday stir-frys your best friend's mom would make when you went over to study. Warm stoves draw everyone to the kitchen and then around the table together.

Cooking consistently (at least three times a week) creates an unmistakable energy in your home that carries you forward in every other aspect of your life. Like a wave. You're part of that cooking story we talked about, so there's now an undercurrent—subconscious attitudes that get embedded in the food you make. There's deep satisfaction and confidence in the knowledge that you can feed yourself (and the people you love). With a single, consistent act, we can create this intangible warm glow, this life-sustaining energy that starts in the kitchen and spills over into every other room.

When we create an environment we love to be in, we will naturally want to take good care of ourselves and invite others into our space. Others who possibly have never experienced the comfort of home. Saying, "Hey, wanna come over for dinner?" is probably the most generous invitation we can extend to another human being.

Make Your Home a Haven

Find a quiet spot for five or ten minutes. Close your eyes. Are your eyes closed? Now forget all the dream homes you've ever seen in magazines and on social media. *Picture the feeling of your dream home instead.*

When you walk through your front door, how do you want to feel? How do you want the people who live with you to feel? How do you want your guests to feel? When they come over, they'll ring the doorbell, then wait. There's that nearly undetectable heart-leaping moment of *I wonder what their house is going to be like* anticipation before you swing the door open. What *is* your house going to be like?

Be like > *look* like.

You might have paint-chipped cabinets, a slightly wobbly dining table, pink tiles in the bathroom from the seventies, and a hand-me-down sofa that follows you to every single apartment even though you swore you'd get rid of it three moves ago. None of these things matter. Here are the things that do:

Energy and Life

BRING NATURE IN: Open the windows wide, and open them often. Not just for the fresh air, but also for those calming nature sounds—thunderstorms, birds, and crickets. Keep fresh flowers on the table. Grow green plants and herbs on the windowsill.

FULL OF LIFE: Then there are the intangible, full-of-life things we bring into our homes as humans. Music, laughter, singing, dancing, traditions, celebrating people, noticing people, good thoughts, and good conversation—all the habits in this book that help us create space for expression, inspiration, and belonging.

SOMETHING ALWAYS BAKING IN THE OVEN OR SIMMERING ON THE STOVE: We talked about the power of a warm stove earlier. Like how, when you're on your way to someone's apartment and smell something from the hallway, you already know you're welcome there and you're invited to stay awhile. You can create this feeling, day in and day out, for yourself and the people in your life.

DECLUTTER: Your stuff lurks. It follows you. If you have too much stuff or if it doesn't have a place, your home will feel cluttered. So will your brain. The solution is this timeless quote from William Morris: "Have nothing in your houses that you do not know to be useful or believe to be beautiful." That means even that decorative plate your mom got you that you don't like. You're not forced to keep stuff, despite that unwritten rule.

CLEAN: House chores. They feel like yet another job you have to do when you get home from your job. No one wants to spend their Saturdays mopping floors. But the piles of laundry, the soap-scummy shower, the oil-splattered stove and slightly sticky countertops . . . You know they're there. Sometimes you even want to leave to get away from it (which leads to spending money you don't want to spend). Here are some ways to not hate housework so much. (1) Make room in your budget and hire someone else to do it. (2) Failing that, get in a whistle-while-you-cook state of mind. Listen to a podcast or audiobook while doing a smaller chore every day. Find a way around your annoyances.

Beauty and Light

Your home should feel like an extension of you. Even if you don't yet have the bigger stuff you're dreaming of, these smaller things make home feel beautiful.

LIGHT: This doesn't cost a thing. Drench your home with sunlight during the day. Everything will look brighter and more cheerful. And at night, fill your home with warm lighting—dimmers (cozy restaurant secret), lamplight, roaring fireplace, candles at the table, candles in any and every room.

ART: It completely transforms a room. Put things on your wall that have meaning. It could be as simple as blowing up a favorite work of art by your favorite five-year-old and framing it.

BOOKS: Books belong in every room. A wall-to-wall shelf of them in your living room, a bedroom nightstand stack, a cookbook collection in the kitchen. They're a visual reminder of everything you've learned and everything you hope to learn. A reminder to notice, stay curious, and be willing to walk in someone else's shoes for a while.

OPEN SHELVING: If you see a lot of the things you own out in the open, you don't need to wonder where they are, where they're hidden. Whatever you're looking for is easier to see, easier to grab, and you'll use your stuff a lot more often. Especially in the kitchen and dining areas, this helps out with the "Unfinished Hospitality" habit.

YOUR OUTDOOR SPOT: This is your home oasis and spot to escape without leaving home. It should receive as much care and attention as the inside of your home. If you've got the space directly outside your house, invest in a table and chairs you absolutely love, hang some twinkle lights, and add plants or even a garden.

Flow

If you're thinking, *I really wish I had a spot to do* _____, sometimes simply defining a space for an activity and rearranging a few things will make it happen like magic.

MORE COZY CONVERSATIONS: Reconfigure your living room so the seating is in a closed formation rather than all facing out toward the TV.

MORE READING: Move a comfy chair to that awkward corner that you haven't been able to figure out what to do with. Add a small side table for your drinks, a cable-knit throw, and a basket for books, and now it's a reading nook.

MORE SOLITUDE AND REST: Assign your closet as your alone-time space (or anywhere you can find consistent, intentional quiet) when you need to hear yourself think. There might be the noise and shuffle of everyone getting ready for the day just outside that door, but your morning meditation is taped on the wall and you sit in there for a few minutes to prepare your mind for the day.

MORE COOKING, MORE EATING TOGETHER: Is everything in your kitchen in a place that makes the most sense as you cook? Are your cutting boards and knives closest to where you usually like to chop? Is your table inviting and cleared of old mail and crumpled receipts? Are your plates and flatware in the most logical place for setting the table? Sometimes things feel more complicated than they should be because of bad flow.

All these details add up to a home you'll love, and one that you will want to cook and eat in.

Element 4:
Be Together

A PUBLIC SERVICE ANNOUNCEMENT THAT OTHER PEOPLE IMPROVE
OUR HUMAN NATURE AND WE IMPROVE THEIRS. THE BEST PLACE TO BE TOGETHER
IS AROUND THE TABLE, EATING GOOD FOOD.

There's a modern health epidemic that has been linked to chronic diseases, mental illness, and even premature death. And it's not related to the food we eat.

It's loneliness.

There is an irony to the loneliness epidemic, of course. At the touch of a button we can FaceTime anyone in any part of the world. We have more friends on social media than the total population of some small towns. But virtual friends are not the same as IRL humans. Our brains are wired for connection, and our bodies pay a price when we are starved of it.

Being a whole (and healthy) person requires something we seem to have forgotten about: other people. You don't just need people to prevent you from dying early. You need them so you can love the life you already have. Here's why:

Other people refine us. Do not buy into the whole "be your own best friend" mumbo jumbo. You can't be your own best friend. Because you have a major blind spot—you. We may admit some of our flaws to ourselves, but usually the ones that are most detrimental are the ones in our blind spot. You can't see them, but another human can, just like they can't see theirs but you can. And therein lies one of the beautiful things about human relationships. We refine each other. Surround yourself with people who love you unconditionally but who are also unafraid to speak the hard truth. Let their love and insight build you up.

Other people inspire us. We need inspiration in our lives, and we need it often. Without it we become stagnant, finding ourselves repeating routines that no longer serve us. We can easily fall into a rut mentally, spiritually, relationally, creatively—the list goes on and on. While we can certainly be inspired by great thinkers and doers, we also need inspiration from people who actually know our name. It could be that you watched your friend train for a marathon and it inspires you to get healthy. Maybe your father's love of history is so ingrained in you that you can't visit a bookstore without picking up another biography of Abraham Lincoln. Recently, your forty-something-year-old cousin decided to take up the cello. Just like that. And it stirred something in you.

Other people allow us to share (and make food taste better). We have an innate desire to share our experience with other humans. The things that spark wonder or stir our hearts are infinitely more enjoyable when there's someone sitting right next to us looking at the same shooting star. Any kind of good news or achievement or life event seems less significant if those we love aren't there to join in the celebration. And if there's one thing we love to share more than anything, it would probably be food. How many times have you tasted something amazing and uttered, mid-bite, "Oh my gosh, you have to try this"? It's our common, essential human need, and it connects us.

But don't wait for the holidays or special occasions—consider incorporating more shared meals and everyday traditions into the other three-hundred-something days of the year: weekday dinner parties, just-because confetti cake, Thursday pasta bowl night, dance-off Sundays. You'll begin to feel the pull of the table. By that we mean you'll want to open up your home to others. Hospitality is a gift we've forgotten about. We've mislabeled it as stuffy, demanding, and anxiety-inducing. But at its core it's as simple as saying, "Stay awhile. I'd love to share some food with you."

Habits

Unfinished Hospitality

The reality is that entertaining at home scares people almost as much as public speaking. We get it. There's pressure: *How do I set the table? What if I overcook the fish? I won't have enough time to clean up the kitchen before guests arrive. I totally underestimated the cooking time for this roast and dinner won't be ready until 10:30—what am I going to do?*

First, breathe.

The goal here is to make this *having people over* thing a regular thing, not a perfect, buttoned-up, every-once-in-a-while thing.

Here's the secret to entertaining without the pressure and anxiety: Don't be ready. Leave things for your guests to do. Don't have them come when dinner is ready; have them come for happy hour. Your job is to get at least some of the food simmering, music playing, and maybe candles already flickering. That's the trifecta for creating an atmosphere where you and everyone else will want to linger until after the candles have burned down to their final minutes. Then, as everyone arrives, delegate. They can mix some drinks, get the cheese platter going, help with chopping, and set the table. Don't stress about the table too much. Google the fork and knife placement if you must, but sometimes go for menus that require zero table setting. A big pot of chili, for instance, where anything other than a stack of self-serve bowls and a grab-your-own bundle of spoons would be bad form. Or simple weekend breakfasts where friends arrive in sweats just as the coffee starts brewing, and there are tulips on the table.

The energy feels relaxed instead of frazzled and rushed, and conversations flow easier when everyone's got a job to do. Your guests are enjoying themselves and so are you.

By the time you're sitting at the table to eat, the conversation has already been going strong and naturally flows into dinner. Allowing this pre-dinnertime makes for fewer awkward pauses and none of that "So the weather's been unseasonably chilly lately, huh?" Hours later, your guests will leave feeling full, and not just because they ate well. They'll leave feeling connected, taken care of, heard, and even loved. There was an intangible can't-put-your-finger-on-it warmth in your home. Could it be the drinks? The food? The music? The dinner? The linens and table setting? The conversation? It's everything and nothing. It's the essence of unfinished hospitality. It's the invitation to be part of the process.

You might be thinking, "Umm, yeah, this sounds nice, but you said you'd help me. And here I am with no clue how to do any of this." Trust us, after a few weeks of cooking three times a week, you will. Pinkie promise. This is another one of those changes that doesn't *poof* happen overnight. But after about two months, not only will you be more comfortable in the kitchen, but you'll even have found some favorite recipes. Those recipes are your golden ticket.

The 7 Elements

And that's how it all begins. Before you know it you'll have six people coming over for Rosemary-Brined Pork Loin with Chunky Pesto-Topped Asparagus & Butter-Basted Potatoes—and feel completely in your element.

Celebrate People!

We all want our birthday to feel like the most special day of the year. We want to be extra noticed. We remember who said a sincere "Happy birthday" to us in real life, and especially those who went a little beyond that:

- With a small, thoughtful gift. Maybe it was literally $5, but they found a special edition of your favorite book in an old bookstore.
- With a super-thoughtful text. Words that kept you smiling the entire day and well into the next.
- With a snail-mail card. Rainbow confetti fluttered out when you opened it, and you never thought a folded piece of paper could feel like a mini party just for you.

Let's not be serial lame obligatory "Happy birthday!" Facebook wall posters. Because, at the end of the day, is there anything more important than seeking out ways to make those around us feel admired, valued, loved?

So let's make celebrating people a regular thing—with grand gestures sometimes, but mostly the everyday kind. In real life. For anything from work promotions to winning soccer games to being born. Even just because you're suddenly struck by how grateful you are for someone on an ordinary day. Life is fuller when there are handwritten notes, hugs, cakes, confetti, champagne toasts, someone cooking you your favorite dinner, and hey-this-made-me-think-of-you gifts.

You know who your people are. Look for simple ways to make them feel interesting, important, and validated. There's no one like them; honor the things that make them uniquely them. Celebrate them to their very core. Get some lecture passes on an obscure topic that interests them. Take old-school dance lessons. Bake them their favorite dessert and stick candles in it (and it doesn't have to be cake). Create a scavenger hunt through all their favorite spots. Plan a surprise potluck picnic. Hire an art student to make a framed, original work of art (maybe a sketch of someone they love and miss). Or snag a print from the weekend art fair that reminds you of them.

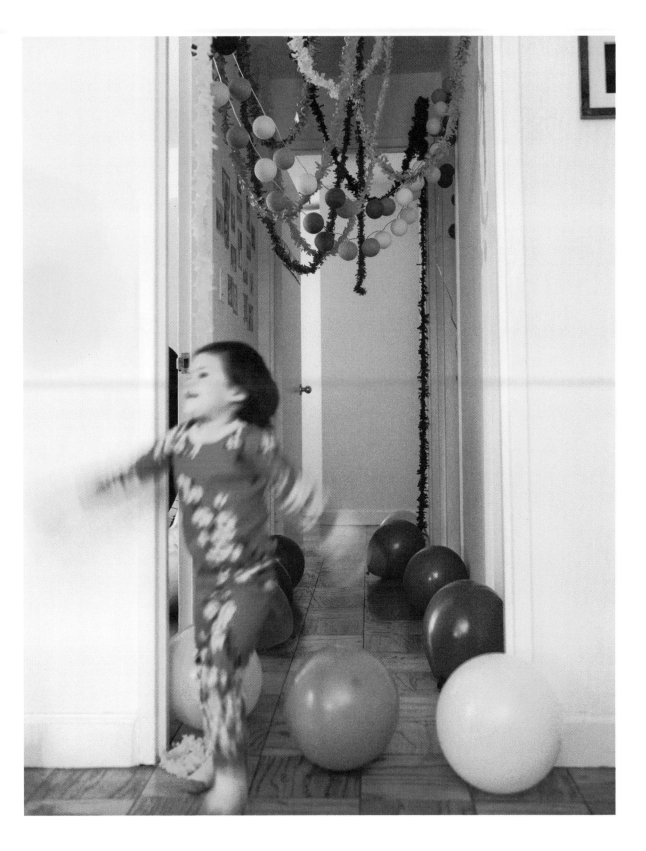

Serve breakfast in bed. Make a late-night balloon birthday wonderland right outside their doorway; it'll feel like they're walking through rainbows first thing in the morning.

They'll remember this forever. And something even better is to tell them exactly *why* your life is better because they're in it. Don't just say, "I'm grateful for you," and leave it at that. Write a note or card or letter with specifics. Tell them in person or make an actual phone call. We can be really rusty at this, so if you need to, use a thesaurus for proper adjectives and adverbs to describe them and what they mean to you. No generic words like *amazing* or *awesome*. Expand your people-celebrating vocabulary.

Plan Priorities

NOW WE START IMPLEMENTING THE FIRST FOUR ELEMENTS.

If you've read up to this point, maybe you're thinking you want to start incorporating some of these habits into your life. Or you want to find new ways to keep improving on them—deeper relationships, a home that refreshes you, being outside more, climbing out of mental ruts. This element is the one that begins to turn all the other elements into reality.

So let's get specific. What do you want? Maybe you want to feel more confident in the kitchen, or to spend more time with family and friends around the dinner table, or to get better at meal planning and shopping.

Write it all down, along with *why* you want these things. Otherwise it'll feel like a fleeting thought or just another New Year's resolution. It'll also be easier to fend off the excuses: Maybe when you have more space, you'll invite people over. You'll feel more confident in the kitchen when you have nicer pots. You'll make weekly meal plans when the kids get older.

You know that waiting—until you're comfortable or have more resources or time or the circumstances align—is never a good idea. You'll be waiting forever.

Start with one specific, small action. Here, we're starting with that goal of cooking three times a week.

Habits

Planner Purge

These specific, smaller actions usually need to be assigned time and day details. If you don't already have a day planner, consider picking one up. There's something about seeing January, February, March, April, May, June, July, August, September, October, November, and December all stretched out in front of you, in a format you can write on. This is one year of your life. These are the only four seasons, twelve months, fifty-two weeks, 365 days, 8,760 hours, and half a million minutes (give or take) you will get in this one year. How will you spend them?

Maybe you do have a planner, but it's in your tote bag, pulsing like Jumanji. Do you hear ominous drumbeats at the very thought of opening it and seeing *everything* you have to do? It rules you.

You're about to feel the most liberating feeling you've felt in a long time. We're purging your planner. Completely. It's only going to have the stuff you absolutely need to do, and lots of stuff you want to do.

1. Transfer all your to-dos and obligations onto a separate sheet of paper, with dates if applicable.

2. Leave everything you *really, truly* want to do, then cross out everything else from your planner pages with a thick Sharpie. You don't *have* to go to your aunt's neighbor's grandkid's fifth birthday party on Saturday morning. You don't *have* to stay at work late. Feel how liberating it is.

3. On those now (mostly) blank planner sheets, create a daily rhythm and routine you would look forward to following. The crucial plot points for making cooking three times a week a habit are: scheduling the Solo Date (page 36); setting meal times and sleep time in stone; having good morning and evening routines so you set yourself up for making good decisions; determining the time you'll start cooking dinner; and deciding which day you'll grocery shop.

4. Next, schedule in the things desperately needed for life to go on (like getting your car fixed or filling out insurance forms before your coverage expires). Everything else, keep on that separate sheet of paper so it doesn't loom and dictate your days. You'll get to it when you get to it, and if you don't, life goes on and you are happier for it.

It's surprising how much ends up on our to-do lists that we don't even need to do or want to do. Things we do because our priorities aren't strong and clear enough, or we're subconsciously afraid of judgment, or we have trouble saying no and establishing boundaries.

So which three days are you cooking this week?

Family Meeting

Okay. There are a lot of vegetable-focused dishes in this book. You might want to eat this way and cook more at home, but you're probably already thinking, *Too bad we won't ever eat this way as a family.* Every time you want a new habit or routine to stick, call a family meeting. During this meeting you will explain why you called it and what changes will be implemented and how it requires everyone to pitch in, even your three-year-old.

Decide exactly what you want to change. Is it family dinner at a certain time? Is it reducing snacks and eating more veggies? Is it family evening reading time? Why do you want to do this?

The *why* is really important, because if you can't clearly explain it to your kids, it won't stick.

Kids are smart, and most of the time, if you take the time to explain what you're doing and why, they'll get on board. Don't plop some Brussels sprouts on their plate after you decided to stop making separate kiddie meals and expect them to chew with a smile. But if, the day before, you briefly explain how vegetables and greens fuel our bodies and make them grow strong, you're taking down a brick in their resistance wall. When you explain that a lot of the junk food we eat tastes good because it's been covered with fake stuff, another brick may not come down, but it'll get wiggly. They need to understand that all the excess fake flavor/sugar/salt confuses their taste buds and blocks subtle flavors. (Try eating a steamed green bean after cheesy chips and soda.) But if we drink mostly water, don't snack, and come to the table hungry, we'll start tasting things better. Sure, you can even talk about how strawberries have a season and how a farmers' market strawberry in the summer tastes *sooo* different from the ones at the grocery store in the middle of February. But for now we're just explaining the *why*.

After you explain the *why*, decide as a family how you'll support this new plan. Write a kitchen manifesto. What are six rules that go on there? Ask everyone for input, including your kids. If they are involved in coming up with the rules, they're more likely to abide by them.

Rules to get you started:

- You have to taste whatever is on your plate.
- If you don't like it, explain why. Is it the texture, the smell, something else?
- Be thankful for all food, because someone worked hard to grow it, someone worked hard to buy it, and someone worked hard to prepare it.
- Whoever cooks doesn't clean up.
- Everyone has a job to do.
- Planning the weekly menu is by committee: everyone picks a dinner.

Less is more. You want something that you can remember. And the more you practice it, the more it becomes part of your daily life.

Element 6:
Whistle While You Cook

DO WHAT YOU SAID YOU'D DO
(WITH LESS COMPLAINING).

Whistling, although you can certainly take it literally, is a state of mind. It's finding a way to enjoy any task. It's going from "Ugh, I have to ＿＿ again" to "I know doing ＿＿ is important. Since I still don't want to do it, I'll listen to some music to make the time go by faster." And then you find yourself kind of enjoying the process after all.

Try these whistle-while-you-cook ideas:

- Listen to your favorite playlist, radio station, podcast, or audiobook
- Or simply savor the silence
- Put fresh flowers or herbs on your windowsill or counter
- Buy cute prep bowls, something cheery
- Savor a glass of wine to feel French-chefy
- Light an unscented candle for mood

It doesn't really matter what you choose to do; all that matters is that it resonates with you. Notice what you need to whistle while you cook.

Habits

Fill the House with Music

Oftentimes the missing ingredient to making cooking an enjoyable habit is music. It has the power to transform your mood and make repetitive tasks, like chopping, something you might even look forward to. Music can calm or energize. It can relieve stress, inspire creativity, help you be more productive, increase focus, trigger memories, make you smile, and help you linger at the dinner table longer. It's the magic in the kitchen. It's your secret weapon for getting dinner on the table consistently and making everyone who sits around it feel special.

Be intentional about when and why you're listening to music. If most of the people in your home are sorta grouchy in the morning, have calming or happy music playing in the kitchen. Go about your breakfast routine like normal and watch the mood begin to shift. Then, later, when the dinnertime hustle approaches, you're ready. You find a playlist (classic vocal jazz is always a cooking favorite: Frank Sinatra, Ella Fitzgerald, Peggy Lee), push play, and absorb the first thirty seconds of music before you go about your chopping. You and the music.

Some days will feel rushed, some sad, some happy, some loud, and some even angry. That's okay—there's a playlist for that.

Rhythm and Routine

HOW THE TRANSFORMATION HAPPENS.

Routine. Is there a word that feels more blah? If routine were a person, it would be Bob from accounting who tells jokes in a monotone voice and then just stares at you, lifeless.

We don't seem to have such a negative reaction to rhythm, though. I mean, rhythm is a dancer. It's a soul companion. You can feel it everywhere. No arguing with that. Rhythm is in every single person, whether we acknowledge it or not. There's a seasonal rhythm we follow from nature; our cues come from the seasons. In spring, there's a spirit of renewal and we're itching to spring-clean. In summer we're looking forward to some R&R&R—rest, relaxation, recreation. Fall's all about apple pies and crisp notebooks. We naturally want to plan and prepare. And then winter comes. We crave coziness and candlelit dinner parties with braises, stews, and roasts. It's time to slow down.

Within these seasons, there's our twenty-four-hour circadian rhythm that can guide us, too, if we let it.

The problem is, we're kind of ignoring these rhythms. Both the recipes and the habits in this book are reminders to sync back up. They consider both your outside rhythm (seasons) and your inside rhythm (circadian) to help you build a routine that finally sticks.

Part 2 is packed with rhythms and routines specifically to make cooking three times a week a habit. Choose one that you're instantly excited about or feels natural to you, or one you know would really help you out in the immediate future. Don't put a time frame on it; do it as often as you can. It should make your life feel easier, not harder. Notice what works, what doesn't, and why. Keep making changes.

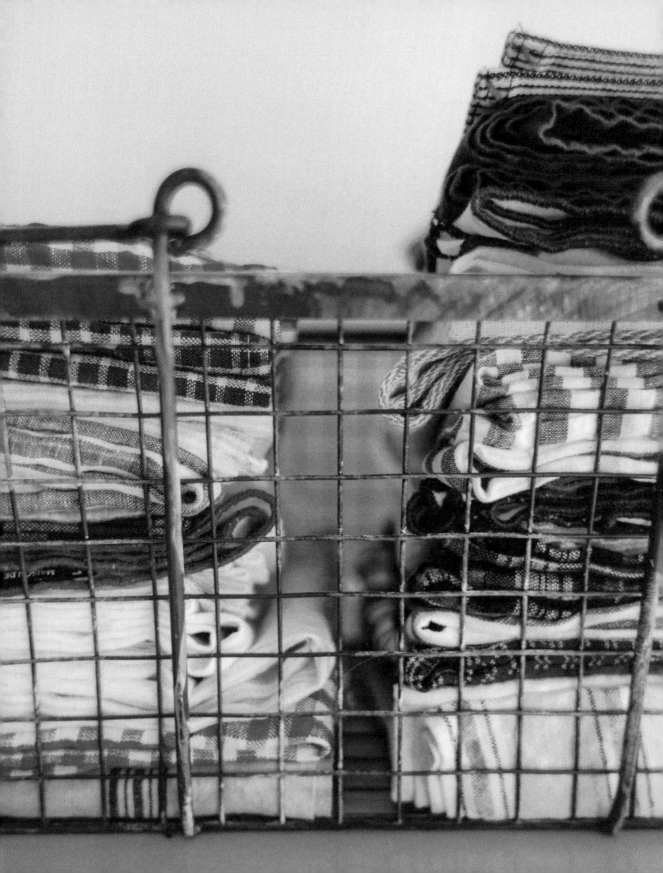

Part 2

Kitchen Habits

SOME RHYTHMS & ROUTINES TO HELP YOU STICK TO COOKING 3X A WEEK.
ADD THEM ONE BY ONE.

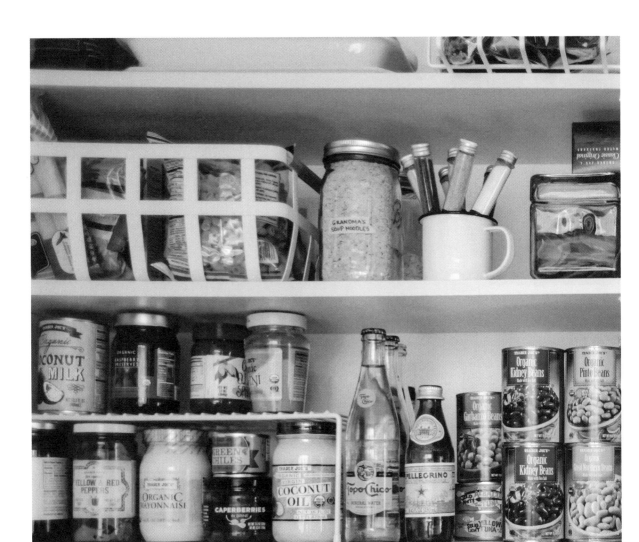
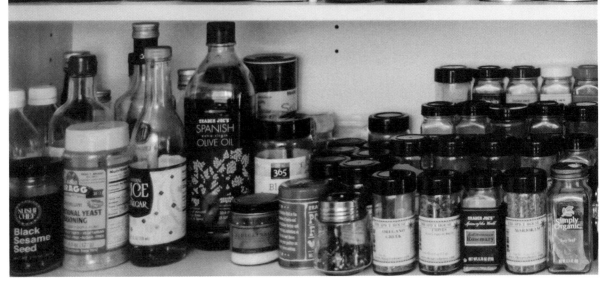

Pantry Purge

There's no definitive pantry guide in this book. Neither of us has ever paid much attention to these lists that commonly appear in cookbooks—even when we were kitchen newbies. So instead of cluttering this book with info you'll likely skip over, we're asking you to trust us. There are zero ingredients in this book that we don't keep on hand regularly and use in multiple dishes. You'll build your pantry as you cook through each season. Gradually, you'll fill jars with all sorts of things you may never have thought you'd stir into two meals in one week. And by the end of this book, we're confident you'll know exactly what *you* like to keep on hand, and why.

But the most important step here is removing things from your pantry, not adding them. If the kitchen is the heart of your home, purging your pantry is like a full-on spring-cleaning of its very core. It will almost instantly give you solid resolve to be a consistent cook and clear up mental space you didn't even know you had. It once completely got rid of a monthlong writer's block.

Here's the Huckle & Goose method for gutting and organizing your pantry:

1. Take all your pantry ingredients off the shelves, out of cabinets, out of the pantry. Every single thing.
2. Check expiration dates and toss all expired stuff.
3. Now make two groups—the ingredients you use regularly, the ingredients you don't.
4. Put the ingredients you use regularly into jars. These can be jars you've purchased or jars you've saved and peeled the label off of. If you'd like, make pretty labels with something as simple as masking tape and a Sharpie. Put the now filled and labeled jars back on the shelf. If you've got open shelving, even better. By seeing everything displayed, you'll be more likely to look up as you're cooking and get inspired. Planning your week and shopping trips will be easier, and you'll use up all the ingredients more regularly.

5. On to the ingredients you don't use regularly. Are there any you want to use but haven't? How can you include at least one in this week's cooking categories (page 35)? Pour these into jars, too, and make sure they're on the plan. Donate the rest.

6. Make a pact with yourself that you won't buy stuff on a whim anymore and clutter your pantry. You'll likely add more items as you cook through this book.

Once you start bringing stuff into your pantry:

- Try to buy as little plastic as possible.
- If you're buying something jarred, bottled, or packaged, turn it over to read the ingredient list. You should know all the words, and they should be real food. If there's anything that sounds like a chemical or preservative, there's a 99.9 percent chance it is. Try to avoid it.
- When you spot a new ingredient that inspires you, go for it. This is the exception to the don't-buy-stuff-on-a-whim rule. But do this with only one thing at a time until you're using it regularly. Otherwise you'll end up with a lot of stuff you don't use and have to do a pantry purge all over again.

Think in Cooking Categories

Having good recipes, and weekday categories for them, solves 99 percent of your cooking problems.

We often don't think about it this way, but the never-ending, universal what-am-I-going-to-eat dilemma has two (kind of three) parts. (1) *What* ingredients am I going to use? (2) *How* am I going to use those ingredients? (Also, I need variety. I don't want to spend too much money, and I want to eat dairy, gluten, and meat in moderation.) Good luck. It's a lot to figure out in just one question, which is why our brains feel like they'll combust while we stare into the fridge. It's too much to compute. Not only is there an overwhelming number of options—cookbooks, Pinterest, magazines, websites, blogs, printed pages—but we're trying to somehow filter all those options into a seven-day plan with a single question (that's not really a single question).

We experienced the exact same burnout having to choose fifty-two weeks' worth of recipes—every. Single. Week. We needed a system. Creating cooking categories eliminated the "*How* am I going to use those ingredients?" question entirely. And it addressed the variety issue, too. The "*What* ingredients am I going to use?" variable was the only one left.

The system unexpectedly became tradition—in our own homes, in our subscribers' homes—and it will for you, too. It's how we've laid out the entire book, week after week. The same categories over and over, in the same format, every season.

MONDAY: hearty bowls—pasta, grains, legumes
TUESDAY: taco-centric—Latin flavors or any cuisine in taco form
WEDNESDAY: light and easy—soup or salad
THURSDAY: keep it simple—meat and side
FRIDAY: a Friday state of mind—pizza, burgers, sandwiches, or comfort food for any mood
SATURDAY/SUNDAY: not in this book, to reflect your days off, night out, takeout, leftovers, or having Sunday suppers or weekend dinner parties

You could follow the designated days as we've categorized them, or switch the nights around to fit your schedule and needs: Monday's Pasta Night on Sunday instead, or Thursday's meat and side on Wednesday. Choose at least three slots each week. Eventually, you might increase the number of cooking days, but either way, plan what you'll be eating those in-between days, too—whether it's takeout, dining out, something premade from the freezer. Maybe some days it's half-and-half—you get something to go and make a crisp salad to accompany it. Or you still cook, but it's the most lightning-fast thing you know how to make in a skillet.

If you stick to your categories, they'll eventually become ingrained in you. A sort of filter through which you'll view every ingredient. Each week you're layering cooking techniques and filing away flavor profiles in your brain; little by little you'll surprise yourself with the kitchen confidence and improvisational skills you've built. Maybe you'll be at the market in late September and see some gorgeous heirloom peppers and immediately think, *You'll be going in my pasta tonight*. You let the ingredients speak to you and decide on the menu after. Everything in your fridge will have a place to go, because you cook in categories.

Kitchen Habits

The Solo Date

The best time and place to begin planning your first cooking category week(s) is the Solo Date. The Solo Date is where you turn your two main human priorities—feeding yourself and finding your purpose—into actual actions in your schedule. Here's how to do it:

1. As far as frequency goes, find what works for you; we like every two weeks. Set aside one to two hours.

2. Choose a somewhat quiet spot where you feel comfortable and creative—it could be a coffee shop, the library, a park bench. Find a way. It probably won't be easy; you've got to push unnecessary obligations out of the way and carve out the space.

3. What to bring: (1) Yourself—this is alone time. (2) A pen, notebook, calendar, and laptop or tablet. (3) This book and/or another cookbook/magazine/your digital sources of recipe inspiration. (4) Any extra stuff, like headphones if you might be in a potentially distracting place or just feel like listening to something.

4. Arrive at your destination, maybe order a latte, get comfy, and start with food planning.

5. Pore over the food inspiration you brought. Figure out which three days you're cooking each week. Dream up at least one extra special day when you'll make a drink or dessert to go along with dinner. Or maybe it's a picnic or Sunday brunch. Choose breakfasts, lunches, dinners for the week. Then think about: Are people coming over? Are you celebrating anything? Are you going to finally schedule in that fancy restaurant date? Cover all the extra bases, and double or triple any recipes as needed. Make a grocery list. Make space in your planner for shopping once a week and cooking on the three or more days you chose. Done with the food planning, on to the life planning.

6. Now, this is where you think far into the future and imagine your life. Are you taking steps toward that future now, no matter how tiny? But really think about it. This is not the same old you who keeps re-resolving New Year's resolutions year after year like a broken record. They're things you want for your life, and they require figuring out a way to finally do them. So grab your notebook and plot out your next steps.

7. Go home feeling refreshed and completely on top of life. Now schedule your next date, and repeat every two weeks on the day that works best for you. For us, Fridays work best so we can plan the weekend *and* the week ahead.

"The Official Declaration of What We're Eating This Week"

When you get home from your Solo Date, plaster your weekly selections, in really big letters, in plain sight somewhere in your kitchen. Monday's pasta, Tuesday's tacos, Wednesday's soup, Thursday's meat and side, Friday's burger. Or whatever cooking categories you decided work best for you.

You've already spent a bunch of time doing the most time-consuming part of this process—planning and maybe even shopping. But it can be easy to get unmotivated about the follow-through. You might even forget what you decided to cook. Fast-forward seven days—you're tossing limp beets, slimy spinach, and questionable meat in the trash. So much time, money, and good intention wasted.

This weekly written declaration is a reminder of your initial plan and all your hard work so far. It's reassurance. It's you telling yourself, "You've got this. Remember?" You'll see it in the morning, when you come home from work, and the fact that you wrote it, in larger-than-usual letters, tells your brain this is important. Typing a phone reminder won't do the trick. Because if it's not posted for all to see, you're not really declaring it.

So grab a large sheet of newspaper from the recycling bin. Scrawl out the plan in super-thick Sharpie. Tape it up. Eventually you can get a chalkboard or something you like better, but you want to start immediately, even if it's not pretty. This is the point of no return. So let it be written. So let it be done.

Okay, now that it's up, let's review. This is not a rigid schedule. It actually helps you be more free and flexible. Here's how:

1. You come home and know what you're cooking. There are no back-and-forth 5 P.M. texts about what's for dinner. You know. Everyone knows. You don't have to deal with hangry

voices asking, either. You can just point and keep chopping. You just added years to your life.

2. The broccoli haters in your crew can mentally prepare for that broccoli dish on Thursday. They know they can't whine their way out. It's posted. It's happening. They'll also be more motivated to be involved in the dinner declaration picks.

3. You can also include any restaurant reservations, to keep you motivated about sticking to the plan. It's a lot easier cooking three or more times a week when you can see the days you gave yourself a break.

4. Life is predictably unpredictable, isn't it? Meetings run late, there are emergency doctor visits and flat tires. There's also the good stuff. A friend calls with exciting news and you drop everything to celebrate. Or you're having an unexpected heart-to-heart with your kid and the moment is way too good to interrupt. Dinner can wait. This is where having a visible version of your plan gives you more flexibility: you can break it when necessary. You can see exactly what to swap and where to swap it.

5. When shopping day comes around, you know what ingredients you have left and for what meal. You don't have to rummage through the fridge. And you know you have to prepare for one less meal the coming week so you can catch up with what you've already purchased. In fact, because you're in the kitchen consistently, you'll develop a photographic memory of what you have in your pantry and fridge at all times. This is a pro home-cook skill, and you now have it.

6. The swappability factor also allows you to invite people over on a whim. Family is coming to town unexpectedly at the end of the week, and the pasta from Monday feeds six, so you'll save that for Friday night and make Friday's dinner on Monday. Or it's a friend's birthday on Thursday, so you'll do tacos on that night instead, and bake a cake, too.

You're now an unfrazzled and gracious host, an expert planner and time saver, and a composed cook dealing with picky eaters—and you have mastered your kitchen. All because you declared it and did it. Over and over.

This is also where you can visually delegate food-related tasks for family members so no one can deny responsibility. Enlist the help of people at home in every department, if possible—cooking, washing dishes, choosing favorites for next week, and so on. Have a family meeting and set expectations, if needed.

The Empty Fridge

The only thing we love more than a full fridge is an empty fridge. Nearly bare, practically nothing in it except the essentials, anything that keeps awhile, and leftover dairy items you'll use up soon. This is what a Huckle & Goose fridge should look like at the end of every week, right before you go shopping and after you've cooked everything on the Official Declaration of What We're Eating This Week.

Why? Once you get the hang of it, having an empty fridge means you estimated your needs for the week well, planned well, and didn't have to run to the grocery store four extra times. You're now in a weekly rhythm that curbs waste, saves money, and prevents the frazzled feeling we tend to get about cooking. You know what to expect and have a better idea of what's in your fridge at all times. You get to start over every week with a clean slate, and you'll never pull weird expired containers from the back of the shelf again.

Here's how to get started:

Before Empty-Fridge Routine:

1. Purge your fridge of any expired stuff. And let it sink in that those containers and bunches of vegetables used to be money.
2. Use whatever you have left to put together meals until you end up with a nearly empty fridge. Make a shopping trip if you need to, for just a few extra ingredients to help bring these meals together.

Empty-Fridge Routine:

1. Now go on a Solo Date to plan food for the upcoming week.
2. Set your weekly shopping day and time in stone. Aim to stick to it most of the time.
3. Before you go shopping, bask in the glory of your empty fridge and wipe it down. Now it's gleaming and ready for the upcoming week's bounty of washed greens, vegetables, trendy yogurt, a jar of homemade dressing.

This takes some practice, but eventually you'll start knowing exactly how much you need to buy. Once you've gone *empty fridge*, you'll never go back.

Kitchen Habits

An Eat-Better, Spend-Less Budget

How much do you *want* to spend on food per month?

How much do you *actually* spend on food per month?

The discrepancy between these two questions is, for many of us, the bane of our existence. Will we ever master this before we die?

The solution is the total opposite of the two things we instinctively do.

1. When we resolve to change our money habits, we often employ sheer will and maybe spreadsheets to spend less. What if we're thinking about it all wrong? Less *spending* might not be the best goal. Less *wanting* is probably a better goal.

2. Then, of all the spending categories, food is the one that gets chopped first. We know that cooking at home should help us save money, but frustratingly, it often doesn't. Then we resort to cheap, quick options or bare-bones meals to save money. And because that makes life feel more unhealthy and/or restrictive (read: miserable), it's tempting to rebel by blowing our budget on an indulgent dinner, continuing the cycle of bad financial decisions.

You might be thinking, "So let me get this straight. Wanting less stuff and spending *more* on food are the answers?"

Yes, and sort of. It's a bit more obvious that contentment would lead to wanting less, and consequently to spending less. But for this idea of spending *more* on food, we have to go through a few layers of mindset shifts, so stay with us here.

This is not about buying food on a whim. This works *only* if you plan and don't waste any food. If you're still reading this habit page, you've already admitted that you spend more on food than you wish to. The amount that we're suggesting probably lies somewhere between want to spend and actually spend.

Let's keep in mind that Americans spend a pretty small percentage of household income on food. We are also home to a staggering obesity rate and rank as one of the unhealthiest high-income countries in the world. Could these things be related? Are you spending more to keep your car running well than to keep yourself running well?

But when we think of better food, $$EXPENSIVE$$ with a bunch of dollar signs flashes in our brains. What we eat affects our well-being *and* our wallet, so we need to find what works for us, without a doubt. But instead of asking, "Why is this item so expensive?" a better question might be "Why is this other thing so cheap?" Because it rarely is. Your tax money might be in there, in the form of government subsidies, or perhaps corners were cut, workers underpaid.

Good food helps you feel good. And when you feel good, you make better decisions. And when you make better decisions, you start confidently living your values. And when you start confidently living your values . . . you find contentment. Full-circle moment.

Spending more on food = spending less in other areas, because you want less.

You can start feeling this shift in just a few weeks. And here's the money application. You're way less likely to impulse shop. You're spending less on snacks, because you don't need them. You bought super-nutritious food that filled you up and you're learning to eat (and want) just enough. You don't feel the need to dine out as regularly, because you know how to make dishes that rival most of the restaurants in town. You invite friends over instead of meeting at restaurants. You're excited about packing leftovers for lunch, because dinner was *actually* good.

This confidence and clarity now shows up in all your money-related decisions.

What to Eat and When to Eat It

———————

You may have heard that there are right and wrong times to eat stuff—you should eat before *this* time. Breakfast is important. Don't eat that food past a certain time or it'll make you fat. But why, *exactly*? And is any of this advice actually true?

Here is the underlying science behind all these rules. This is basically a crash course in how your body digests. Ready?

Remember how the circadian clock in your brain responds to light? When you wake up in the morning, if you listen to your body, it's basically saying, "The sun is up, you're up. Please feed me well, we've got important work to do today. And whatever you eat, I'm going to burn energy so you can do that work." It's asking for vegetables, eggs, good fat, protein, and fiber that will give you optimal focus and energy. That's the ideal fuel, and it's burned as energy. If you feed it a coffee and a muffin, you get a temporary, jittery, crash-and-burn type of energy. So a treat is fine, but it comes with a cost. We usually save them for days when we can afford to be lazier. You get to choose. How do you want to feel today? Do you want to stay sharp and motivated? Or is it an indulgent day?

As the day goes on and you're approaching lunchtime, your body assumes you'll still be up for a while, continuing to work. So it burns those calories as energy, too. But as you approach dinnertime, you're treading a finer line. The sun is on its way to setting, and your body will start preparing to shut down for sleep. Toward the tail end of this transition, your body is saying, "Aaaand that's a wrap on today," and beginning to store calories as fat. Five to seven is the ideal window for dinnertime (because nine to ten is the ideal bedtime, and the earlier within that window you can swing it, the better).

This also means that with not-so-great-for-you foods—refined stuff, sugar, flour, starchy things that are not as easily digested—the earlier in the day you eat them, the better you'll digest them. Your body is in higher gear.

What happens if you skip breakfast or have irregular meal times? Breakfast controls your hunger and blood sugar for the rest of the day. It sets the pace and gives your body hope that you'll eat according to its ideal digestive rhythm. When you don't eat every three or four hours, you leave your body in limbo, wondering how to process your next meal—as fat or energy. Pair this with an out-of-whack sleep schedule and good luck trying to feel well or stay at a healthy weight. Your body has zero clue what you're doing. It can't follow along. And when that happens, your insulin (fat-storing hormone) level spikes. This is even worse for your body than eating unhealthy foods. Creating a predictable eating and sleeping pattern that syncs with your circadian rhythm is surprisingly important.

Here's what an ideal day might look like:

7:30 A.M.: Breakfast
12:00 noon: Lunch
3:15 P.M.: Snack—and maybe some afternoon tea, too
6:45 or 7:00 P.M.: Dinner

So if life allows, eat the biggest meals earlier in the day and the lightest later on. Try to shift your dinnertimes more toward six rather than toward eight if you can. Set your meal times and sleep times in stone. And, most important, don't skip breakfast.

The Grown-Up Lunchbox

Have you ever pulled back the plastic cover on your Tupperware and thought, *I guess sad lunches are my life now*? What happened? The haze of adulthood, that's what. We're here for you like lunch fairy godmothers. We've been intentional about creating recipes that aren't just great dinners but can also be enjoyed for lunch the next day. You've just gotta pack it.

Here are just a handful of favorites to get you started, but any soup, salad, grain bowl, pasta, wrap, or sandwich in this book would be great.

Roasted Romanesco & Toasted Farro with Warm Cherry Pepper Vinaigrette (page 298)
Spiced Lamb Wraps with Ramp Raita (page 82)
Neighborhood Café Frittata Sandwich with Early-Autumn Fruit (page 245)
Greens & Grains Bowl with Rosemary Roasted Garlic Dressing (page 212)
The Chicken Caesar Salad Wraps (page 268)

Now that you know what to pack, get rid of those pitiful lunch containers. You know which ones. The one with mystery stains on the bottom that will never come out. The one with the cover that just. Won't. Close. No matter how hard you press. Toss them all out. Instead, invest in glass and stainless steel containers. You want quality + function + design. Get some jars with wide mouths for toting soups or salads, smaller jars for dressings, and don't forget about the utensils.

And before you say "Spending $25 is just too expensive!" just add up your weekly lunch allowance (that salad or wrap place you love) and we promise you'll be taking a salad that's ten times better and cheaper than what you buy.

Okay, you've got the food and the container all figured out. Don't waste it. And by "Don't waste it" we mean you've got a lunch hour, so use it. If the weather allows it, go outside as often as you can. Have a conversation with a co-worker or decompress a bit by listening to music or a podcast. Point is: lunch is lunch. And it'll spark creativity for whatever you work on after lunch.

Netflix & Do Dishes

TV sucks hours from our days and weeks. If we're not mindful about how much screen time we consume, we'll find ourselves reading fewer books at bedtime, spending less time with family, and slacking on chores.

Reality for most of us: Once you're on the couch, it's very hard to stop at one episode. Sometimes after dinner we'd relax and then attempt to clean up after *just* one episode. What ended up happening was that either the dishes were being done waaaaay too late or we'd give up and say, "We can tackle them tomorrow."

Only problem is that there's nothing worse in the morning than waking up to regret in the form of dirty plates with cement-like food stuck to them. Good luck starting your day all bright-eyed and bushy-tailed when your favorite mug is lost somewhere in the depths of the sink. Now you have to settle for one of the ugly mugs that make your coffee taste bad. Great.

And now you're spiraling—ugh, maybe you'll just get your coffee from the coffee shop next to work. But you remember you already spent your week's coffee budget. Now you're debating whether four bucks will really be that bad. And if you're going to get the coffee, you can't not get the scone. Now you really have to fit in the workout today, since you binge-watched last night and overslept. This inner dialogue had you staring at the wall, but now you see the dirty dishes again. *Dang it, when am I going to do these?! When I get home. But if I work out, it will be later, and then I can't make dinner. I'll just order pizza and do the dishes after.* You look at the clock and realize you'll be late for work if you don't leave the house in fifteen minutes. And that is how we fail at life. And it's a good lesson on how one bad decision leads to another.

But there is a solution, TV lovers: On weeknights, watch TV only while you're doing the dishes. Your kitchen will be spotless every night, and you won't binge-watch. All you need is a tablet or laptop. Set it on top of a sturdy container—the jar you keep sugar in, anything to give it some height for optimal viewing. Find your show or movie and push play. And voilà! You'll find yourself wishing there were more dishes to wash.

Happy Hour at Home

If you've never been a glass-half-full person, this is our secret to becoming an optimist: Drink fancy drinks. We're not talking about the priciest wine on the menu. But just as a glass of chilled rosé feels like it was bottled with a gulp of carefree, sophisticated French air, other colorful, sparkling, or boozy drinks have a similar strong sense of place. Somewhere simpler. A sip can instantly make you feel like you're swinging on a porch swing or sitting on a breezy café patio.

There's a whole range of fancy drinks you can make at home—from aguas frescas that transport you to legit taquerias to cocktails with a dash of swanky Manhattan speakeasy. We've made sure to include some of our foolproof favorites in every category here.

Some you'll sip in slo-mo, soaking up the afternoon sun with your kids. Others will make you feel like James Bond, mixologist extraordinaire. And let's be honest: There's a certain *je ne sais quoi* to expertly mixing a couple of ingredients and pouring them into a chilled glass. We want you to get so expert-level that you eventually have your very own legendary "house" cocktail you can make with your eyes closed. It'll get requested at every party. The basic formula: two parts spirit, one part sour/citrus/freshly squeezed lemon or lime, one half part sweet, and any extras like herbs, spices, garnishes, and bitters (we love bitters).

So, ya know, once or twice a week, pour yourself a glass of something for your mood. A crisp white wine while you cook during golden hour. Shake up a Green Gemini to celebrate—cheers to nailing that interview. Sip an Apricot Bourbon Smash in your favorite chunky sweater while you read by firelight; spectacles optional. Other times, the happiest of happy hours are shared. And for these times you need ain't-nobody-got-time-for-that pitcher drinks like Pear Pitcher Margaritas, Doublemint Mojitos, and Summer Orchard Sangria with Elderflower & Basil.

Friends, some habits are easier to keep than others. Cheers!

The Herb Box

If you ever see "1 teaspoon fresh parsley, minced, for garnish" in a recipe, triple-check to make sure that amount makes sense for what you're cooking, or *ruuuuuun.*

Such inconsequential quantities of herbs are silly. Herbs aren't garnishes—that's why they're sold in bunches. Either cook with 'em like you mean it or don't bother, you know?

You could start at the supermarket with the mini packaged herbs to get the hang of it. Then walk through the market whenever you're ready. Those way bigger, fragrant bunches will practically call your name and you'll feel the pull to use them throughout the week. Your mojitos will taste infinitely more minty. Boring salads will be a distant memory. Herbs will thoroughly invigorate and inspire your cooking. The flavors are pure, verdant magic; you'll learn to look for creative ways to use them instead of stressing about wilting herbs.

Eventually, having two to four herb bunches in your fridge, at the same time, will be totally normal. But how do you keep them from dying on you?

Here's the Huckle & Goose foolproof storage method that works for basically everything. First, give them a good wash—especially cilantro, because it's usually got extra grit. Spin, and let them sit out a bit to fully dry. Basil is needy and unpredictable, so use that early in the week and quickly. But every other herb will be content wrapped in a dry paper towel or cloth (to absorb and wick away accumulating moisture) and tucked together in a big glass box (airtight). Some even keep for up to two weeks.

Almost every single recipe in this book has fresh herbs. Dill, tarragon, cilantro, mint, basil, parsley, chives, thyme, sage, summer savory, Thai basil, rosemary. They're in everything from cocktails to pastas to tacos to dressings to spreads to burgers. And we've selected the recipes for each week based on the herb, so you can use up your bunches quickly and easily. It's all built into the pages. From now on you'll cook every meal and make every drink thinking, *How can I make this better with herbs?* And you'll know exactly what to do.

Something Sweet Every Week

Have you ever read those articles about eating whatever you want as long as you *pay attention*? And then thought, *Right. But hoooow*?

Embodying a spirit of moderation and enjoying positive results makes sense in theory. But it seems like there's some sort of special switch or secret trick that suddenly initiates the self-control you've always wanted and allows you to effortlessly make perfectly balanced food choices simply by paying attention. Maybe the secret is being French . . . ?

Short of moving to Paris, there is a switch you can flip. And this book was created to activate this deep-down-discipline switch for you.

It starts with an unwavering commitment to baking or cooking something sweet every week so that it becomes a rhythm for you.

As you cook and bake from this book, you'll start noticing that when you salt well, use good ingredients, add abundant herbs and bold flavor, and keep everything in the right proportions, food tastes surprisingly good at home. Probably more than you ever imagined it could. You can now make really informed mental comparisons about the food you eat. For instance: "Our usual takeout is pointlessly greasy, but I really love how the stir-fry I make at home is lighter and just as flavorful." Or "I really love this cake, but it's a bit too sweet. I'm going to attempt something similar at home with less sugar." As you venture out of your comfort zone with new ingredients and cooking methods, your palate becomes more *discerning*. Which is a nice way of saying: secretly snobby about your food. Once you notice the snobbery, fully embrace it. It's the main ingredient in activating those nonchalant yet calculated food choices. It'll make saying no to things a breeze. Because, seriously, the scones at your usual coffee place skimp on the berries, so you might as well wait till you make them on Saturday morning. Your mindset shifts from "I can't have that," which sends deprivation signals to your brain, to "I'm choosing not to have that because there's something better I'm looking forward to."

Your state of mind matters here because it influences your metabolism, too. Confidence and zero guilt about indulging help your body break down the food better so you can fully enjoy it. So if you ever tread into mindlessly-wiping-out-half-a-sheet-pan-of-cookies territory, remember that your digestion is already syncing up with your future regret.

Which is why the Something Sweet Every Week routine is important. Since none of the recipes yield a single serving, you'll have to share them with other people and throw dinner parties so you don't eat an entire cake or tray of cookies. Plus, you'll be the person who always has a delicious slice of cake to serve at a moment's notice or has cookies to bring in to work. The best part about food is sharing it, and this is one of the easiest places to start.

The Greens Box

You open your fridge and pull out a wilted, soggy, all-out nasty bag of forgotten greens from the crisper. The kind of nasty that requires just two fingers holding the corner of the bag. You throw it in the garbage, along with any self-worth, clenching your fist à la Seinfeld—wilty greens are your Newman. No matter how good your intentions were when you bought them earlier in the week, you're back to square one. You basically paid money to waste food. Ugh.

Let's work on keeping your trash can from eating any more of your greens.

1. First, you need a box. It can be plastic, but aim for glass if you can. It has to have an airtight lid and be big enough to fit a good bunch of greens. (Anywhere between one and two gallons is the perfect size.)
2. Now turn your (clean) sink into a giant bowl. Spray it down with a mix of half vinegar, half water, then rinse. Fill it with water and add all your greens (leaves separated if in head form, e.g., romaine, radicchio, frisée). Swish them around with your hands. The dirt should sink to the bottom and say hello to any friendly bugs that emerge from the greens. Some might need two changes of water.
3. Remove the clean greens, add them to your salad spinner, and spin, spin, spin. Dry greens are happy greens. You want as little moisture as possible in your Greens Box or they'll get wilty, slimy, or moldy a lot faster.
4. Wrap greens in kitchen towels, flour sack towels, or paper towels (again, to absorb moisture) and nestle in your box.
5. Close and keep in the fridge until you're ready to use them. Repeat next week.

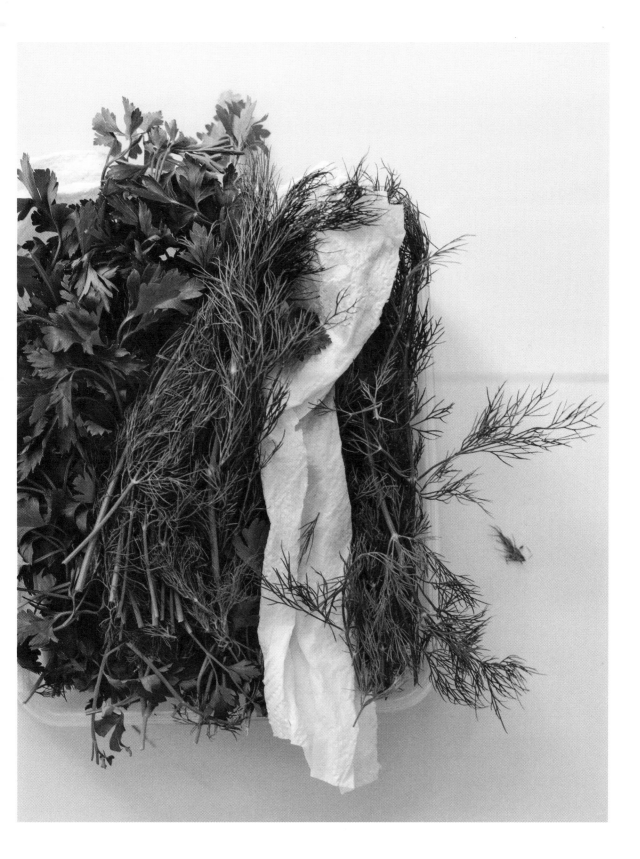

Spoiler alert: You're never gonna love washing, drying, trimming, and storing your greens weekly. But you're gonna do it anyway, because the surest way to actually eat more salad is by having it waiting for you. You're tired of the trash can winning.

Okay, now you've got them in your fridge. You should be eating them every day in different ways. Don't freak out about the "every day" part. This doesn't mean salad for dinner each night. It means that a variety of greens are used in various ways throughout the day. Sometimes it's more of a garnish on top of a sandwich, other times you'll stuff handfuls in a blender for a smoothie. Don't just buy kale and romaine; try mâche, frisée, rainbow chard, arugula, mizuna, or spinach. Adorable microgreens and sprouts count, too. If you're trying new greens, buy a smaller amount and ask the farmer. They'll tell you their favorite ways to eat them. Here are some of ours: the quintessential raw salad; morning smoothies; frittatas and scrambled eggs, next to an omelet—just a little handful that doesn't even need dressing; wraps and sandwiches; soups and stews (most soups could do with some chopped, wilted greens); quick sauté with garlic and oil (the perfect side for any meat or fish); quesadillas and tacos; pasta tossed with chopped greens; stuffed in meatballs, meatloaf, or burgers (veggie burgers included); any and all grain bowls. Now get out there and find your Greens Box.

The Dressing Jar

You've got one more step: dress those greens well.

Homemade dressings took us from "I *have* to eat some greens" to "I can't believe I'm actually eating a second serving of salad!" Salad never took center stage. That was something people on a diet did, not us. But if you've ever bought beautiful baby greens from the market, you know that dressing them with that month-old bottle of store-bought ranch is kind of a crime. Like wet cement being poured on a bed of flowers. There are really good, simple dressings throughout this book that you can whip up in less than five minutes, shake-shake-shake in a jar, and keep in the fridge for a week, always ready. Welcome to the "I love greens" side of life!

You've Got Restaurant Reservations

There's nothing like being wined and dined. And it's absolutely necessary if you're going to keep up a cooking-at-home habit.

Make a list of six to twelve restaurants for the year—the ones you've dreamed about, read about, heard about. The ones you'd really love to try but don't because—not enough dinero. It's not in your budget, except maybe once a year for your birthday or an anniversary. It's reserved for the few, the proud, the wealthy. Make the list; don't look at the $$$ signs for now.

You might be thinking, "But wait, I thought this book was about eating out less, and I'm already spending too much on food. And now you want me to book five-star restaurants?"

We want to help curb *unplanned* dining out. Because one of two things happens when we impulsively dine out: (1) The food is delicious and you're happy you treated yourself, but when the going-over-budget reality hits later on, it's instant regret. Or (2) the food is mediocre and you know after one bite that you could've had something better at home. Regret, once again.

Spending money on the wrong meals out can be almost completely avoided if you plan well, make a habit of cooking three times a week, and feel giddy about eating at a spectacular place you set aside money for. You stuck to it and didn't blow that $120 on last-minute lo mein orders, pizza deliveries, or at the café that usually burns the coffee and has dry muffins. You're trading all that for memorable food at home and eating at the best places in town.

So write this month's restaurant in bold letters on a piece of paper and tape it to the wall next to your Official Declaration of What We're Eating This Week. Maybe you need it next to the take-out menus. Doesn't matter where—it's there to remind you to stick to your plan and your budget.

And then reservation day arrives! It's at 7:45 P.M.—you've already checked the menu online. You're also debating between two outfits—that dress with the tags still on it and the usual contender for nights out. Go for the tags. When you're finally at the restaurant, make it count. It was your discipline that got you here. Order a cocktail at the bar before heading to your table. Have a conversation over candlelight (no phones). Order dessert with tea or cappuccino and linger, linger, linger.

You'll leave refreshed, inspired, and willing to do this again so you can experience another cool spot. It might even spark ideas for recipes to replicate at home—your next lunch salad or a vegetable you previously disliked but ordered anyway and realized you could be cooking it differently.

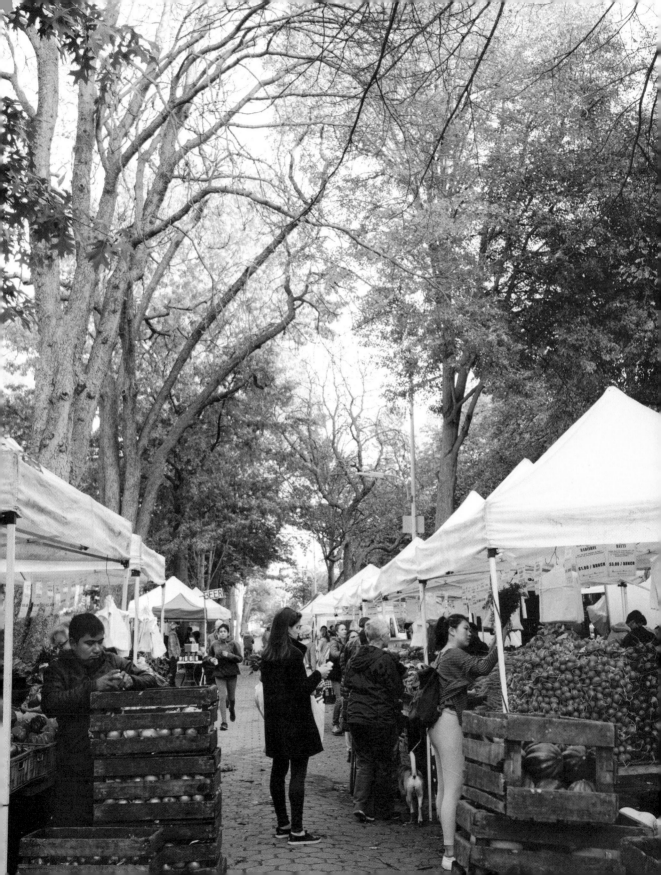

Part 3

Cook 3x a Week

———

The Recipes

NOTICE WHAT'S HAPPENING OUTSIDE (NATURE)

AND INSIDE (HUMAN NATURE).

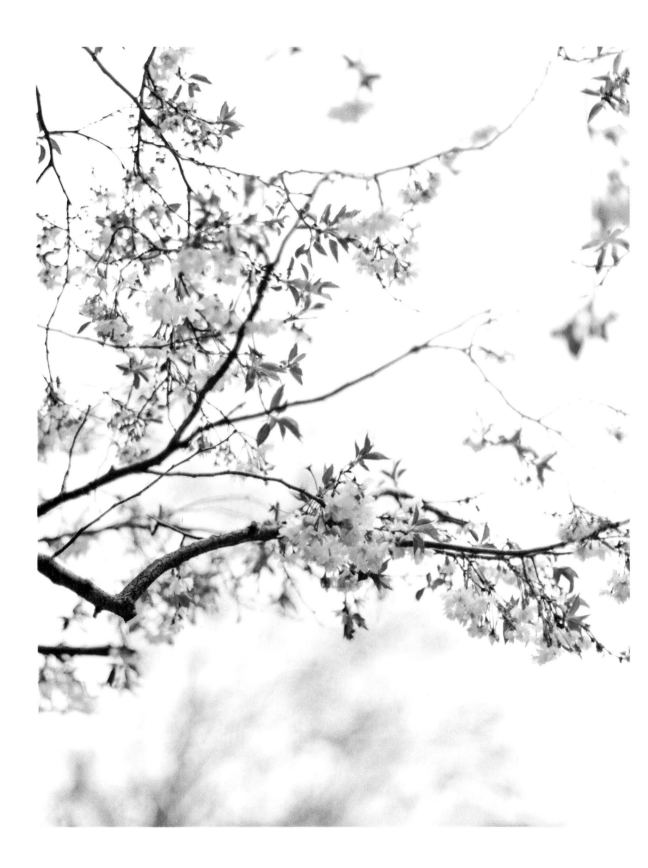

Spring

NOTICE WHAT'S HAPPENING OUTSIDE (NATURE) . . .

If you've forgotten how to notice—really notice—then any moment, any time of year, is the right time to start. But spring is the sweetest time. Cold to warm, dead to alive, sleep to awake. There's snow, snow, snow, then you discover a patch of new green sprouting through. Birds chirp again, bees buzz. Trees are still bare, still bare, still bare, then they're suddenly speckled with buds and blossoms. These are nature's daily baby steps toward growth after a long winter. A way to remember—one that's all around you and under your feet—that blooming happens little by little, and hard work happens in the dirt. It's messy, but that's the beauty of it.

. . . AND INSIDE (HUMAN NATURE)

The newness of spring days helps us sense the promise of fresh starts. It's when we feel the strongest tug to grow ourselves. Make nature's pace yours, too. Slow, sure, steady.

HERE'S WHAT TO LOOK FORWARD TO:

Bunches and bunches of fresh herbs, first asparagus, peas, rhubarb,

picnics, cherry blossoms, magnolia trees, tulips, daffodils, violets, flying kites,

the smell of freshly cut grass, blowing dandelion puffs, strawberry picking,

rainstorms, jumping in puddles, cherries.

Your Spring Kitchen Plan

COOK 3X A WEEK:

Choose three dinners.

Add on breakfasts, something

sweet, and a drink, too, if you'd

like. Make a grocery list.

Remember to think in
cooking categories (page 34)
and add a new kitchen habit that
will help you stick to your
plan (pages 31–51).

After 4 weeks, mix and match
favorite recipes to cook the rest
of the season.

Week 1

Monday	Garden Lentil Soup with Lemon & Dill
Tuesday	Brilliant Roasted Beets with Arugula & Jalapeño-Feta Sauce
Wednesday	Spring Chopped Salad with Tarragon-Shallot Vinaigrette
Thursday	Chicken Yakitori & House Salad with Miso-Ginger Dressing
Friday	Be the Babushka Beef Stroganoff

Week 2

Monday	Market Lentil Salad with Coriander-Roasted Roots, Mint & Goat Cheese
Tuesday	Lucky No-Sear Korean Short Rib Tacos with Quick-Pickled Root Slaw
Wednesday	Asparagus Soup for Rich People
Thursday	Beer-Braised Chicken with Peas & Bacon
Friday	Spring Fever Pizza with Crumbly Sausage & *Raaamps!*

Week 3

Monday	May Day Pasta Bowl
Tuesday	Spiced Lamb Wraps with Ramp Raita
Wednesday	Ensalada Primavera
Thursday	Herb-Butter Fish in Parchment with Tender Spring Veggies
Friday	Actual Garden Burger with Herbs, White Beans & Peas

Week 4

Monday	Shortcut Ramen with Spring Vegetables
Tuesday	Skirt Steak & Charred Green Onion Tacos with Chipotle Crema
Wednesday	Herb Box Salad with Kale, Chickpea Croutons & Lemony Sumac Dressing
Thursday	A Proper Spring Supper
Friday	Spring Afternoon Picnic Quiche with a View

Breakfasts, Drinks, Something Sweet

Breakfast	Soft-Boiled Eggs with Herb Butter Toast Dips
Breakfast	Hello Spring Egg Salad Sandwich with Chive Blossoms
Breakfast	Super Good Spelt Crepes with Strawberries
Breakfast	Warrior Three-Egg Omelet
Happy Hour	Doublemint Mojitos
Sweet	Party Like It's 1999 Compost Cake
Sweet	Ode to Rhubarb Cornmeal Cake
Sweet	Strawberry-Basil Granita
Sweet	Pistachio Blondies with Berry Collision à la Mode

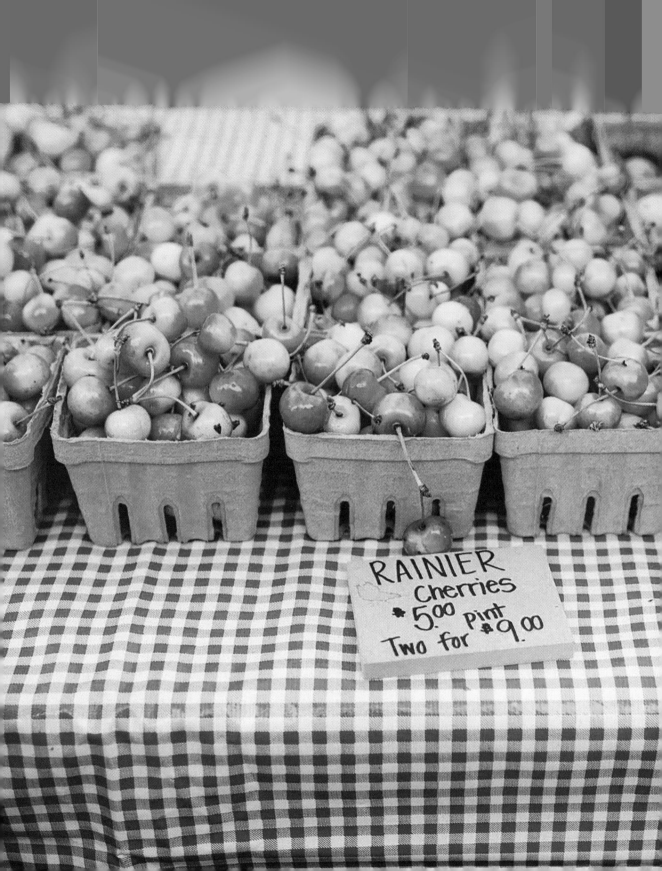

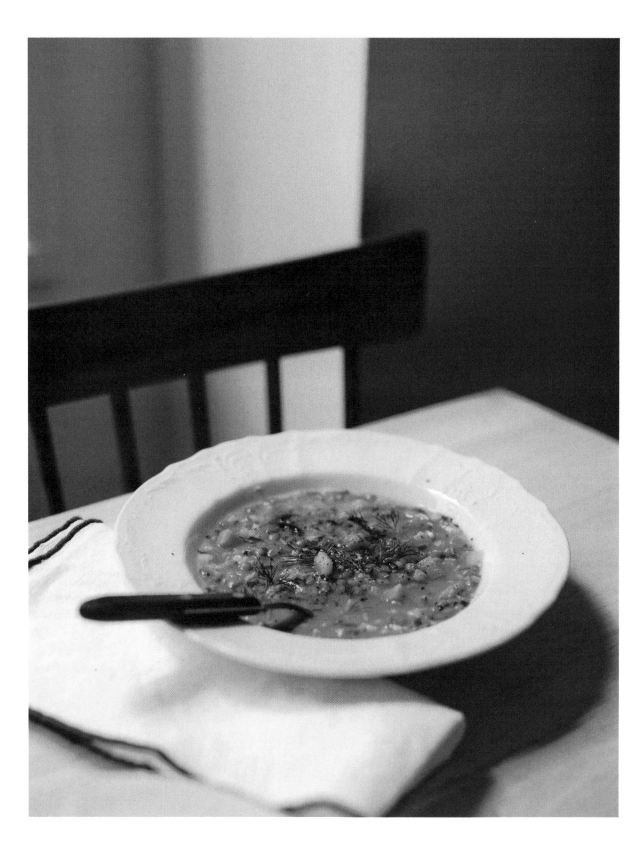

Garden Lentil Soup with Lemon & Dill

Serves: 6

_____

3 tablespoons extra-virgin olive oil, divided

2 tablespoons unsalted butter, divided

I yellow onion or a small bunch of spring onions, diced

2 stalks celery, diced

2 carrots, diced

3 cloves garlic or green garlic, minced

¼ teaspoon each: dried basil, rosemary, thyme, marjoram, oregano, or I heaping teaspoon herbes de Provence

I teaspoon lemon pepper seasoning

½ teaspoon crushed red pepper

4 cups low-sodium chicken or vegetable stock

2 cups water

I bay leaf

¾ cup French green lentils, soaked overnight for max nutrition

½ cup long-grain white rice

Juice of I lemon, plus zest of ½ lemon

¼ cup fresh dill, minced, plus more for garnish

Parsley and chives, optional; if you have either on hand, mince up a handful to stir into the soup

Salt

Pepper

The lentils from your winter pantry have a spring in their step. With the addition of early spring market finds like fresh herbs, spring onions, and green garlic, it's a bright and warming supper for a dreary March day. It's also a lesson in layering a soup with a generous amount of all the things that make it taste hearty and complex: two types of fat (butter and oil), acid (lemon and zest), aromatics (garlic, onion, celery, carrots), and herbs (both fresh and dried).

1. Set a soup pot over medium heat and add in a tablespoon each of oil and butter.

2. Once the butter is melted and bubbly, add onion, celery, and carrots. Sauté for 5 minutes, until softened, then add garlic, herbs, lemon pepper, crushed red pepper, and ½ teaspoon salt, and stir for 30 more seconds.

3. Pour in the stock and water with another ½ teaspoon salt and some cracks of pepper; drop in bay leaf.

4. Bring to a boil, then turn the heat down to a low simmer; add lentils and rice, giving everything a good stir.

5. Partially cover and simmer for 20 minutes (assuming they both need about 20 minutes to cook). Check the rice package instructions and adjust time if needed. Add another cup or so of water if needed for your desired liquid-to-other-ingredients ratio. Taste for salt, check lentils and rice for doneness, then turn off heat.

6. Pour in remaining 2 tablespoons of oil, and swirl in remaining tablespoon of butter, lemon zest and juice, and minced dill. Cover and let the flavors meld for 5 minutes, then ladle into shallow bowls with a drizzle of olive oil and a sprinkle of parsley or chives, if desired.

_____

Note: Also, if you anticipate having leftovers, the rice absorbs a lot of the liquid pretty fast; cooking it separately and adding it to the soup bowls as you serve solves the issue of the soup thickening.

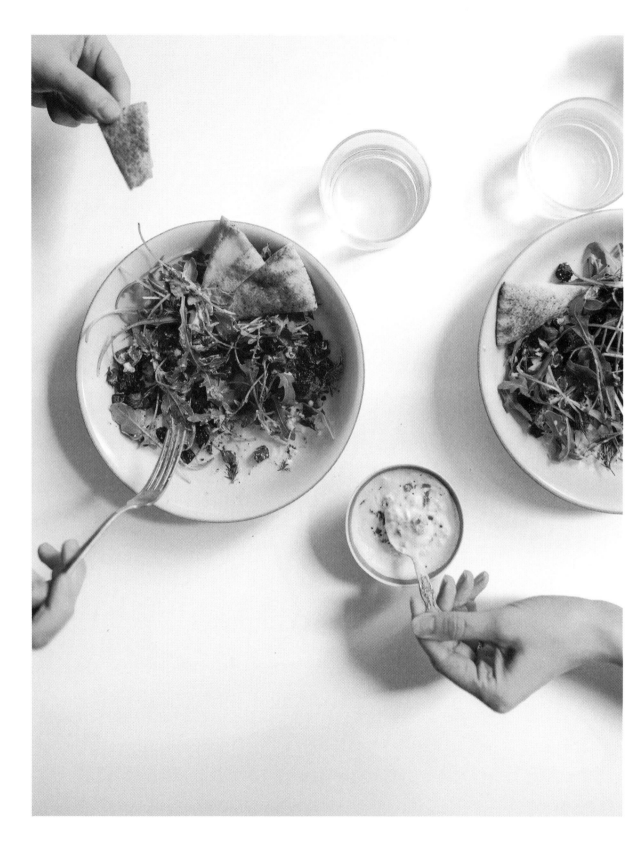

Brilliant Roasted Beets with Arugula & Jalapeño-Feta Sauce

Serves: 4

Beets

2 tablespoons grapeseed oil

2 teaspoons granulated garlic

2 teaspoons dried oregano

1 teaspoon dried marjoram

½ teaspoon dried thyme

¼ teaspoon ground nutmeg

1 teaspoon salt

¾ teaspoon pepper

1¾ pounds beets, a mix of red, golden, and Chioggia, scrubbed or peeled

Juice of ½ lemon

Sauce

4 ounces feta cheese

¼ cup pickled jalapeño brine, plus a few pickled jalapeños if you'd like

2 teaspoons extra-virgin olive oil

For serving

1 package pita, lavash, or thick flour tortillas

3 cups baby arugula

Grapeseed oil

Beets get a bad rap. If you've ever eaten a poorly seasoned beet with unappetizing texture—rubbery on the outside but still slightly firm in the middle—we don't blame you for writing them off. Here's the trick to becoming a beet lover: tiny cubes. They should be no bigger than a quarter inch, you have to season them generously with salt, herbs, and spices, and you've got to roast them until they're caramelized and jammy all the way through.

1. Preheat oven to 425°F.

2. In a very small bowl, whisk together the oil, herbs, spices, salt, and pepper with a fork. Set aside.

3. Slice off the tops and bottoms of the beets; chop into tiny ¼-inch cubes. Pile onto a baking sheet and drizzle on the herbed oil. Toss with your hands to coat, then spread them out evenly. Slide in the oven for 30–40 minutes, flipping halfway through. When they're soft and slightly browned, squeeze lemon juice over and stir right on the baking sheet. Set aside.

4. Meanwhile, place feta, jalapeño brine (and jalapeños, if using), and olive oil in a blender; blend until smooth. Add more brine to adjust consistency if needed. Set aside (or refrigerate in a jar for up to a week).

5. To serve, stuff beets and greens into pitas, lavash, or flour tortillas, like tacos, and drizzle with sauce. Or pile beets onto a bed of arugula and drizzle generously with sauce for one of the best salads of your life. To make homemade pita crisps: Slice pitas into wedges or strips, brush with a bit of oil, and slide into a 400°F oven on a sheet pan for 5–10 minutes, until crisp.

Spring Chopped Salad with Tarragon-Shallot Vinaigrette

Serves: 4

Dressing

¼ cup extra-virgin olive oil

3 tablespoons white wine vinegar

2 tablespoons red onion, shallot, or spring onion, very finely minced

2 tablespoons fresh tarragon, minced or snipped with kitchen shears

½ teaspoon salt

½ teaspoon pepper

Salad

1 head crisp lettuce, chopped or torn into ½-inch pieces

½ cup mixed fresh herbs: dill, chives, basil, and/or mint, chopped or snipped with kitchen shears

½ bunch radishes, thinly sliced

½ cup snow peas, very thinly sliced

2 ounces sharp cheddar cheese, chopped into tiny cubes

Chopping up greens and veggies in small, uniform, bite-size pieces and tossing with an herby vinaigrette and some creamy cheese makes salad eating not so bad. (It's easier for kids to eat, too.)

We used tarragon for the dressing here because it's underused and spices things up with its anise-like flavor, but you could swap for a totally different herb, like chives or parsley. Get creative with other veggies, too—roasted asparagus or peas. If you have any cured meat in the fridge—mortadella, prosciutto, salami—thinly slice and add. You could swap out the cheddar for another cheese you like more—Parm, feta, or goat cheese would all work well.

1. Combine dressing ingredients in a small jar and shake, shake, shake (about one minute) until it looks thickened and well combined.

2. In a large bowl, toss chopped lettuce, herbs, radishes, and snow peas with the vinaigrette and divide among shallow bowls, topping with cheese (and meat, if using). Or you could let everyone dress their own salad, especially if you're packing it for lunch or a picnic.

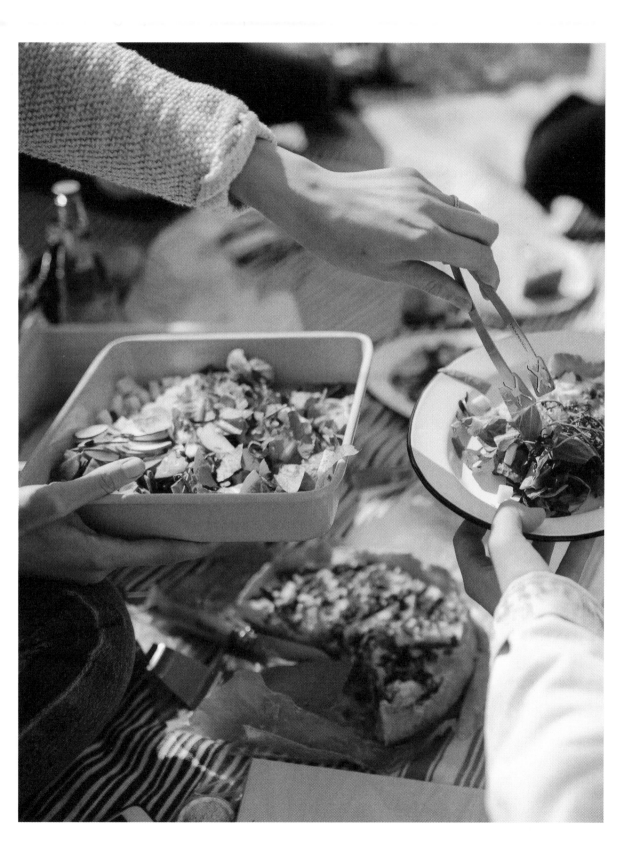

Chicken Yakitori & House Salad with Miso-Ginger Dressing

Serves: 4

_____

Chicken

2-inch piece fresh ginger, thinly sliced (no need to peel)

4 cloves garlic, minced

3 tablespoons coconut sugar or maple syrup

½ cup soy sauce

½ cup mirin

1 teaspoon cornstarch

1 tablespoon water

1¼ pounds boneless, skinless chicken thighs, cut into 1-inch pieces

1 bunch scallions, cut into 1–2-inch pieces

Wooden skewers (soaked in water for an hour)

2–3 cups cooked white or brown rice, to serve

We love our neighborhood Japanese joint. Gyoza, chicken yakitori, miso soup, and house salad are must-orders. And since our favorite bright orange dressing is raw pureed carrot with miso and ginger (basically salad on top of salad), we had to try it at home.

1. In a small saucepan, combine the ginger, garlic, coconut sugar, soy sauce, and mirin. Bring to a boil, then simmer for about 15 minutes, until slightly thickened. In a small cup, whisk together the cornstarch and water until cornstarch is dissolved; pour into the sauce. Simmer another minute or so, until thickened. Turn off heat, remove ginger, and set aside.

2. Reserve 3 tablespoons of the sauce to serve on the side later.

3. Pour the rest of the sauce over the chicken, using your hands to massage it in, making sure to coat all over.

4. Preheat broiler.

5. Grab your skewers and begin by threading a piece of chicken, followed by 2 or 3 scallion pieces; repeat until you've filled up most of the skewer. Squish everything together so the scallions don't burn and chicken stays juicy.

6. Transfer skewers to a foil-lined sheet pan. When you've used up all the chicken and scallion, brush on some of the remaining sauce the chicken was marinating in. Slide in the oven (about 4 inches from broiler) for 10 minutes.

7. In a high-powered blender, puree the dressing ingredients—everything from carrots to sesame oil with a good pinch of salt and pepper—until smooth. Transfer to a jar and refrigerate for up to 3 days.

8. When the chicken is a bit charred and cooked through, remove from the oven and serve immediately with the reserved sauce and rice.

9. Serve the romaine lettuce with dressing drizzled over, or lightly toss the entire salad and serve with extra dressing on the side.

Salad

2 medium carrots, peeled and roughly chopped

½ shallot, cut into quarters

2 tablespoons white miso

2 tablespoons coconut sugar or maple syrup

½ cup grapeseed oil, or any neutral-tasting oil

1-inch piece fresh ginger, chopped

3 tablespoons rice wine vinegar

1 teaspoon sesame oil

Salt

Pepper

1 head romaine lettuce, chopped

Kitchen note: When in season, cucumbers, radishes, and tomatoes would be delicious in this salad as well. It's perfect for a packed bento box lunch the next day. PS: Miso is super healthy–it's fermented and packed with gut-healthy nutrients like enzymes and probiotics.

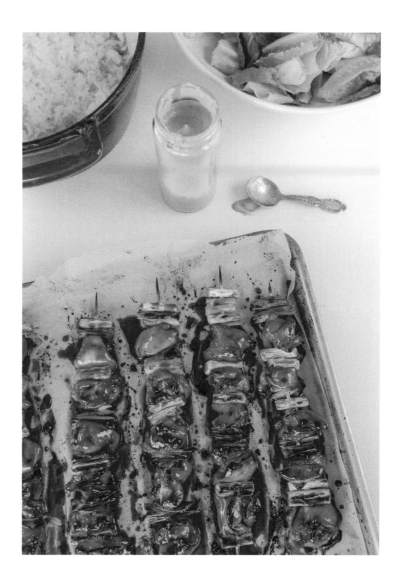

Be the Babushka Beef Stroganoff

Serves: 4

_____

3 tablespoons unsalted butter, divided

10 ounces shiitake mushrooms, stems discarded, sliced

¾ pound egg noodles

3 tablespoons fresh Italian parsley, chopped, divided

1 pound top round, hanger steak, or boneless rib eye, thinly sliced

1 large yellow onion, sliced

¼ cup vodka, cognac, or brandy

6 cloves garlic, minced

1 tablespoon paprika

1 tablespoon Dijon mustard

½ cup chicken broth or water

½ cup sour cream

2 tablespoons fresh dill, chopped

Salt

Pepper

Maybe you've been snappy, hurried, and stressed this week. The whole family feels it, and tempers are short. Dinner together has been an afterthought. You need to get yourself and everyone else back on track. This is when you channel your inner babushka. The babushka is the thread that holds the family together. She is no-nonsense in her approach to the things that matter most. Sometimes love needs to be full force and determined, so she makes a dinner full of comfort. Take a swig of vodka like she would, and let's get to work.

1. Heat a large skillet over medium-high heat. Add 1 tablespoon of butter and, when melted, add the mushrooms. Cook 2 minutes without stirring so they get nicely browned. Then shake the pan or stir, sprinkle with a few pinches of salt, and cook another 2 minutes. Transfer to a bowl and set aside.

2. Bring a large pot of salted water to a boil. Add the egg noodles and cook according to package instructions. Drain and add back to the pot or a large bowl. Add 1 tablespoon of butter and 1 tablespoon of chopped parsley; toss to combine.

3. Meanwhile, season the sliced beef with salt and pepper. Then, in the same pan used for the mushrooms, melt another tablespoon of butter over medium-high heat. Add the beef in a single layer (do it in 2 batches if needed). Cook 1 minute, then flip and cook another 30 seconds. Using tongs, transfer the beef to the bowl with the mushrooms and set aside.

4. Lower heat to medium, add more butter if needed, then the onions. Sauté for 10 minutes, until soft, and pour in vodka to deglaze (fancy term for scraping up the browned bits on the bottom of the pan after adding liquid). Stir well and cook until the vodka is almost all evaporated.

5. Stir in the garlic, paprika, a few pinches of salt, mustard, and pepper to taste. Cook for a minute, then pour in the broth or water. Stir well, then add the sour cream and turn heat to low. Add the mushrooms and beef to the sauce and stir gently to coat. Add the dill and remaining parsley and give one last stir. Serve immediately over noodles.

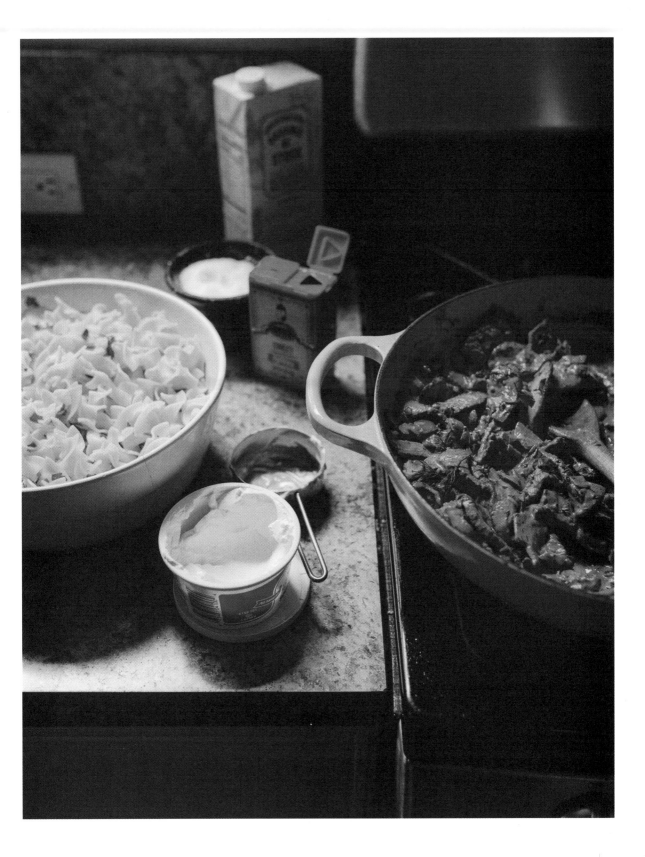

Market Lentil Salad with Coriander-Roasted Roots, Mint & Goat Cheese

Serves: 6

Lentils and vegetables

½ cup French lentils, soaked overnight for max nutrition

2 bunches of beets, peeled or scrubbed; swap in some turnips if you'd like

5 large carrots, or 1 bunch of spring carrots

1–2 tablespoons grapeseed oil

1½ teaspoons granulated garlic or garlic powder

1½ teaspoons ground coriander

½ red onion, minced

Dressing and salad

2 tablespoons rice wine vinegar

¼ teaspoon crushed red pepper

2 tablespoons grapeseed oil

1 cup chopped fresh mint, cilantro, and parsley, packed

2 ounces goat cheese or feta, optional

1 cup toasted pepitas

Salt

Pepper

It's easy to skip over lentil salads. They're often predictable or just too lentil-y. It can be like eating cold, bland, soft pebbles. The key here is spiced and well-roasted roots, a way higher vegetable-to-lentil ratio, and a slightly unique acidity from the rice wine vinegar. Cilantro and parsley are nice supporting herbs, but mint is crucial—be generous with it. And the pepitas are necessary for that final crunch. Add a handful of lacy greens, too, if you'd like.

1. Cook the lentils like pasta. Fill a medium pot with lots of salted water, add the lentils, and cook until they are tender and hold their shape but are still slightly creamy—about 20 minutes. Drain and set aside.

2. Meanwhile, preheat oven to 425°F.

3. Slice beets into those magical ¼-inch cubes (page 61). If you've got market carrots with green tops, scrub them really well and slice a few in half lengthwise. Cube the rest like the beets. On a sheet pan, toss with a tablespoon or two of oil, 1 teaspoon of salt, some cracks of pepper, granulated garlic, and coriander.

4. Okay, here's how you arrange everything. The carrots sliced lengthwise will need a little steam to roast all the way through, so pile them together in a huddle on one corner of the sheet pan. Spread out the beet and carrot cubes. Slide into the oven for 30–40 minutes, tossing halfway through, until everything is tender and soft and cubes are caramelized and jammy. Set aside.

5. While lentils are cooking and veggies are roasting, make the vinaigrette in your serving bowl. Combine vinegar, crushed red pepper, a pinch of salt, and a few cracks of pepper. Gradually stream in oil as you whisk.

6. Add drained, warm lentils and onion to the dressing and toss. Set aside to marinate.

7. When ready to serve, toss marinated lentils with roasted vegetables, chopped herbs, little goat cheese plops, and pepitas.

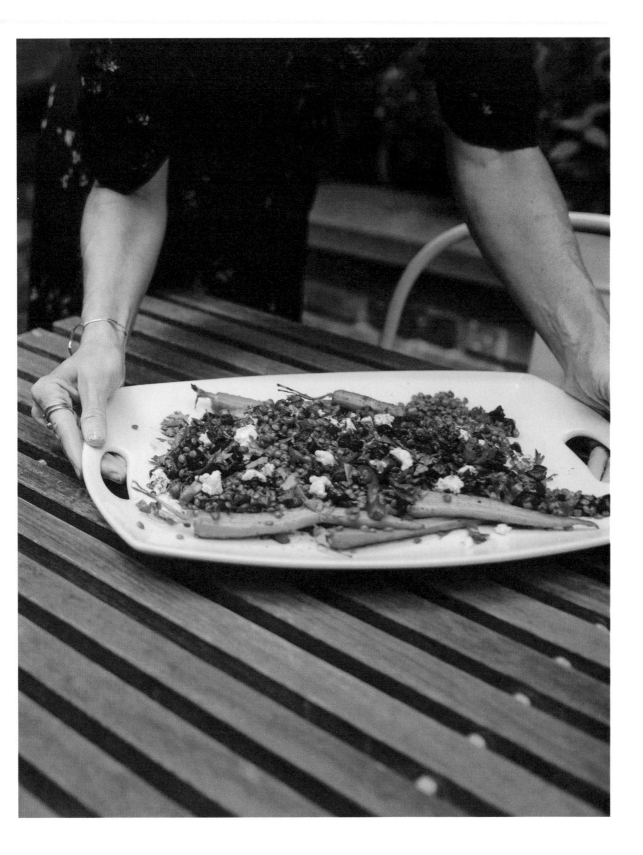

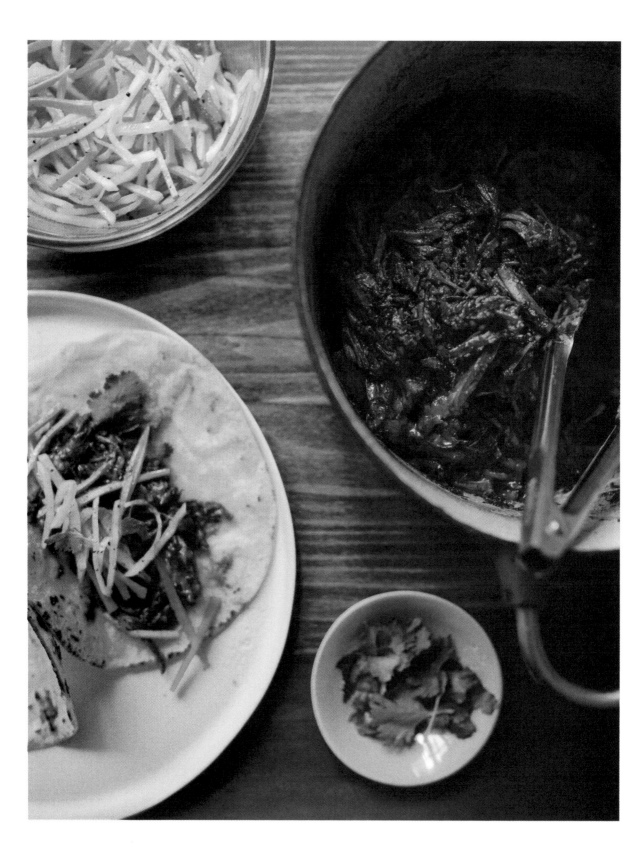

Lucky No-Sear Korean Short Rib Tacos with Quick-Pickled Root Slaw

Serves: 4

_____

Ribs

3 pounds beef short ribs

6 cloves garlic, minced

2 tablespoons fresh ginger, minced

½ cup soy sauce

¼ cup rice wine vinegar

1 tablespoon sesame oil

2 teaspoons sriracha, more if you like it spicy

3 tablespoons coconut sugar or honey

Root slaw

3 carrots, peeled and cut into thin matchsticks

1 turnip, peeled and cut into thin matchsticks

½ white onion, thinly sliced

¼ cup fresh cilantro, chopped

1 tablespoon rice wine vinegar

1 tablespoon lemon or lime juice

2 teaspoons honey

1 tablespoon grapeseed oil

½ teaspoon salt

⅛ teaspoon pepper

For serving

8 soft corn tortillas

2-3 tablespoons fresh cilantro, chopped

You know when you sear meat on really high heat and oil splatters everywhere, and then you have to open all your windows and disarm the smoke detectors? It's no fun but you do it because you love the result: flavorful, seared meat. But what if you could skip the drama and get the same results? We tried it. Pricey short ribs tossed in a pot with all the remaining ingredients. Covered and transferred to the oven. No grease, no smoke, and after leaving them in the oven for three hours, we gasped. Incredible, crispy, succulent meat.

1. Preheat oven to 325°F.

2. Place the short ribs in an oven-safe pot (we love to use enameled cast-iron ones).

3. In a small bowl, whisk the remaining ingredients and pour over the ribs.

4. Cover and transfer to the oven. Roast for 2½–3 hours, until the meat is falling off the bone and has caramelized around the edges.

5. Meanwhile, make the root slaw. Put all veggies in a medium-size bowl.

6. Whisk the remaining slaw ingredients in a measuring cup and pour over the slaw. Toss to combine. Refrigerate until needed.

7. Remove the short ribs from the oven. Transfer meat to a bowl and, when cool enough to handle, shred with a fork. Add the meat back to the pot and toss in the sauce. You can skim some of the fat off if you'd like.

8. Serve with root slaw, more cilantro, and really good tortillas.

_____

Kitchen note: You can also braise the short ribs in a slow cooker on low for 7-8 hours.

Asparagus Soup for Rich People

Serves: 4–5

2-3 tablespoons unsalted butter

I yellow onion, chopped

6 cloves garlic, minced

¼ teaspoon crushed red pepper, optional but adds a nice heat

I bunch asparagus, tough ends removed, cut into 2-inch pieces

I quart chicken or vegetable stock

I teaspoon salt

½ teaspoon pepper

½ bunch fresh basil, chopped; basically you can make this soup as basil-y as you want

Juice of ½ lemon (you'll probably need only a teaspoon or two)

Chives, optional, for garnish

You know the kind of soup we're talking about here. Shallow fancy soup bowls, and you eat with your pinkie up. Conversations center around where to take the yacht this year. But really, behind the scenes, this soup takes twenty minutes and requires just a handful of ingredients. It's so velvety, light, and delicious that you can't help but feel high society eating this.

1. Melt the butter in a small soup pot over medium heat.

2. Add the onion and sauté for 5–7 minutes, until it is soft and translucent. Stir occasionally to prevent the onion from browning too much.

3. Add the garlic and crushed red pepper and cook for another minute, until garlic is fragrant, but not burned.

4. Add the chopped asparagus and pour in the stock. Season with salt and pepper and bring the soup to a boil. Reduce to a simmer and cook for 10–15 minutes—you want the asparagus just cooked through, not mushy and overcooked. The more vibrant the color, the better.

5. Add basil to your liking, but it really makes the soup, so be generous. Puree the soup with an immersion blender or transfer to a blender and blend until silky smooth. Give it a taste. If you can barely taste the basil, add some more. A squeeze of lemon juice will also brighten up the soup. If it tastes bland, season with more salt as well.

6. Serve hot, cold, or at room temperature. It's super light and perfect in a pretty soup bowl. Channel *Downton Abbey*.

Note: Proper soup-eating etiquette is to dip the spoon into the soup and scoop away from you. Yeah, the opposite of how we've all been eating.

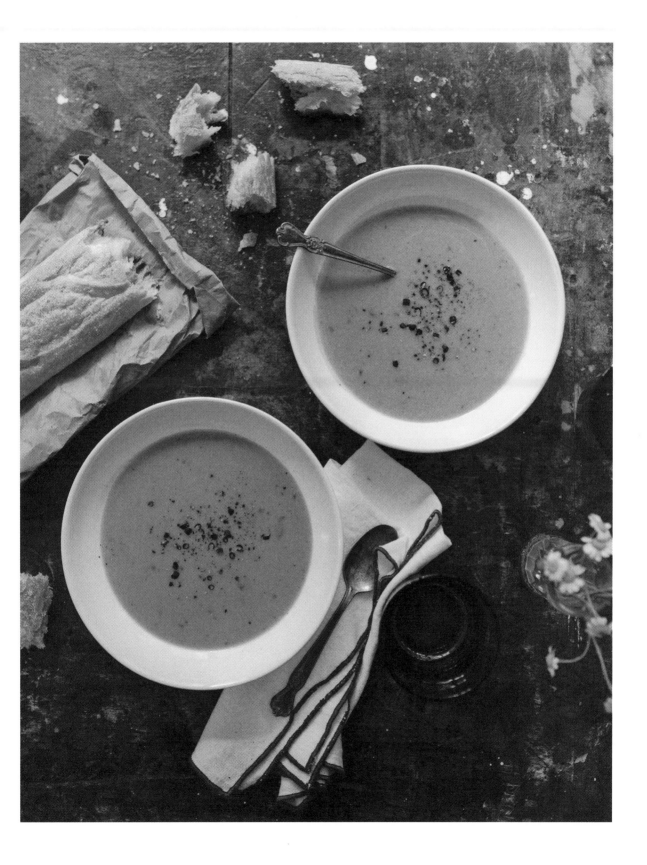

Beer-Braised Chicken with Peas & Bacon

Serves: 4

Chicken

4 slices raw bacon, chopped

1¼ pounds boneless, skinless chicken thighs

8 ounces cremini mushrooms, halved or quartered, depending on size

1 yellow onion, finely chopped

4 cloves garlic, minced

1 cup beer

3 tablespoons leftover mixed fresh herbs (thyme, sage, dill, oregano, basil), chopped

1½ cups fresh peas

½ cup heavy cream

⅓ cup Parmesan cheese, freshly grated

1 teaspoon cornstarch, optional

2 tablespoons fresh Italian parsley, chopped, for garnish

Herbed potatoes

1½ pounds potatoes (new potatoes, whole and unpeeled, or larger potatoes peeled and cut into 1-inch pieces)

3 tablespoons unsalted butter

2 tablespoons fresh chives, finely chopped

2 tablespoons fresh Italian parsley, chopped

Salt

Pepper

March, April. It's technically spring on the calendar, but outside it can feel as if Mother Nature has one foot in winter and one in spring. Cling to the promise of April showers bringing May flowers while this braise is in the oven. It's rich and comforting, with peas thrown in for specks of hope.

1. Add bacon to a large skillet and cook over medium-low heat for 5–7 minutes, until crispy but not burned. Remove bacon with a slotted spoon to a large bowl and set aside.

2. Season chicken on both sides with salt and pepper and add to the pan. Raise heat to medium-high and cook on each side for 2 minutes. You want some browning, but it doesn't need to be fully cooked. Using tongs, transfer to the same bowl as the bacon.

3. Add mushrooms and onion to the pan and cook for 10 minutes over medium-high heat, or until onion is soft and mushrooms are cooked and brown. Add garlic and cook for an additional minute.

4. Pour in the beer and scrape the bottom of the pan to release all the brown bits. Add the herbs, chicken, and bacon (reserving a couple of tablespoons for garnish), gently stir, then cover. Reduce heat to a simmer and cook for 15 minutes.

5. Add the peas to the pan, cover again, and cook for 5 minutes, until peas are just tender.

6. Transfer chicken to a plate. Whisk heavy cream and Parmesan into the pan. If the sauce is too thin, mix the cornstarch in a small ramekin with 1 tablespoon of the sauce. Pour cornstarch into pan and simmer for 2 minutes, until sauce thickens. Return chicken to pan and garnish with reserved bacon and parsley.

7. While chicken is simmering, make the potatoes. Place them in a pot of well-salted water. Bring to a boil, then reduce heat to a simmer for 15 minutes or until potatoes are cooked through.

8. Drain potatoes, then add them back to the pot, along with butter, herbs, ¼ teaspoon black pepper, and ¼ teaspoon salt. Gently stir until butter is fully melted. Taste and season with more salt and pepper if you'd like. Serve immediately with the chicken.

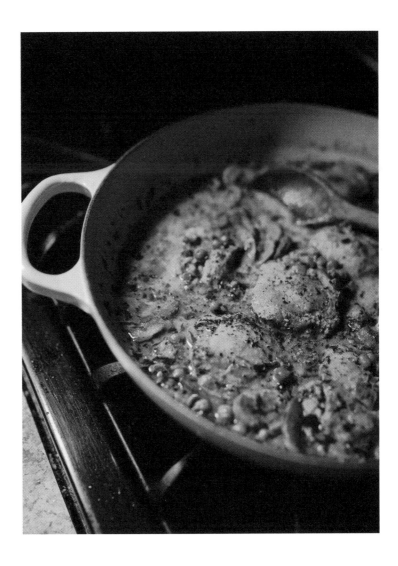

Spring

Spring Fever Pizza with Crumbly Sausage & *Raaamps*!

Serves: 4

Sauce

½ cup heavy cream, very cold

¼ teaspoon red pepper flakes

3 cloves garlic or green garlic, grated or finely minced

¼ cup yellow onion, minced

¼ cup fresh basil

Salt

Pepper

Toppings

½ pound Italian sausage, casings removed

1 tablespoon extra-virgin olive oil, plus extra for brushing crust

½ bunch asparagus, woody ends snapped off

½ bunch ramps, garlic scapes, or spring onions

8 ounces low-moisture mozzarella cheese, shredded

3 tablespoons fresh chopped herbs: basil, chives, chive blossoms, parsley, dill

Crust

16-ounce ball of homemade or store-bought pizza dough

1 tablespoon cornmeal, plus more if needed

After a long winter, and an even longer early spring, when it takes everything nearly forever to grow again, ramps and asparagus finally appear—officially sending everyone into a frenzy here on the East Coast. No ramps where you live? Consider moving or use garlic scapes or spring onions instead.

Note: There are three methods for cooking pizza in this book: sheet pan, baking stone, and baking steel. Here we're using the baking stone. Be sure to preheat it for at least 30 minutes to ensure a crispy crust.

1. To make the sauce, pour heavy cream into a glass measuring cup. Add in red pepper flakes, garlic, onion, basil, ½ teaspoon salt, and a few cracks of pepper. Use an immersion blender to make whipped cream; it should take 15 seconds or less. It's amazingly fast. Refrigerate until you're ready to top pizza.

2. Now prep the sausage. Heat a skillet over medium-high heat and swirl in oil. Once it's hot, add sausage and immediately start breaking it up into the tiniest bits with a wooden spoon. Cook for 6–8 minutes, until browned in some spots.

3. Next, chop the asparagus into coins, about ½-inch thick, but keep the tips whole. Everything will cook crisp-tender directly atop the pizza this way.

4. Thinly slice all the ramp whites and greens.

5. Preheat oven to 475°F and move the oven rack to the bottom of the oven. Preheat baking stone for 30 minutes.

6. Divide pizza dough in half to make two pizzas. Holding the first piece in your hands, begin to gently stretch it into a round or oval shape. Stretching rather than rolling allows those delicious bubbles to form.

7. Spread 1 tablespoon of cornmeal onto a pizza peel (see note), then place the stretched pizza dough on top and continue stretching until

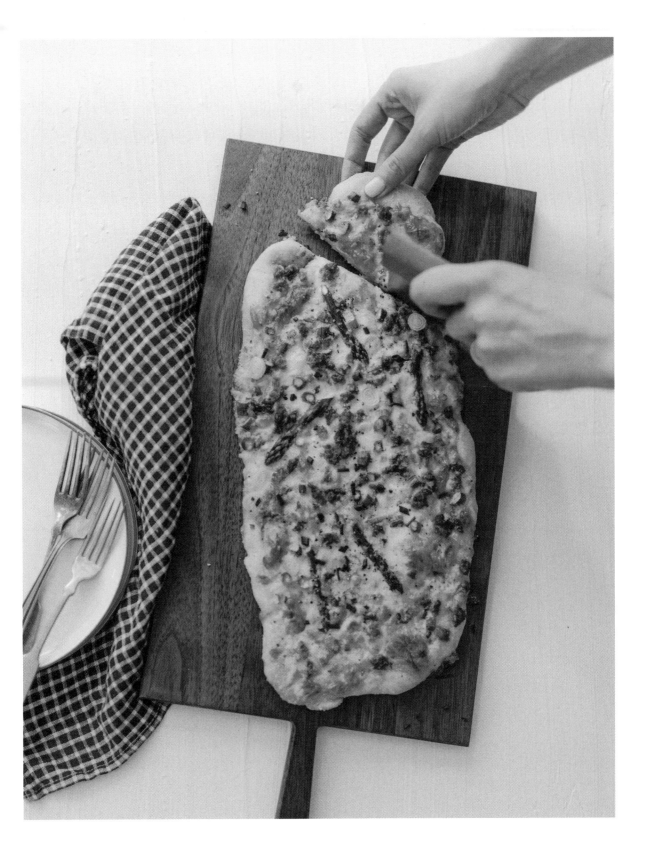

it's very thin. Throughout the topping process, make sure the dough can move around on the peel. Lift and add more cornmeal wherever it's sticking.

8. Spread half the white sauce onto the dough, leaving a border. Brush the border with a little oil and top the pizza with half of the other toppings: cheese, then sausage, asparagus, and ramps.

9. Working quickly (but carefully), slide the pizza onto the baking stone. Bake for 10–12 minutes or until crust is golden brown and cooked through and cheese is bubbly. Top with the fresh herbs.

10. Prepare the second pizza while the first one is baking. Cut and serve hot as they come out of the oven.

————————

Note: A pizza peel is an unrimmed wooden paddle with a long handle for transferring pizza into an oven without burning yourself. That thing you've seen at brick-oven pizzerias. If you don't have one, you can put the pizza dough on a large piece of parchment paper set on an upside-down sheet pan and slide that directly onto the baking stone.

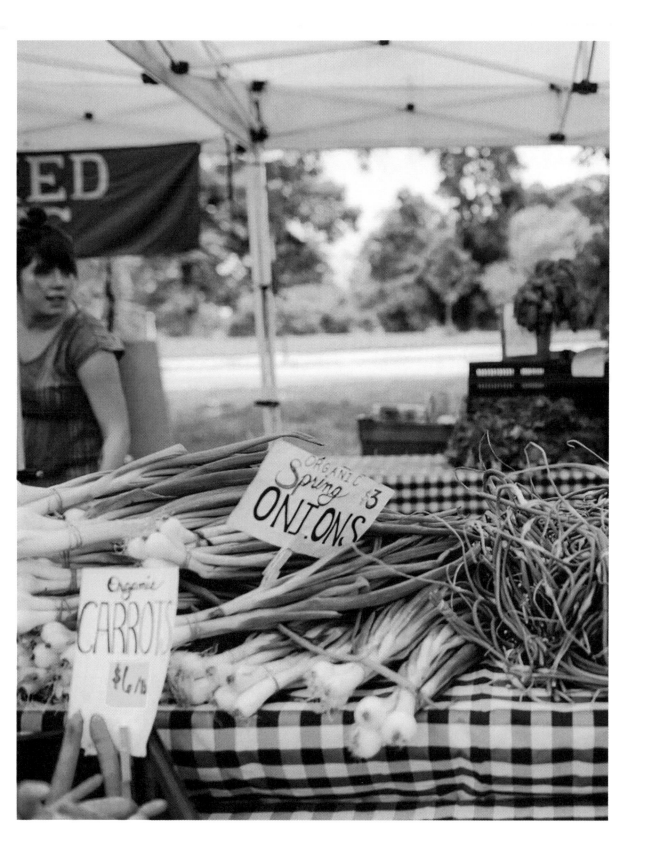

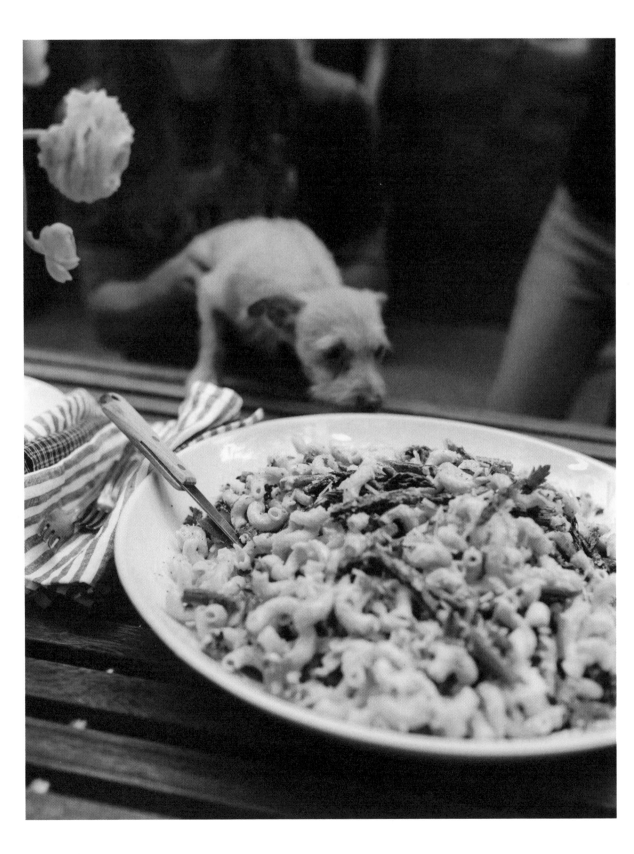

May Day Pasta Bowl

Serves: 4

———————

¾ pound pasta
(get creative with the
shapes, and go
gluten-free if you'd like)

l bunch asparagus, tough
ends removed, cut into
2-inch pieces

½ pound snap peas,
cut in half

2 tablespoons unsalted
butter

l yellow onion, diced

6 cloves garlic, minced

8 ounces mascarpone

½ cup Parmesan cheese,
freshly grated

½ bunch fresh basil,
chopped

¼ bunch fresh Italian
parsley, chopped

Salt

Pepper

Mid-May market days mean heaps of bright green stuff. Bring home a couple of vegetables that catch your eye and showcase them in a May Day Pasta Bowl tossed with a simple garlicky sauce. This is perfect for a crowd, especially on a massive showstopping platter.

1. Bring a large pot of salted water to a boil. Add pasta and cook according to package instructions until al dente. Drain and transfer cooked pasta to a bowl, keeping the water at a boil.

2. Blanch all the veggies in the boiling water until just tender but not mushy. The asparagus needs 2–3 minutes, the snap peas need 1 minute. Add them to the pasta bowl as you go. Reserve 1 cup of the water.

3. Meanwhile, in a skillet set over medium heat, melt the butter. Add the chopped onion and sauté for 5–7 minutes, until softened. Add the garlic and cook another minute.

4. Lower the heat and whisk in the mascarpone, ½ cup reserved pasta water to start, and Parmesan cheese. Season to taste with salt and pepper. Add more pasta water if the sauce is too thick.

5. Toss the pasta with mascarpone sauce, basil, and parsley. Extra Parmesan, too!

———————

Note: We've introduced blanching as a vegetable cooking method here, but you could also roast or sauté your favorite spring vegetables (asparagus, fiddleheads, snap peas, fava beans, garlic scapes) instead.

Spiced Lamb Wraps with Ramp Raita

Serves: 4

_____

Lamb

1 pound ground lamb

½ cup yellow or red onion, finely chopped

2-3 cloves garlic, minced

2 teaspoons fresh ginger, finely grated

1 teaspoon garam masala

1 teaspoon curry powder

1 teaspoon paprika

Salt

Pepper

Ramp raita

8 ramps, just the greens, minced

2 tablespoons extra-virgin olive oil

2 teaspoons lemon juice

½ cup yogurt

Wraps

4 large flour tortillas or wraps

2 Persian cucumbers, sliced very thin on a mandoline

½ red onion, thinly sliced

Fresh cilantro sprigs, about ¼ bunch

Greens or microgreens

We drop the word *flavor* around here unabashedly. And these lamb wraps are pretty high on our flavor dial. The lamb's bursting with spices and herbs and is served with a raita that deserves some global recognition. We make these babies in the oven, but they would also be amazing cooked on a grill.

1. In a medium bowl, mix the spiced lamb ingredients with 1 teaspoon salt and ½ teaspoon pepper. Cover and refrigerate.

2. Next, combine the ramp raita ingredients with a couple of pinches of salt and give it a good stir. Cover and refrigerate that too.

3. Remove the lamb mixture from the fridge and uncover. Shape into elongated patties, about 5 inches long, and flatten slightly; you should have 10 total.

4. Turn broiler to high and place the lamb patties on a small sheet pan. Broil for 10 minutes. Do not turn them halfway through cooking—it will ruin the texture. Remove from the oven and set aside.

5. Heat the tortillas (either in the microwave or using tongs to hold them over an open flame for a few seconds) to make them more pliable.

6. On a piece of wax paper, place a tortilla, spread some raita on it, then top with a few slices of cucumber, onion, 2–3 lamb patties, a couple of sprigs of cilantro, and microgreens. Roll the tortilla pretty tightly using the wax paper. Twist the edges so all the ingredients are snug inside (like a Tootsie Roll). Let it sit 5 minutes before slicing in half.

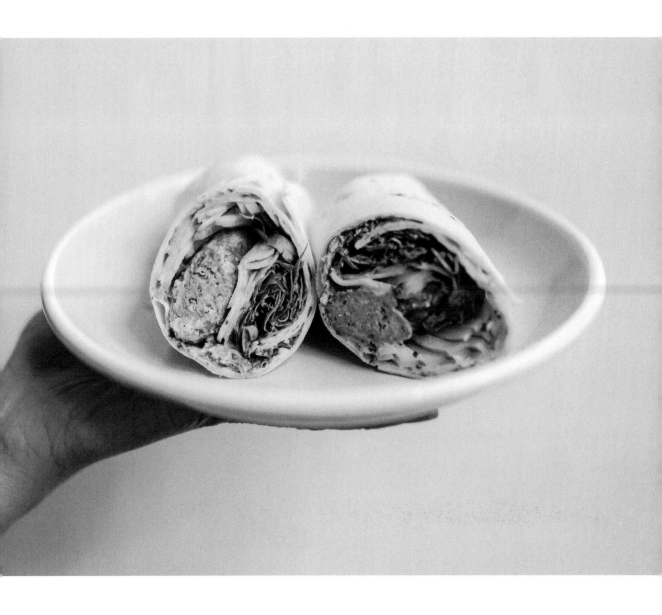

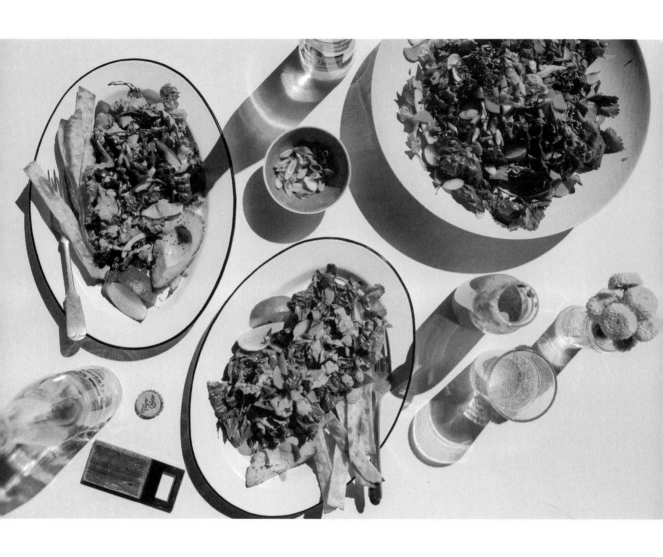

Ensalada Primavera

Serves: 4

Dressing

½ cup mayonnaise

I cup fresh mint

½ cup fresh Italian parsley

¼ cup fresh chives

I or 2 cloves garlic, grated or chopped; you could also use a few garlic scapes or a very small spring onion

I teaspoon anchovy paste, or I anchovy

I tablespoon red wine vinegar

I teaspoon lemon juice from ¼ lemon

I tablespoon water, plus more to adjust consistency

Salad

2 heads romaine lettuce, chopped into bite-size pieces

I small kohlrabi or ½ head cabbage, thinly sliced

2 carrots, thinly sliced or chopped into tiny cubes

½ bunch radishes, thinly sliced

¼ bunch cilantro, leaves and stems

I avocado, sliced into 4 wedges

I lime, sliced into wedges for serving

Optional, but ideal: thick strips of crispy corn tortillas (see page 154)

Optional, for carnivores: bacon, crumbled chorizo, or salami

Salt

Pepper

This mostly mint dressing will stop you dead in your tracks. It's the more sophisticated, flamboyant cousin of the Southwestern Summer Salad on page 154. Since summer vegetables usually get the delicious Tex-Mex treatment, spring vegetables and herbs are setting the record straight here with these vaguely Latin flavors.

1. Place dressing ingredients with ½ teaspoon salt and a few cracks of pepper in a blender and blend until completely smooth. Give it a taste and add more garlic, herbs, acid, or salt if you think it needs a little more of something.

2. In a bowl, combine lettuce, kohlrabi or cabbage, carrots, radishes, and cilantro.

3. Divide onto plates with wedges of avocado and lime, plus tortilla strips and meat, if using.

4. Before you dig in, squeeze lime on the avocado and the rest of the salad. Season the avocado with a sprinkle of salt and pepper. Add a thick pour of dressing across your salad, toss with your fork, and go for it.

Herb-Butter Fish in Parchment with Tender Spring Veggies

Serves: 4

---

3 tablespoons unsalted butter, softened

2–3 tablespoons mixed fresh herbs: basil, parsley, tarragon, chives, cilantro, whatever you have on hand

1 small zucchini or squash, cut into thin slices

1 large shallot, thinly sliced

4 cod or halibut fillets, 6 ounces each

1 large carrot, cut into matchsticks

⅓ cup fresh peas

12 asparagus stalks, ends trimmed and cut into thirds

1 lemon, half zested and sliced for packets, the other half cut into wedges for serving

Salt

Pepper

4 parchment sheets, 12 × 16

If ever there was a wow-factor dinner, it's fish that's baked in some paper. While cooking en papillote, as the French say, looks intimidating, the truth is it couldn't be easier. And the best part? The packets can be made hours before guests arrive and popped into the oven while you're shaking up come cocktails. Your hospitality game just went to expert level.

1. Preheat oven to 375°F.

2. In a small bowl, stir together the butter, ½ teaspoon salt, pepper, and herbs.

3. Make some room on the counter. Fold the parchment pieces in half to create a crease down the center, then open them all up on the counter.

4. Now, on the right half of each sheet, about 2 inches from the crease you made, make a little bed of zucchini and shallot slices; sprinkle with salt and papper.

5. Top with fish fillets.

6. Divide the carrots, peas, and asparagus and nestle around the fish fillets.

7. Sprinkle the fish with lemon zest, salt, and pepper.

8. Spread the herb butter on top of the fish. Add a lemon slice anywhere (on the top, on the side, near the edge).

9. Fold parchment in half again over the fish and veggies; crimp or fold so it's like a tightly sealed empanada packet and no steam can escape. Repeat for all the packets.

10. Transfer the packets to a sheet pan and bake for 12 minutes.

11. To serve, place each packet on a plate with lemon wedges. The fun is having each person tear or cut through the top of their own packet.

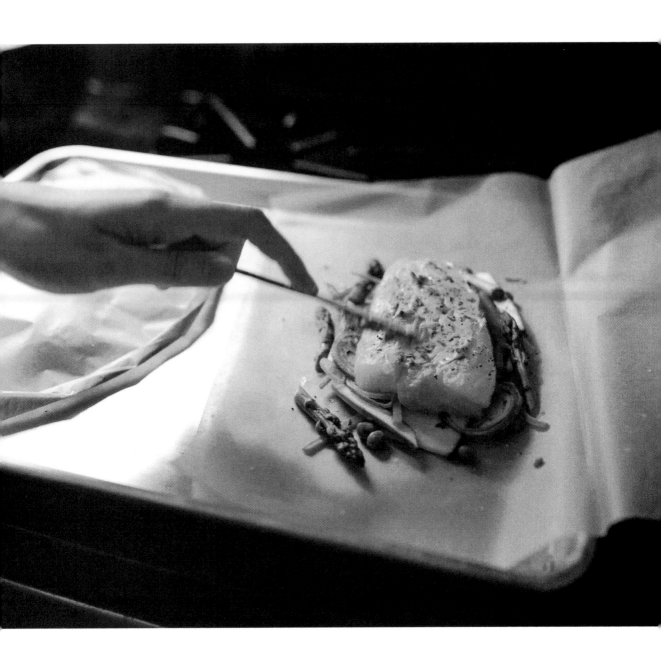

Actual Garden Burger with Herbs, White Beans & Peas

Serves: 6

Garden burger

1½ cups canned or cooked cannellini beans

2 cups fresh or frozen peas, cooked if fresh, thawed if frozen

¼ bunch Italian parsley, chopped

¼ bunch cilantro, chopped

3 tablespoons chives, chopped

½ small onion, finely chopped

2 large eggs, beaten

1 cup panko breadcrumbs; if you want it gluten-free, use a heaping ½ cup of oat flour instead

Extra-virgin olive oil, for pan

6 brioche buns, sliced in half

3 tablespoons unsalted butter, softened

1–2 avocados, sliced

1 bunch microgreens or watercress

Salt

Pepper

Pickled jalapeño schmear

½ cup mayonnaise

½ small red onion, finely chopped, 3 tablespoons total

2 cloves garlic, minced

2 tablespoons chives, finely chopped

¼ cup pickled jalapeños, chopped

½ teaspoon lemon juice

This recipe came to be because one day I (Anca) craved an unfamiliar craving. A veggie burger. I never ordered them at restaurants or made them at home. I mean, why would anyone eat a veggie burger over an actual burger?! But out of nowhere, the Huckle & Goose Effect happened—I craved something I never thought I'd want. So here it is, friends. It could convert you, too.

1. In a large bowl, mash the beans with a potato masher until they're half mushy, half chunky, about a minute. Add the peas and mash a little more. You'll want the mixture to be pretty chunky but clearly sticking together.

2. Add herbs, onion, eggs, and breadcrumbs (or oat flour) and season with 1 teaspoon salt and ½ teaspoon pepper. Mix everything until combined.

3. Form into six patties (try to make them the size of your burger buns). If they're not sticking together, really smoosh them; overworking here is not an issue. Refrigerate for 15 minutes (this helps them keep their shape).

4. In a small bowl, whisk together all the schmear ingredients along with ¼ teaspoon each salt and pepper. Refrigerate while you cook your burgers.

5. Set a skillet over medium-high heat. When hot, add about a tablespoon of oil and swirl to coat the bottom. Add half the patties to the pan. Don't touch them for at least 2 minutes or they'll stick and break. You can take a peek after that with a spatula to see if the bottom is crispy and brown; this usually takes 3–4 minutes total. Gently turn the patties over and cook another 2–4 minutes, depending on how crispy you like them. Transfer to a plate and cook the remaining patties, adding more oil if needed. In another pan, toast your buns in a little butter.

6. Slather your bottom bun with the pickled jalapeño schmear, top with a crispy patty, avocado, watercress, some more schmear, and then the top bun. Eat immediately; everyone else can fend for themselves.

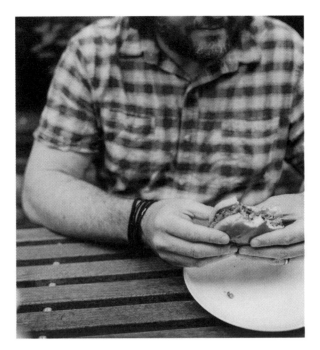

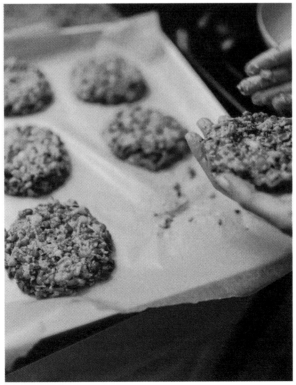

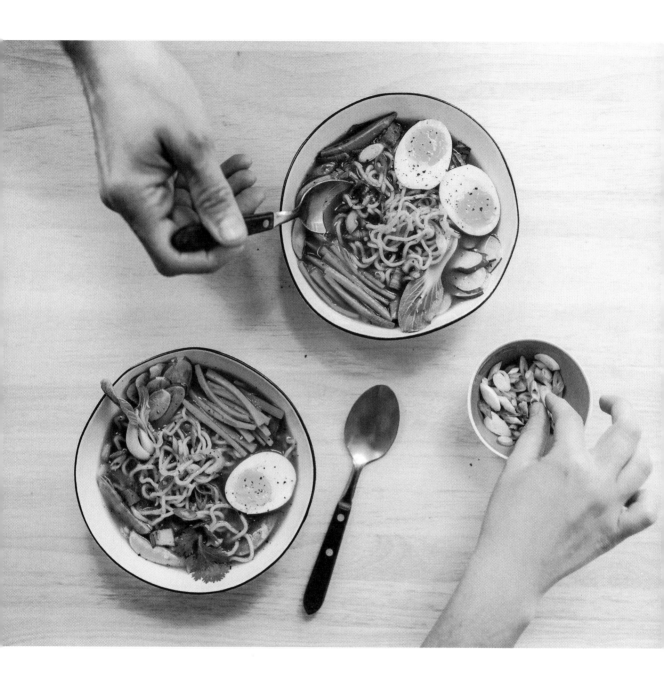

Shortcut Ramen with Spring Vegetables

Serves: 4

_____

4 cups low-sodium chicken or vegetable stock

4 cups water

½ teaspoon crushed red pepper

2 inches fresh ginger, thinly sliced

6 cloves garlic, thinly sliced

1 leek, well cleaned and thinly sliced

¼ cup soy sauce or liquid aminos

1 tablespoon sugar

1 teaspoon sesame oil

5 ounces fresh or dried ramen noodles, give or take (the packages may not end up being perfect)

1 cup sugar snap peas

1 small bunch bok choy

1 carrot, peeled and very thinly julienned

2 scallions or garlic scapes, thinly sliced

3 tablespoons fresh cilantro, chopped

Optional: 1–2 large eggs for whoever wants some in their bowl (see note)

Optional: thinly sliced chiles or hot sauce for serving

This is one of our favorite ways to eat spring vegetables. The broth is so good you could drink it straight up. Eat at a table full of your favorite people, accompanied by loud slurping.

1. Pour stock and water into a soup pot and bring to a boil.

2. Meanwhile, prep the aromatics—crushed red pepper, ginger, garlic, leek, soy sauce or liquid aminos, sugar, and sesame oil—and just toss/pour them in as the liquid heats. Once boiling, turn heat to low and let everything simmer for 30 minutes, partially covered.

3. While the broth simmers, prepare all the vegetables. Thinly slice the bok choy, keeping the stems and leaves separate, and chop the snap peas into bite-size pieces—you'll cook those later in the broth. Reserve the carrot, scallions or garlic scapes, and cilantro for garnish.

4. Using an Asian spider strainer, remove all the aromatics from the broth and discard. Add in the noodles and cook according to the time on the package. Using the strainer again, remove the noodles from the broth and transfer to a bowl to prevent mushiness. If they sit in the soup, they absorb a ton of the broth and overcook. Toss with a little neutral oil to prevent them from sticking together; set aside.

5. Next, cook the vegetables in the broth. Since the snap peas take longest, add those to the broth first and cook for 2 minutes. Next, in go the bok choy stems for another minute or so, then the bok choy leaves. Cook for 1–2 more minutes, stirring once.

6. To assemble the ramen bowls, ladle in broth and green veggies and add lots of reserved noodles, or just a little. Garnish with carrot, scallions, and cilantro. Top with half a soft-boiled egg if you made them. Slurp away.

_____

Note: You could also add peas, asparagus, thinly sliced daikon radishes, kohlrabi, or shredded cabbage. For soft-boiled eggs, see page 181.

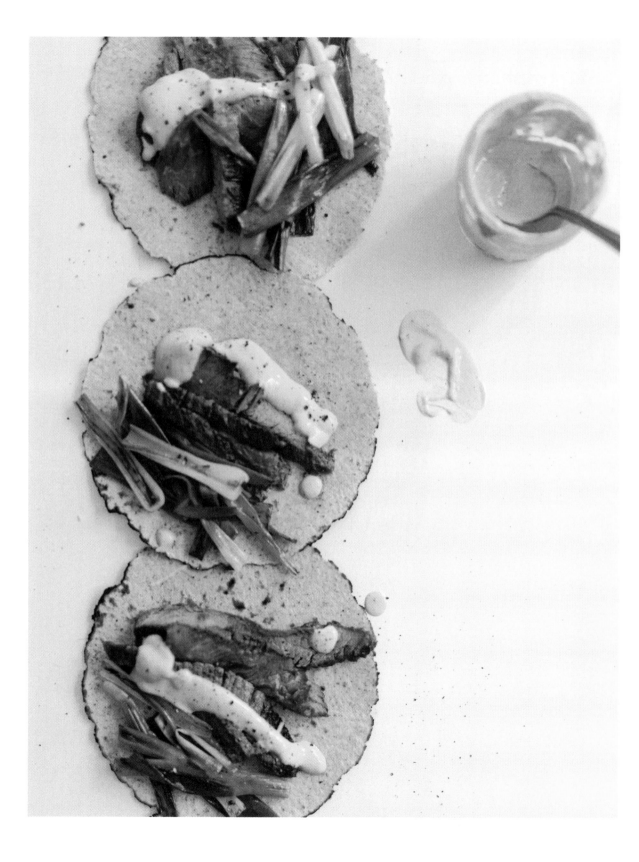

Skirt Steak & Charred Green Onion Tacos with Chipotle Crema

Serves: 4

Marinade and steak

Juice of 2 limes

6 cloves garlic, chopped

½ bunch fresh cilantro, stems included

¼ cup grapeseed oil, plus more for pan if needed

1¼ pound skirt steak

Salt

Pepper

Chipotle crema

½ cup sour cream

½ cup plain yogurt

2–3 canned chipotle peppers in adobo sauce

For serving

2 bunches green onions

1 package soft corn tortillas

We love the first grill of spring. It may not be hot out yet, but it's definitely warm enough to stand in front of your grill without a coat on. A big slab of marinated meat and lots of green veggies is our tradition of welcoming back grilling season.

1. In a blender, combine the marinade ingredients (everything but the steak), with 1 teaspoon salt and ½ teaspoon black pepper; puree until smooth. Transfer marinade to a shallow dish or a large Ziploc bag and add the meat. Marinate at room temperature for 30 minutes or refrigerate for up to 8 hours.

2. Using a blender, puree the crema ingredients with a few pinches of salt and pepper until smooth. Refrigerate for up to 5 days.

3. Remove meat from the fridge about 45 minutes before cooking and preheat an outdoor grill to medium-high.

4. Pat steaks dry and transfer to the grill. Cook without touching for 3 minutes and turn over for another 3 minutes for medium-rare, longer if you want more doneness. Remove to a cutting board and allow it to rest for 5–10 minutes.

5. While steak is resting, grill the green onions, turning frequently, for about 4 minutes, until nicely charred and softened.

6. Thinly slice steak against the grain and serve with the charred green onions, chipotle crema, and tortillas.

Note: If you don't have an outdoor grill, make this in a large cast-iron pan or grill pan.

Radish, Cilantro & Chive Salsa

1 bunch radishes, about 6, chopped into thin quarters or tiny cubes

1 jalapeño pepper, diced

3 tablespoons fresh chives, chopped

2 tablespoons fresh cilantro, chopped

1 teaspoon grapeseed oil

Juice of ½ lime

Salt

Pepper

In a medium bowl, stir together all the ingredients with one huge pinch each of salt and pepper. Serve with tacos.

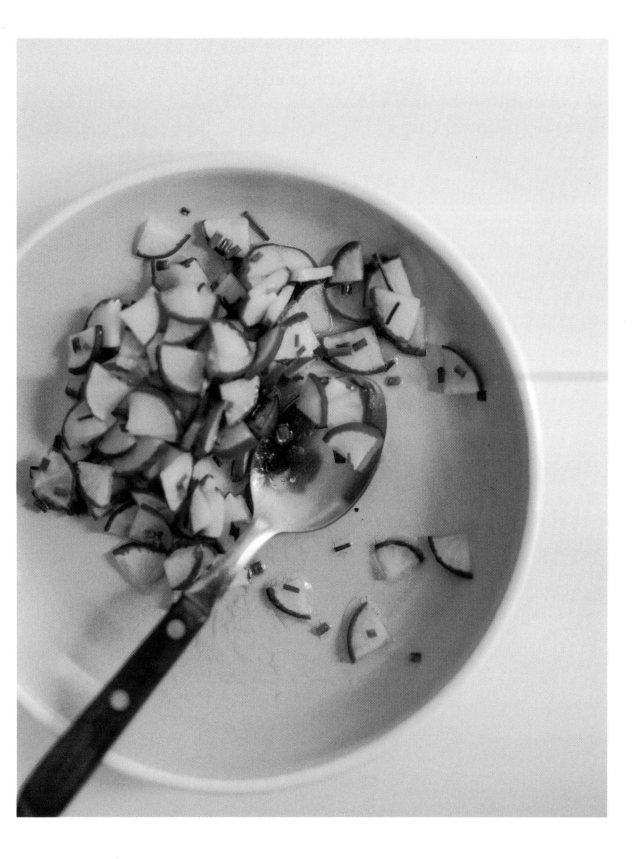

Herb Box Salad with Kale, Chickpea Croutons & Lemony Sumac Dressing

Serves: 4

---

30 ounces or 3 cups canned or cooked chickpeas, rinsed

1 tablespoon grapeseed oil, plus more for breadcrumbs

2 teaspoons smoked paprika

1 heaping teaspoon tahini

1 clove garlic, minced

2 tablespoons lemon juice from ½ lemon

1 teaspoon sumac

4 tablespoons extra-virgin olive oil

1 bunch kale, de-stemmed

1½ cups stale bread cubes (or crushed pita chips)

1–3 cups fresh cilantro, mint, dill, parsley, and chives; don't stress about the amounts, just dump everything you've got in there, leaves left whole with some tender stems

Salt

Pepper

This salad has lots of personality—zesty, crunchy, exotic, a little spicy, and bursting with verdant flavor. Kale is playing a supporting role here, and the herbs are the main event. Use up everything in your herb box so you can have an empty fridge before the next shopping trip. It's the ultimate pantry dinner—when all you have is that kale bunch you've been avoiding, herbs threatening to wilt any day now, some stale bread, and a can of chickpeas.

1. Preheat oven to 425°F. Dry chickpeas with a dish towel or paper towel. Pile them onto a baking sheet, drizzle with grapeseed oil, generously salt and pepper, and sprinkle on smoked paprika. Toss well with your hands, then spread them out and bake for 30–35 minutes, until crispy, giving them a good shake halfway through. This is a great place to play around with more spices each time you make it—try turmeric, coriander, chili powder, granulated garlic.

2. In the bowl you'll be serving the salad in, whisk together tahini, minced garlic, lemon juice, sumac, and a big pinch each of salt and pepper. Gradually whisk in olive oil and set aside.

3. Now for the kale. The secret is in the chop. Stack the de-stemmed kale and slice the thinnest possible kale slivers you can. It should look like bite-size confetti.

4. Place the kale in the bowl with the dressing and toss, coating well. Let it marinate a bit while you prepare the homemade breadcrumbs.

5. In a food processor, pulse stale bread cubes. Not too fine; slightly bigger crumbs are perfect here. Wait until the chickpeas are done, place them in the bowl with the kale, then use the same baking sheet to toast the crumbs a bit (by drizzling on some oil, mixing around with a wooden spoon, and baking for just a couple of minutes, until golden brown). Don't be tempted to use store-bought breadcrumbs here. They're just not the same. These homemade ones are worth the effort, but crushed pita chips are a good stand-in.

6. Toss in herbs and breadcrumbs and dig in.

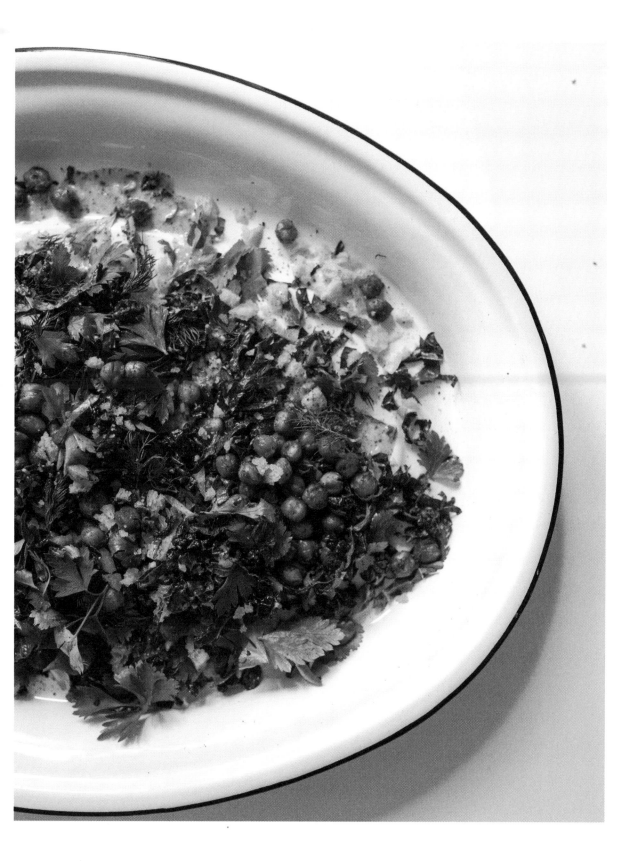

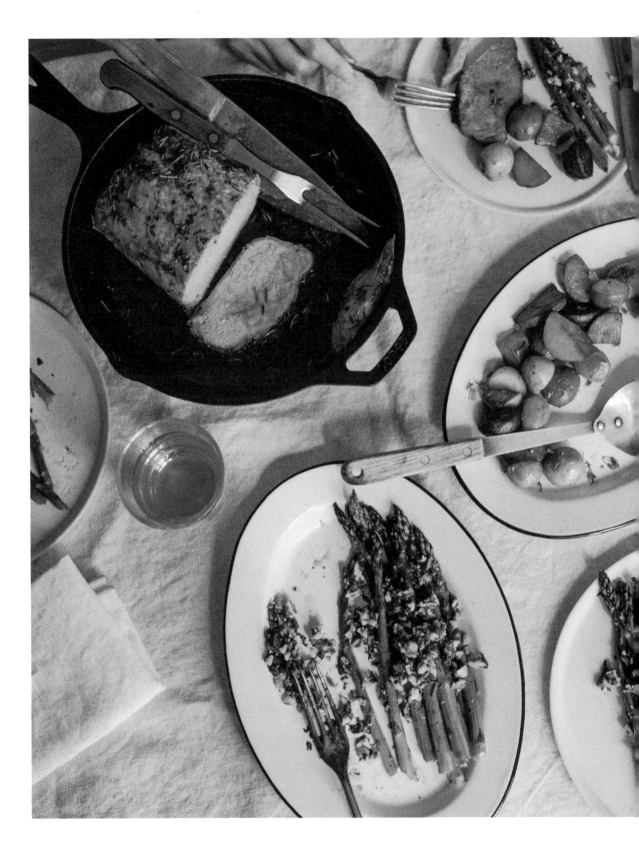

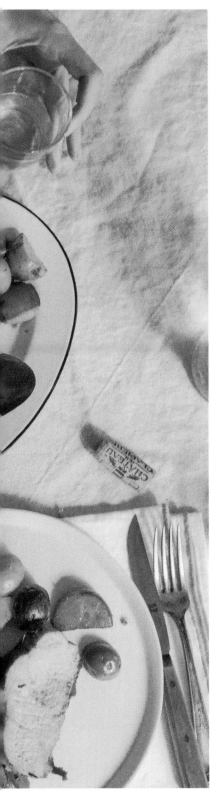

A Proper Spring Supper

Dry brine will change your life. You basically rub some salt on meat and let it sit in the fridge for hours. The result here is super juicy pork that you almost can't overcook. Paired with pesto-topped asparagus and delicate buttery potatoes, this is a dinner to celebrate warmer evenings.

Serves 4

_____

Rosemary-brined pork

3 cloves garlic

1 tablespoon fresh rosemary, minced

2-2½ pounds pork loin

Chunky pesto asparagus

1 bunch asparagus, ends trimmed

¼ cup Parmesan cheese, 3-inch chunk

½ cup mixed fresh herbs: basil and a little parsley

Extra-virgin olive oil

½ lemon

Butter-braised potatoes

4 tablespoons unsalted butter

1¾ pounds baby or fingerling potatoes, scrubbed clean

⅓ cup chive blossoms, optional, torn into smaller pieces

Grapeseed oil, for pans

Salt

Pepper

1. Pork: Mince garlic with ¼ teaspoon of salt (helps garlic to form a paste). Using the flat part of your knife, smash the garlic and drag it a little. Scrape the garlic off the knife and repeat until you have a garlicky paste. Place the paste into a small ramekin, along with the rosemary and 1 tablespoon salt.

2. Rub pork all over with the rosemary salt. Put the pork on a plate and transfer to the fridge, uncovered (the outside of the meat will be crispier when cooked). Let it chill for 4–6 hours.

3. Bring pork to room temperature about an hour before you're ready to cook it.

4. Preheat oven to 400° F. Heat a cast-iron pan over medium-high heat; drizzle in 1 tablespoon grapeseed oil. Sprinkle 1 teaspoon of pepper on the loin, place it in the pan, and sear for 3–4 minutes on the side without the layer of fat. Flip and slide into the oven for 30 minutes or until a meat thermometer reads 142°–145°F. Don't overcook—a little pink color in the middle is what you want. Remove from the oven and let it rest at least 10 minutes before slicing.

5. Asparagus: On a sheet pan, toss the asparagus with 1 tablespoon grapeseed oil and ¼ teaspoon each salt and pepper. Slide on an oven rack under the pork for 15–20 minutes, giving it a shake halfway through, until the asparagus is tender.

6. Roughly chop Parmesan and fresh herbs together to make a chunky mix. Transfer to a small bowl and mix with a drizzle of olive oil and a squeeze of lemon juice to taste. Add a pinch of salt if needed; set aside.

7. Line up the asparagus on a platter and spoon the pesto across the middle to serve. This can stay at room temperature.

8. Potatoes: After the asparagus is in the oven, heat a large high-sided skillet with a tight-fitting lid over medium heat. If you can't fit all the potatoes in one layer, use two pots.

9. Add butter and, when melted, add potatoes and season with ½ teaspoon salt and ¼ teaspoon pepper. Cover and braise for 20–30 minutes, shaking the pan occasionally so potatoes don't burn. But don't remove that lid before 20 minutes. Test a potato to see if it's fork-tender. If not, cover and cook for 5–10 minutes longer.

10. Transfer to a warmed bowl with chive blossoms, if using. Serve right away with pork and asparagus.

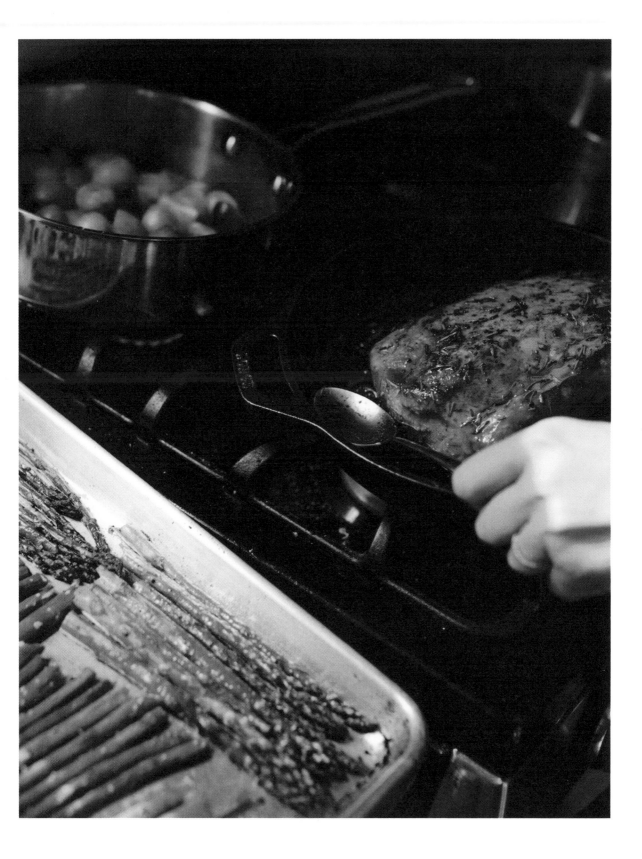

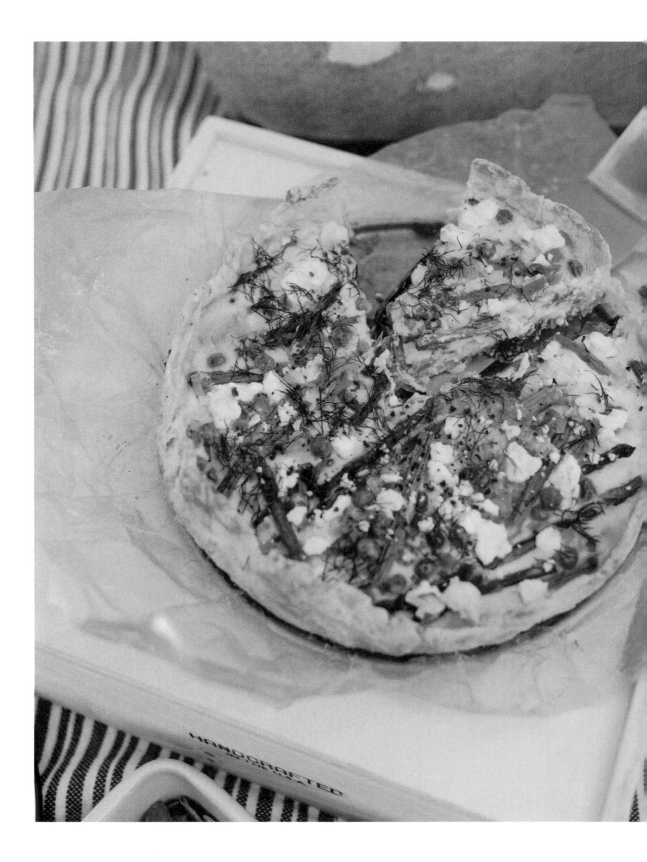

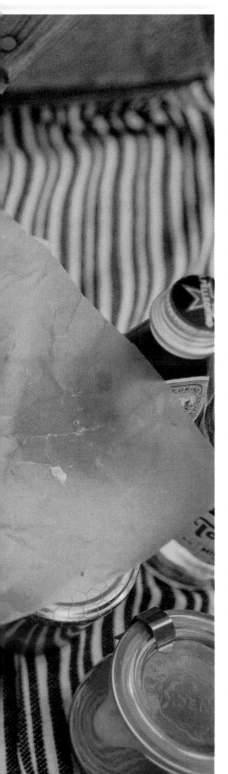

Spring Afternoon Picnic Quiche with a View

This is the type of food that helps you soak in spring to the fullest, especially if eaten outside while sipping a pink drink. The thought of making quiche can be met with equal parts joy (the getting-to-eat-it part) and intimidation, but a quiche is a thing of love. So let's get to work—you have a picnic to attend.

Serves: 8

1¼ cups all-purpose flour

½ teaspoon sugar

8 tablespoons unsalted butter, chilled, cut into small cubes

4-5 tablespoons ice water

1 tablespoon extra-virgin olive oil

¾ cup spring alliums (ramps, green garlic, spring onion, leeks), chopped

½ bunch asparagus, woodsy ends snapped off, then chopped

½ cup fresh or frozen peas

4 large eggs

½ cup heavy cream

4 ounces feta cheese, finely chopped or crumbled

3 tablespoons fresh dill, and a bit of basil, too, if you have it

1¼ teaspoons salt, divided

½ teaspoon pepper

1.   Make the crust: In a large bowl, place the flour, ½ teaspoon salt, and sugar; whisk with a fork. Let it sit in the freezer for 15–30 minutes, along with the cubed butter.

2.   Now scatter the chilled butter over the chilled flour mixture and use a pastry cutter or your fingers to break the butter cubes up into evenly distributed, pea-size bits. Sprinkle on 4 tablespoons ice water and stir/press the dough together several times with a large spatula. Grab a small handful and squeeze. If it sticks together, it's ready. If not, sprinkle on another tablespoon of water.

3.   Without overworking it, press all the dough together into a thick disk, wrap tightly with plastic wrap, and refrigerate for about an hour or up to 2 days.

Spring

4. Remove dough from the fridge 10 minutes before you're ready to roll it out. Meanwhile, prepare a 9-inch springform or cake pan by greasing the bottom and sides and lining it with parchment.

5. Lightly dust flour on clean counter and, with a floured rolling pin, roll into a 13-inch circle (just a couple of inches larger than your pan). Make sure the surface is floured enough that the dough can move around and not stick as you're rolling it.

6. Carefully transfer dough to pan (you can drape it over the rolling pin, then unroll), gently pressing it into the bottom and sides, which you want to come almost all the way up to the top. Trim any overhang and patch up holes. This doesn't have to be perfect. In fact, jagged and imperfect makes it look even better.

7. Place the pie crust in the freezer for 30 minutes. Preheat oven to 425°F.

8. Now par-bake the crust. Why the extra step? 'Cause we're filling it with something very liquidy, and this helps it hold up and not get soggy.

9. Place another sheet of parchment over the crust and set in pie weights or an 8-inch cake pan so the crust doesn't puff or buckle while par-baking. Bake for 15 minutes, then remove parchment and weights and bake for another 5 minutes; crust should feel set. Set aside and reduce oven temperature to 350°F.

10. Meanwhile, prepare the filling. Swirl olive oil in a sauté pan set over medium heat. Once oil is hot, add in chopped alliums and asparagus and stir every couple of minutes, 5–6 minutes total. Season with ¼ teaspoon of salt and some cracks of pepper. Turn off heat, stir in peas, then set aside.

11. In a large glass liquid measuring cup, beat the eggs and heavy cream really well with the remaining ½ teaspoon of salt and a few cracks of pepper.

12. Grab your par-baked crust. Scatter half the cheese evenly on the bottom, then scrape in the vegetables, keeping a few spears for the top. Sprinkle the herbs in, pour in the custard (leaving a bit of crust showing), then top with remaining cheese. Pop in the oven for 40 minutes, or until filling is set and the crust is golden brown. Behold your work of art. Let it rest for at least 20 minutes; serve warm or at room temperature with a tender baby greens salad.

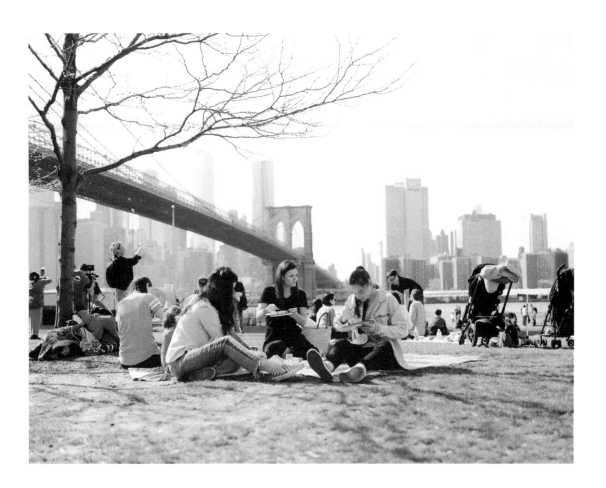

Spring

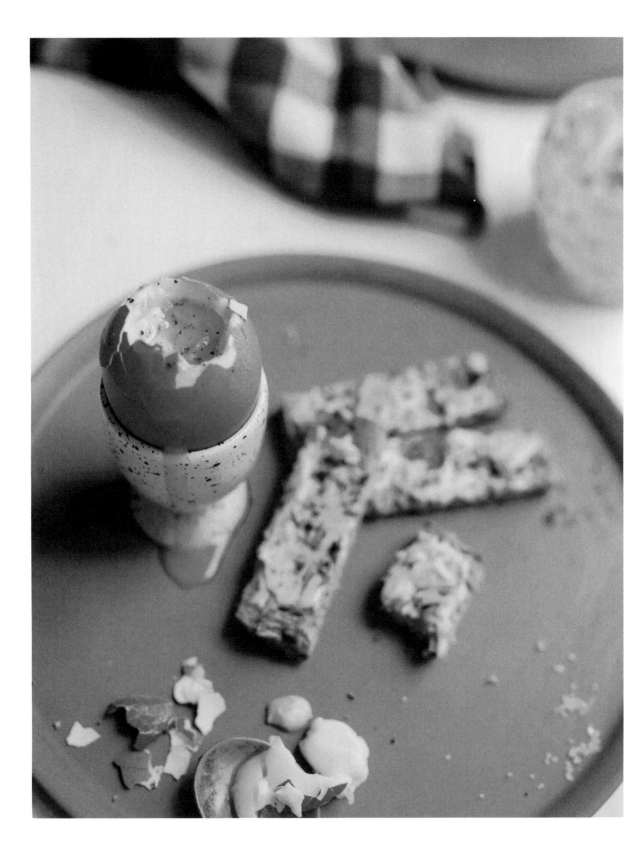

Soft-Boiled Eggs with Herb Butter Toast Dips

Serves: 2–4

---

4 large eggs,
the best you can find

2 tablespoons unsalted
butter, softened

2 tablespoons mixed
fresh herbs, chopped

4 slices bread

Salt

Pepper

This is the cheeriest of breakfasts. First you get to nestle your eggs in adorable egg cups, then crack open the tops and dip butter-slathered toasts into the yolks. You can't have a bad day when you start it this way.

1. Fill a saucepan ¾ full with water. Set over high heat and bring to a boil. Once boiling, reduce to a simmer.

2. To help keep the eggs from cracking, place them all together on a slotted spoon or spider strainer and hold them just over the hot steam for 30 seconds. It brings their temperature up slightly and prevents the dreaded cracks. Gently lower the eggs into the water and set timer for 6 minutes.

3. While eggs are boiling, mix the butter and herbs in a small dish. Season with salt and pepper.

4. Toast bread to your liking, then smear the herb butter on top. Slice bread into strips.

5. When 6 minutes have passed, remove the eggs using a slotted spoon. Let cool slightly or run under cold water, then place in egg cups. Using a small spoon, start tapping the top of each egg to crack the shell. Now you can use your hand to remove the top of the egg. The mess is half the fun.

6. Serve with the buttered toast to dip into the yolks and use the spoon to scoop out the white part of the egg.

Kitchen note: Make extra herb butter and keep it in the fridge–for a sandwich or a sizzling steak or herb-butter fish (page 86) later in the week.

Hello Spring Egg Salad Sandwich with Chive Blossoms

Serves: 4

---

4 large eggs, the best you can find

2 tablespoons mayonnaise (you can even go with less if you prefer)

1 teaspoon Dijon mustard

1 teaspoon champagne vinegar

¼ teaspoon hot sauce

½ teaspoon Worcestershire sauce

½ teaspoon salt, plus extra

¼ teaspoon pepper, plus extra to taste

2 tablespoons chopped mixed fresh herbs: basil, dill, chives and chive blossoms, parsley

4 croissants, sliced for stuffing, or 4 slices of crusty bread for tartines (open-faced sandwiches)

A couple of handfuls of microgreens or baby greens

Sliced radishes, optional

Garlic scapes, optional

Egg salad doesn't have to be mayo-y mush. If you leave the eggs in bigger chunks and don't overcook them, they'll be creamy enough to toss with only a tiny bit of mayo. They don't need much, but they do need really good bread or croissants for max egg salad enjoyment.

1. To boil the eggs, fill a small pot ¾ of the way with water and bring to a boil.

2. Gently lower in eggs with a large spoon as quickly and carefully as possible. Set a timer for 8 minutes—the water should be at a low boil the entire cooking time.

3. Remove eggs and plunge into an ice bath; once they're cool enough to handle, peel them. Slice each egg in half, then quarter each half—so 8 pieces total from each egg. The egg yolks should be jammy rather than hard-boiled, so you can fully appreciate them and so that their creaminess contributes to the binding of the salad (which means less mayo).

4. Meanwhile, in a medium bowl, whisk together the mayo, mustard, vinegar, hot sauce, Worcestershire, salt, and pepper. Fold in the herbs and leave a few pinches for garnish.

5. Add the quartered eggs to the mayo mixture and gently toss, using a spatula. You want the egg yolks and whites to stay together as much as possible.

6. Now it's time for sandwich or tartine assembly. Plate the croissants or bread slices; spoon on egg salad. Crack some pepper over if you'd like, then top with a heap of herbs and microgreens. If you've got radishes and/or garlic scapes on hand, add in some thin slices.

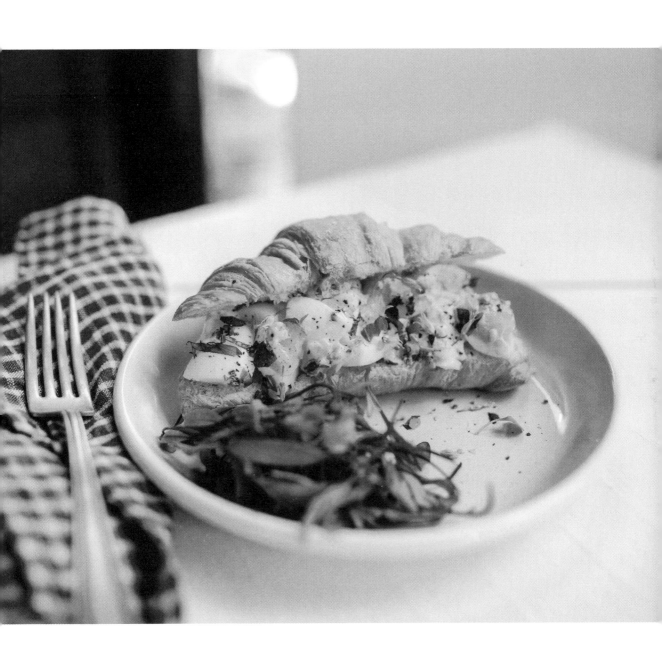

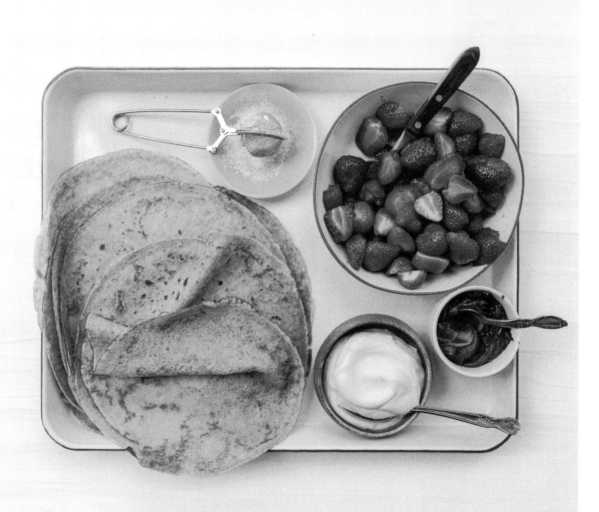

Super Good Spelt Crepes with Strawberries

Serves: 4–6 (makes 12–14 crepes)

———————————

3 large eggs,
room temperature

2 cups milk,
room temperature

1–2 tablespoons sugar
(use 1 tablespoon if you want
a hint of sweetness, 2 if you
want them sweeter)

¼ teaspoon salt

1½ cups spelt flour

3 tablespoons coconut oil,
melted

1 quart strawberries, sliced

Chocolate hazelnut spread,
to serve

Whipped cream, optional,
to serve

When those aqua-colored pints of strawberries show up at the market, we buy as many as our budget allows and rush home to make crepes. Usually we make our grandma's classic recipe, but one afternoon a bag of spelt flour kept staring at us as if to say, "Please let me partake in this strawberry festival." We're glad we obliged, because these crepes are so fragrant, nutty, and textured. Moral of the story: Some days you need a little spin on a classic.

1. Whisk together the eggs, milk, sugar, and salt in a bowl. Add the spelt flour and whisk until completely smooth, without any lumps. Pour in coconut oil and whisk a few times until combined. (You can also whir all the ingredients in a blender, which we do sometimes, contingent upon our *Do I want to wash a blender?* mood.)

2. Let the batter rest on the counter for at least 30 minutes, or refrigerate for a couple of hours.

3. Heat a small or medium-size nonstick pan (or a crepe pan) over medium-high heat. Brush on some coconut oil.

4. Pour ¼–⅓ cup (depending on pan size) of the batter into the pan and tilt it with a circular motion so the batter coats the surface evenly. Cook for about 1 minute. Gently flip crepe and cook an additional 30 seconds. Transfer to a warm plate, then repeat until all the batter is turned into a pile of delicious crepes.

5. Serve with berries, chocolate hazelnut spread, and whipped cream.

Warrior Three-Egg Omelet

Serves: 2

———————

2 tablespoons unsalted
butter, divided

3 asparagus stalks,
cut into ¼-inch rounds,
woody ends removed

3 large eggs

2 tablespoons chives,
chopped

2–3 tablespoons chopped
mixed herbs: parsley, basil,
cilantro, dill–any herbs you
have on hand

3 tablespoons aged cheddar,
crumbled or shredded

Salt

Pepper

This is a get-your-game-face-on kind of omelet. You've got a big interview or presentation at work. A doughnut and last-minute coffee from the corner won't suffice. You need fuel for the day. So you make a wicked-good three-egg omelet, because two eggs are for average days. Today you conquer!

1. Melt 1 tablespoon butter in a nonstick pan over medium heat, add asparagus, and sprinkle with salt and fresh black pepper. Sauté until asparagus is cooked through, about 5 minutes. Transfer to a plate and wipe out pan.

2. Beat the eggs, chives, herbs, salt and pepper to taste, and 1 tablespoon water in a small bowl until foamy. Place pan back over medium heat and add remaining butter. When butter is melted and bubbling, beat the egg mixture again and add to the pan.

3. Using a spatula, swirl the eggs to cover the entire pan. Allow eggs to set slightly. Gently tilt pan while lifting an edge of the omelet to allow uncooked egg to run down and fill that side. Continue with other edges, until omelet is barely dry.

4. Add asparagus and cheese on one side and gently slide onto plate while folding over. Cut in half if you want to share with someone.

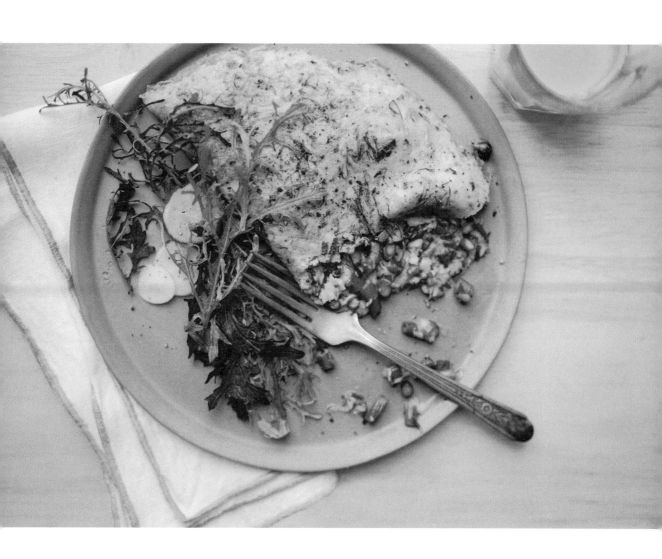

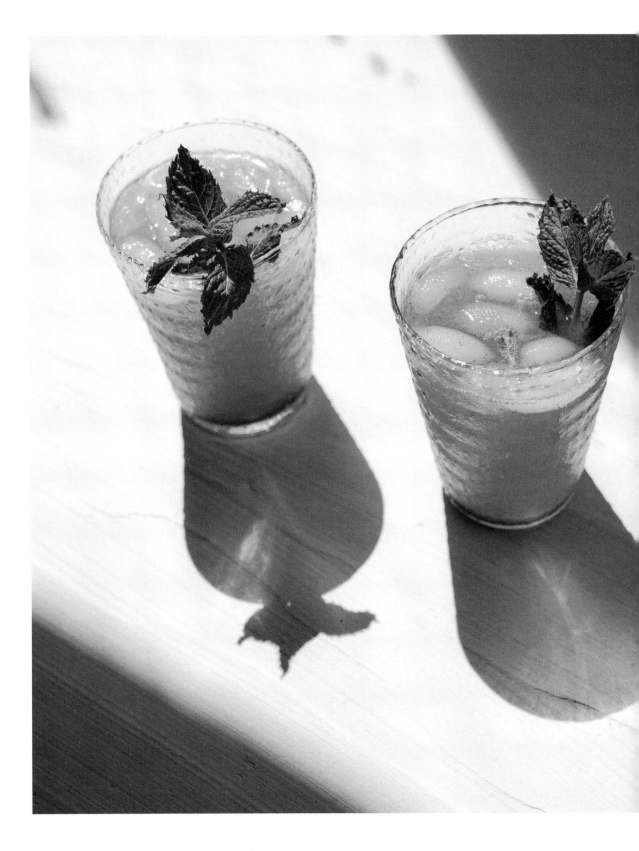

Doublemint Mojitos

We tried multiple methods to yield the mintiest, greenest mojitos. Muddling, blanching for a simple syrup, blanching plus ice bath, but nothing lived up to the promise of preserving flavor or color. And if you're going to drink mojitos, they should be a breeze to prepare, ideally for multiple people at once. We know of no better way to kick off a spring or summer get-together than with a bottomless pitcher of these extra-minty, extra-fresh mojitos.

Serves: 4

½ cup lime juice from
6–8 limes

5 tablespoons cane sugar,
brown sugar, or maple syrup

I cup white rum

I cup fresh spearmint leaves,
plus extra sprigs for garnish

½ cup seltzer or soda water

1. In a blender (or big jar with an immersion blender), blend everything except seltzer water until the mint is just tiny flecks.

2. Strain immediately into 4 ice-filled glasses and top each glass with bubbly water.

Party Like It's 1999 Compost Cake

Serves: 12

---

2 cups whole milk

2 large egg yolks

1½ teaspoons vanilla extract

½ cup sugar

2 tablespoons cornstarch

⅛ teaspoon salt

8 ounces cream cheese, softened at room temperature

¼ cup powdered sugar

1½ cups heavy cream, very cold

16 ounces organic chocolate sandwich cookies ("Oreos")

Gummy worms and artificial succulents, for serving

Is your first childhood encounter with dirt cake forever Etch-a-Sketched in your memory? Served in a flowerpot with gummy worms and a giant fake sunflower?

Fast-forward twenty years. We saw organic chocolate sandwich cookies at the store and knew what they were destined for. So here it is, friends: a dirt cake for the new generation: organic Oreos; grass-fed, free-range, non-GMO everything; no instant pudding. And lose the flowers—plant a succulent terrarium in your compost cake instead.

1. Vanilla pudding: In a large glass liquid measuring cup, whisk milk, egg yolks, and vanilla very well. Set aside.

2. Whisk the sugar, cornstarch, and salt in a medium pot over medium heat.

3. As the sugar mixture heats, slowly stream in ½ cup of the milk mixture. Whisk until sugar is dissolved, then begin streaming in more of the milk mixture, gradually, whisking continuously until everything is well combined.

4. Now wait a few minutes, until the milk mixture begins to steam and ever so slightly bubble. Whisk every 30 seconds for about 10 minutes or until it's thickened and looks puddingish but is still a bit runny. Remove from heat and set aside. Let it cool completely or refrigerate for up to a day.

5. Whipped cream cheese: In the bowl of a stand mixer (or using a handheld mixer), beat softened cream cheese and powdered sugar until well combined, 4–5 minutes.

6. In another bowl, beat heavy cream until stiff peaks form. Gently fold whipped cream into the cream cheese mixture until well combined.

7. Cookies: While the pudding and whipped cream cheese are chilling, turn the cookies into dirt-like crumbs using a food processor fitted with an S-blade. If you've got a regular-size one, do this in

3 batches. Transfer the crumbs to a bowl and set aside until needed. You can do this a day in advance, too; keep covered at room temperature.

8.   Cream filling: Now carefully fold the whipped cream cheese mix into the pudding, stirring gently until well combined.

9.   Final assembly: Grab a bowl or deep-sided round baking dish, about 9 or 10 inches in diameter and at least 3½ inches deep (though you can make any size work; little individual ramekins would be adorable, too). Starting and ending with the crumbs, alternate layers of crumbs and cream in 3–4 total layers, evening them out if necessary with a spatula. Let this set overnight in the fridge, then decorate with artificial flowers or succulents and gummy worms.

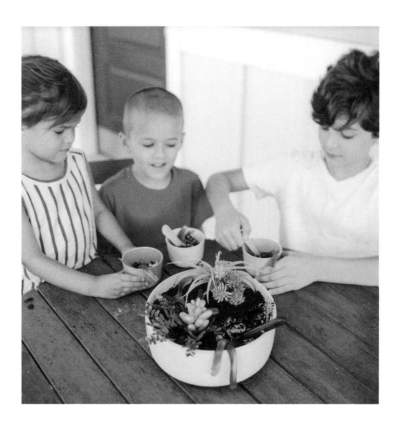

Ode to Rhubarb Cornmeal Cake

Serves: 8

———————

8 stalks rhubarb, chopped into 1-inch chunks (we've tried lots of sizes and this is the best), about 4 cups in all

2 teaspoons cornstarch

1 cup sugar, divided

1 cup almond meal

¾ cup fine cornmeal

1 teaspoon baking powder

¼ teaspoon salt

½ teaspoon ground cardamom

Zest of 1 lemon

8 tablespoons unsalted butter, softened

2 large eggs, at room temperature

½ cup full-fat canned coconut milk, room temperature

2 teaspoons vanilla extract

There are a gazillion things you can make during rhubarb season, but this cake should probably be the first and most frequent. It turned us into hardcore rhubarb lovers. Our spirits were dampened by recipes that called for maybe three stalks max, so we set out to create a cake that would do it justice. If someone doesn't ask you, "What are you doing with all that rhubarb?" you might not be buying enough.

1. Preheat oven to 350°F. Butter a 9-inch cake pan and line with parchment paper.

2. Toss the rhubarb, cornstarch, and ⅓ cup sugar in a bowl. Set aside.

3. Whisk the almond meal, cornmeal, baking powder, salt, cardamom, and lemon zest together in another bowl. Set aside.

4. In a stand mixer (or with a handheld mixer), beat the butter and remaining ⅔ cup sugar until light and fluffy, about 2 minutes. Add the eggs, one at a time. Pour in the coconut milk and the vanilla. Beat for another minute, until well mixed.

5. Add the dry ingredients to the wet all at once and mix on low speed until combined.

6. Transfer the rhubarb to the cake pan. You want to have a good, thick layer of it so you can't see the bottom of the pan anymore. Pour the cake batter over the rhubarb, scraping down the sides of the bowl with a rubber spatula and smoothing the top of the cake when done.

7. Transfer to the oven. Bake for 50–60 minutes or until cake is set and a toothpick comes out (mostly) clean. Let it rest on a cooling rack for 15–30 minutes, run a knife around the edges to loosen, and then carefully invert onto a serving plate. Let it cool completely and serve at room temperature or slightly chilled. A dollop of sweetened whipped cream with a tiny splash of rose water is a good idea, too.

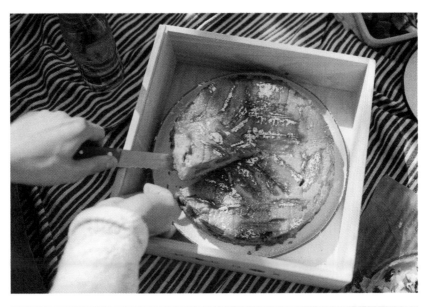

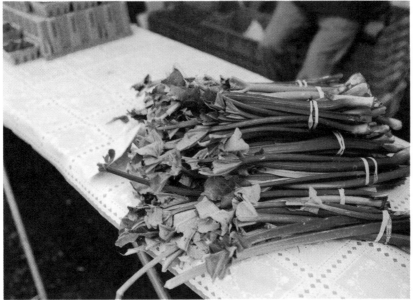

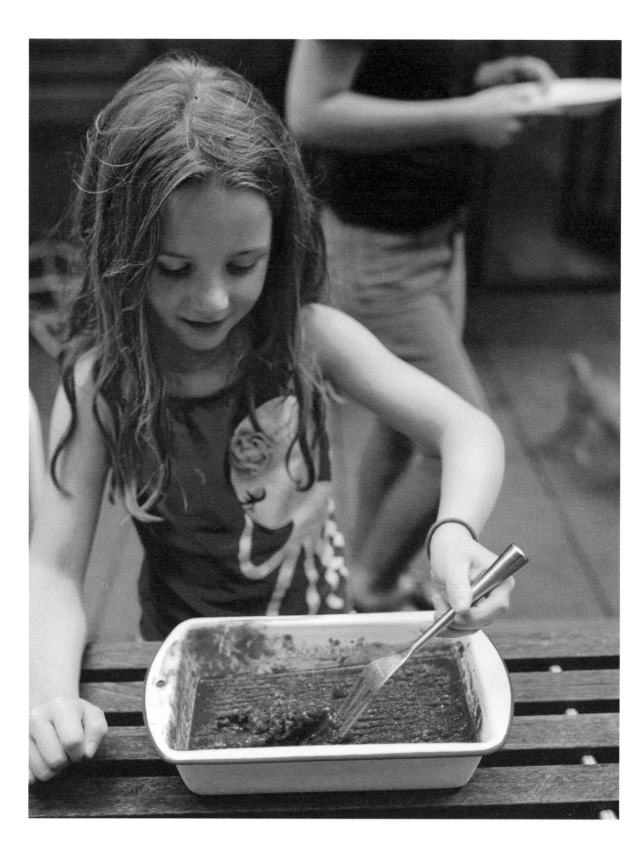

Strawberry-Basil Granita

Serves: 6

———————

1 pound strawberries

3 tablespoons coconut sugar

⅓ cup water

6 basil leaves

This refreshing granita is the perfect ending to any spring meal, but especially heavier ones like pizza, pasta, or fish tacos. It's super easy to make, but you'll need to scrape the puree every so often to prevent ending up with one massive ice cube. Kids *love* to do this (set a timer for them!). And when we serve it to guests, they take all the glory for it. Rightfully so—they did all the work.

1. Hull the strawberries and halve or quarter, depending on size. Add them to a blender, along with sugar and water. Puree until completely smooth. Add the basil and pulse until there are specks all throughout.

2. Pour the mixture through a sieve into an 8-by-8-inch pan. Transfer to the freezer for 1 hour.

3. After an hour, remove the pan from the freezer and use a fork to scrape up the icy mix, making sure to break up any big pieces. Place back in the freezer and repeat the process every 30 minutes. It should take another 2 hours for the granita to reach perfection.

4. You can serve immediately, divided into glasses, or cover and store in the freezer until needed.

Pistachio Blondies with Berry Collision à la Mode

Serves: 8

Pistachio blondies

8 tablespoons unsalted butter

6 ounces raw pistachios, 1½ cups ground

½ cup all-purpose flour

½ teaspoon salt

2 large eggs

1 cup powdered sugar

Berries and cream

1 quart seasonal berries and stone fruits: strawberries, cherries, raspberries, blackberries, blueberries, black raspberries

1 pint vanilla bean ice cream or sweetened whipped cream (with a tiny splash of rose water or a sprinkle of dried lavender)

There's a tiny but glorious window, usually in June, when spring and summer berries overlap. They're ripe and ready at the market, waiting to be combined together in a memorable dessert like this. The pistachio blondie is extra pistachio-y and so easy you could make it in your sleep. Make it look super fancy simply by the way you slice and serve.

1. First, brown the butter (it's worth it). Add butter to a saucepan and set over medium heat. Let it simmer for 5–10 minutes, keeping a close eye on it and stirring occasionally. When it's a light caramel color, you see dark solids on the bottom, and it smells fragrant and nutty, it's done. Remove from heat and set aside to cool in the pan.

2. Preheat oven to 350°F and set a rack in the middle of the oven.

3. In a food processor fitted with an S-blade, grind pistachios just until they resemble a coarse nut flour; do not overprocess or you'll end up with pistachio butter. Transfer to a bowl and combine well with flour.

4. In another bowl, whisk the salt, browned butter, eggs, and sugar until smooth and the texture of molasses.

5. Fold dry ingredients into the wet until well combined.

6. Using a rubber spatula, scrape batter into a greased 8-by-8-inch pan. Smooth it evenly on top and slide in the oven for 17–19 minutes, until set and slightly golden brown around the edges.

7. Transfer pan to wire rack and let it cool completely, at least 30 minutes. When cooled, slice blondies into long rectangles and serve with berries on one side, ice cream on the other.

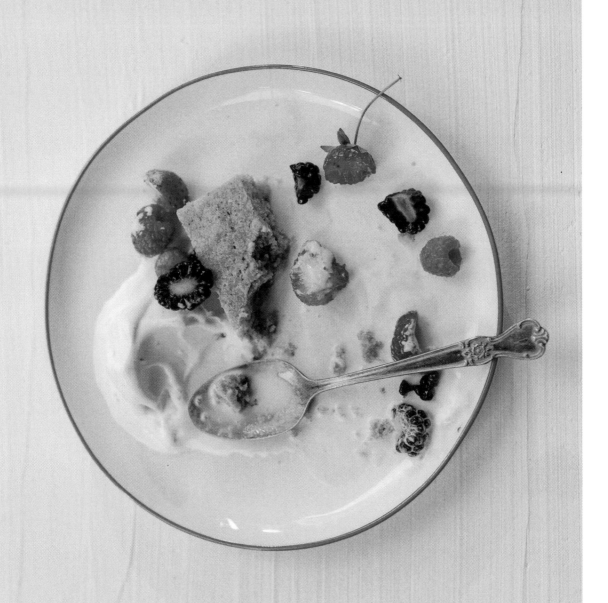

Summer

NOTICE WHAT'S HAPPENING OUTSIDE (NATURE) . . .

Summer is the abundance and culmination of all things good—sun, water, farm trucks overflowing with watermelons, gardens bursting with ripe-and-ready everything to harvest. Nature's one big playground.

. . . AND INSIDE (HUMAN NATURE)

Be wrapped up in childlike wonder. If we don't let go of our grown-up-ness a little, we miss it. Schedule a time for no schedule. Pencil in no-agenda time. Sit in the sun with a book, spend lazy afternoons just eating corn on the cob and ice cream sandwiches on the front steps, run barefoot through the sprinkler. Don't bring your work home. Your job at home is to have some fun. If it's hard to get there mentally and emotionally, just observe the kids in your life. They'll show you the way. They know the best places and the best things that stir wonder in us. It might take some practice; it's been decades. Be freely in the moment. Fully.

HERE'S WHAT TO LOOK FORWARD TO:

Peaches, fireworks, epic sunsets, backyard cookouts, heirloom tomatoes, stargazing

on the grass, chasing ice cream trucks, blackberries and raspberries, summer rain,

napping in a hammock, reading a book on the beach, swinging on the porch sipping iced

tea, picking wildflowers, floating in a pool, getting in a boat, catching fireflies,

making every kind of fruit pie.

Your Summer Kitchen Plan

COOK 3X A WEEK:

Choose three dinners.

Add on breakfasts, something

sweet, and a drink, too, if you'd

like. Make a grocery list.

Remember to think in

cooking categories (page 34)

and add a new kitchen habit that

will help you stick to your

plan (pages 31-51).

After 4 weeks, mix and match

favorite recipes to cook the rest

of the season.

Week 1

Monday	Pattypan & Corn Cavatelli with Ricotta
Tuesday	Charred Corn Tacos with Tomatoes, Cotija & Basil-Jalapeño Drizzle
Wednesday	I Left My Heart in Santorini Salad
Thursday	An Israeli Grilled Lamb Dinner
Friday	Backyard Burgers & Classic Potato Salad

Week 2

Monday	Quick-Marinated Eggplant & Poblanos with Herbed Barley
Tuesday	I Make You (Best) Lamb Taco
Wednesday	Brooklyn Pizzeria Summer Salad
Thursday	A Platter to Feed Them All
Friday	Classic B-L-Double-T with Rosemary Mayo

Week 3

Monday	Pappardelle de Francese
Tuesday	Southwestern Summer Salad with Jalapeño-Cilantro Ranch
Wednesday	Market Corn Chowder with Summer Savory
Thursday	An Intro to Okra with Asian Marinated Flank Steak
Friday	Rooftop Shishito & Corn Pizza with Garlic-Basil Oil

Week 4

Monday	Cajun Potluck Platter with Warm Bacon-Jalapeño Vinaigrette
Tuesday	Thai Basil Chicken Wraps with Peanut Sauce & Cucumber-Carrot Slaw
Wednesday	Transylvanian Herbed Squash & Tomato Soup
Thursday	Basil-Lemon Fish with a Sunny Sauté
Friday	Philly Cheesesteaks with Heirloom Peppers

Breakfasts, Drinks, Something Sweet

Breakfast	Almond Blender Pancakes
Breakfast	The Dilly Dally
Breakfast	A Tale of a Countryside Breakfast Board
Breakfast	French Farmhouse Skillet Hash with Sunny-Side-Up Eggs
Happy Hour	Melon Jubilees
Happy Hour	The Green Gemini
Happy Hour	Summer Orchard Sangria with Elderflower & Basil
Sweet	Bakeshop Blackberry-Lavender Scones
Sweet	Corndoodle Ice Cream Sandwiches with Raspberries

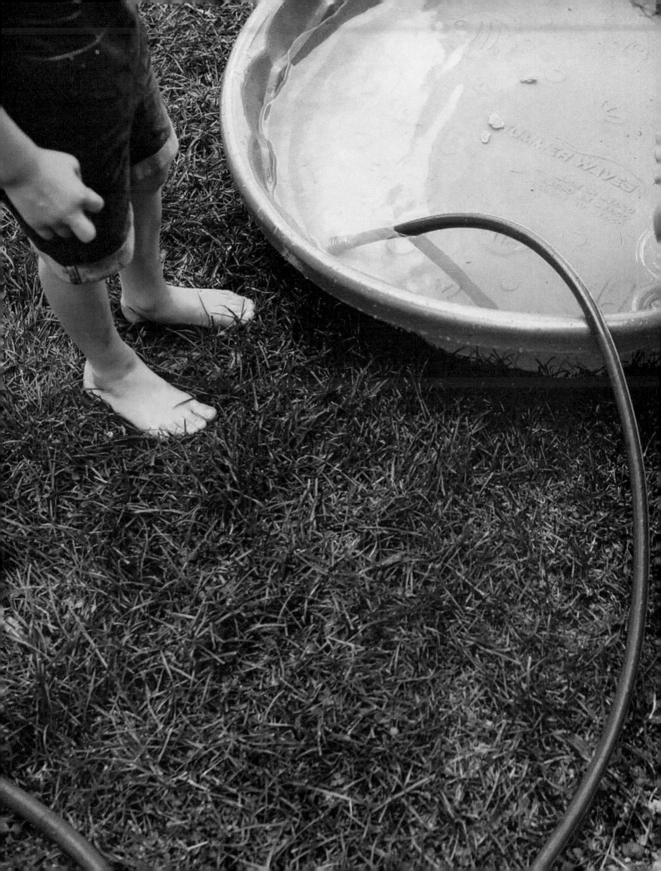

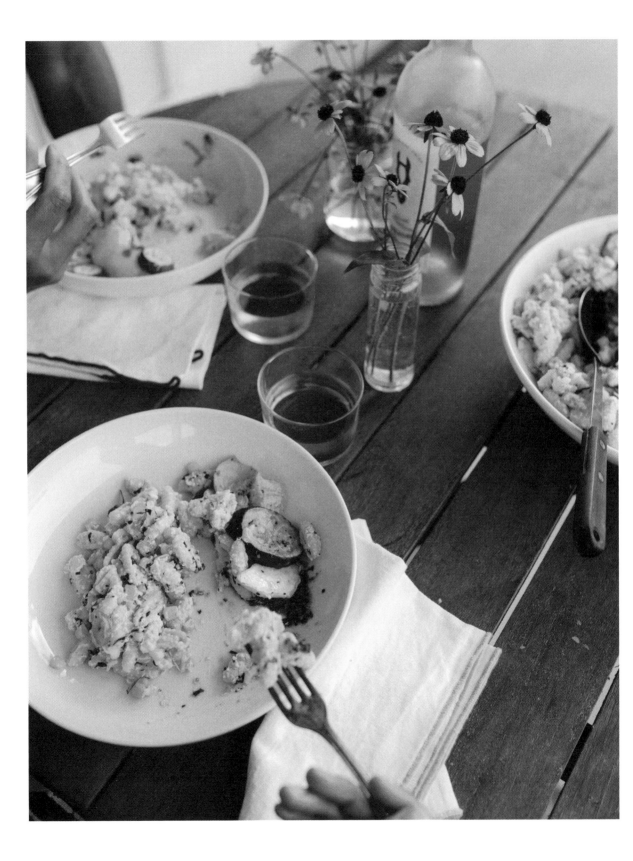

Pattypan & Corn Cavatelli with Ricotta

Serves: 4

1½ pounds pattypan squash, zucchini, or summer squash, ideally a heap of baby ones

Extra-virgin olive oil

1 cup fresh corn kernels, from 2 ears of corn

1 large leek, just the white and light green parts

¼ teaspoon crushed red pepper

½ pound cavatelli pasta, good quality; we love Sfoglini

1 cup ricotta cheese, good quality

Zest of 1 small lemon

1 bunch fresh basil

2 cloves garlic, minced, or 3 garlic scapes, chopped

¾ cup Parmesan, grated, divided

Salt

Pepper

There's nothing quite like this combo on a summer Pasta Night. Ricotta, basil, corn, and summer squash varieties. It's good warm, but it's really, really good at room temperature, when all the flavors have a chance to meld. So tonight's a night when it's okay if dinner gets cold—pour a glass of crisp rosé, set the table outside, and let everyone leisurely make their way to dinner.

1. Preheat oven to 400°F. Slice pattypans into ¼-inch rounds. Drizzle with a tablespoon of oil, season generously with salt and pepper, toss, and arrange in one layer on a sheet pan. Roast for 25–30 minutes, flipping halfway through. Add corn and roast for another couple of minutes; set the sheet pan aside.

2. Slice the leek in half lengthwise, then slice into very thin half-moons. Place in a large bowl filled with water, swish well, and break apart the pieces so the grit falls to the bottom of the bowl. Pull out the leeks and drain; pat dry.

3. Drizzle a tablespoon of oil in a large sauté pan and set over medium heat. When oil is hot, add in leeks and crushed red pepper. Stir from time to time until soft, about 5 minutes.

4. Bring a large pot of well-salted water to a boil and cook pasta a minute shy of package directions until very al dente. Drain, reserving a cup of the pasta water for later, and transfer pasta to the pan with leeks.

5. In a small bowl, mix ricotta with ½ teaspoon salt, a few cracks of pepper, and lemon zest. In a small food processor, give the basil leaves a whir along with the garlic, 3 tablespoons oil, ¼ cup Parmesan, and a pinch of salt.

6. Turn heat back on to medium-low, stir the ricotta into the pasta, coating well, and add splashes of pasta water as needed. Cook for another couple of minutes, then turn off the heat and stir in basil pesto and remaining Parmesan. Taste for salt and crack in lots of pepper. Let the dish rest for at least 10 minutes, then serve with roasted veggies.

Charred Corn Tacos with Tomatoes, Cotija & Basil-Jalapeño Drizzle

Serves: 4

Basil-jalapeño drizzle

1 cup fresh basil

1 jalapeño, roughly chopped

Juice of 1 lime

2 cloves garlic, chopped

⅓ cup mayonnaise

Tacos

2 cups fresh corn kernels, from 4 ears of corn

Extra-virgin olive oil

1 yellow onion, diced

1 red bell pepper, diced

8 corn tortillas

2 tomatoes, diced

½ cup cotija cheese

Salt

Pepper

What we imagine walking through the colorful streets of any Mexican city during late summer would taste like. Authentic street corn in taco form.

Kitchen note: This sauce is so dang good, we've used it on roasted chicken, fresh-mozzarella-and-tomato salad, morning eggs, and epic sandwiches. The possibilities are endless, so make a double batch.

1. In a blender, puree the drizzle ingredients with ¼ teaspoon each salt and pepper, until completely smooth. If it's too thick, add 1–2 tablespoons of water and blend again. Refrigerate until tacos are ready.

2. Set a dry sauté pan over high heat and toast the corn kernels until golden with some brown spots, 5–7 minutes, stirring occasionally. Sprinkle with ¼ teaspoon salt. Transfer to a bowl and set aside.

3. In the same pan, lower heat slightly, and add a good drizzle of oil. Sauté onion and bell pepper for 5–7 minutes; season with ¼ teaspoon each salt and pepper. When soft, add to the bowl of corn and set aside.

4. Char the tortillas over an open flame and set aside on a plate.

5. Serve family-style, letting everyone make their own tacos with the corn filling, cheese, tomatoes, and basil-jalapeño drizzle.

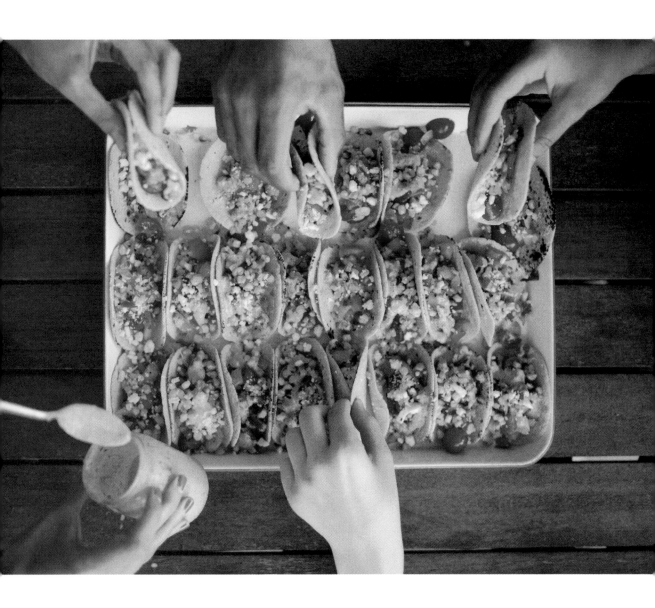

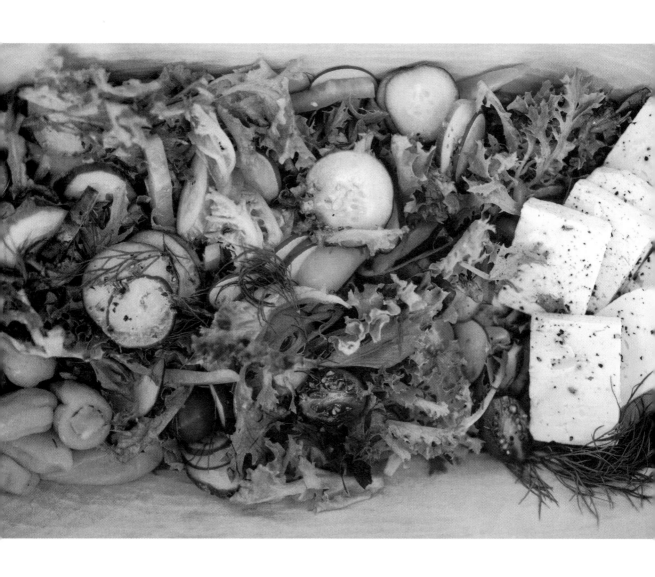

I Left My Heart in Santorini Salad

Serves: 4

_____

Dressing

Juice of 2 lemons,
about 4-5 tablespoons

⅓ cup extra-virgin olive oil

1 teaspoon dried oregano

¾ teaspoon salt

½ teaspoon pepper

Salad

1 head crisp lettuce, torn into
bite-size pieces

1 bunch radishes, thinly sliced

2 medium-size cucumbers,
thinly sliced

2 bell peppers, diced

1 pint cherry tomatoes, halved

¼ cup fresh dill, chopped

½ cup feta cheese, crumbled,
or more to taste

It's been almost a decade since I (Christine) honeymooned in Greece, and it's more breathtaking than any photo can capture: the white-and-blue houses, the windmills, the steep, winding village steps, the sunsets, the black pebble beaches with turquoise water, freshly grilled calamari. Until I can save up to go again, this salad is the next best thing. Make it in your kitchen, too, and you'll instantly be sitting at a cliffside café in Santorini watching the sun go down.

1. Whisk together the dressing ingredients or shake in a jar, about 1 minute.

2. Combine salad ingredients in a large serving bowl and toss with vinaigrette to taste. Enjoy!

An Israeli Grilled Lamb Dinner

Serves: 4

Rack of lamb with spiced brine

1 teaspoon ground coriander

1 teaspoon ground cumin

2 tablespoons extra-virgin olive oil

6 cloves garlic, minced

2½ pounds rack of lamb, or lamb chops, loin or rib

Grilled vegetables

3 zucchini, summer, or pattypan squash, sliced into thick rounds

3 poblanos, sliced

2 tablespoons grapeseed oil, or any neutral oil

Juice of ½ lemon, about 2 tablespoons

Toasted turmeric couscous

2 tablespoons extra-virgin olive oil

½ teaspoon ground turmeric

2 cups Israeli couscous

3 cups low-sodium chicken stock

¼ cup fresh parsley, cilantro, and/or mint, minced

Salt

Pepper

A simple, plentiful summer feast on the grill. The kind where everyone casually sits on the porch, polishing off their lamb bones, talking between sips of wine way past sundown.

1. Lamb: In a tiny bowl, combine spices, oil, and garlic with 2 teaspoons salt and 1 teaspoon pepper to form a garlicky brine paste.

2. Slice a bit between each chop so you can slather paste inside with your fingers, in between each chop, so the meatiest parts get the flavor. This will also help the rack cook faster and more evenly. Let meat sit at room temperature for 45 minutes to 1 hour.

3. Meanwhile, fire up your outdoor grill. You want medium-high heat. (If your grill has a thermometer, about 400°F. If using the hand test, hold your hand about 5 inches above the grates. When you need to move your hand after 5–6 seconds, it's ready.)

4. Have your meat thermometer handy. Cook the lamb rack for about 15 minutes over direct heat, then move to a cooler part of the grill (the outer edge, or you can create hot/cool zones by banking more of the coals on one side of the grill) to cook over gentler heat for 15–20 more minutes or until the thickest part registers just under 150°F for medium. If the bones start to char, cover with foil.

5. Transfer to a plate or wooden board, tent with foil, and let chops rest for 5–10 minutes before slicing and serving with vegetables and couscous.

6. Vegetables: You'll need a grill basket for this; cook alongside the lamb if there's room.

7. Toss zucchini and poblanos with grapeseed oil and generously salt and pepper (roughly ½ teaspoon of each).

8. Place half into the grill basket. You'll work in 2 batches so all the pieces get some color and flavor from the fire (also so they don't steam too much). Cover and grill until soft and slightly charred, using tongs to flip once or twice. Squeeze on a little lemon and transfer to your serving platter.

9. Couscous: In a medium pot or Dutch oven, drizzle in olive oil and sprinkle in the turmeric. Once hot, add couscous. Stir occasionally, 3–4 minutes, until fragrant and nutty.

10. Pour in chicken stock with ¾ teaspoon salt, reduce heat to low, cover, and simmer according to the time given on the package directions (about 10 minutes, usually). Fluff the couscous with a fork and fold in herbs. Add to your platter and feast!

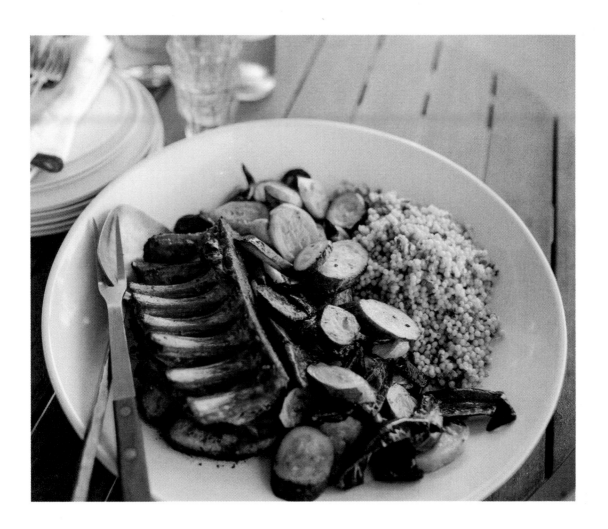

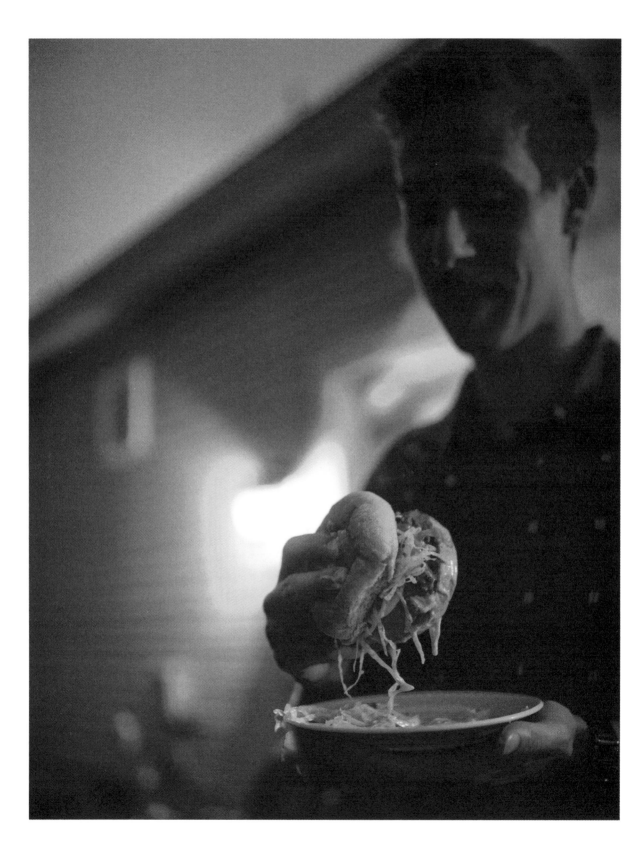

Backyard Burgers

Serves: 4

―――――――――

Awesome sauce

½ cup mayonnaise

2 tablespoons sour cream

2 tablespoons ketchup, or sriracha if you like it spicy

2 tablespoons sweet pickle relish

2 tablespoons red onion, grated

1 teaspoon Worcestershire sauce

2 teaspoons lemon juice

Burgers

1 pound ground beef with at least 20 percent fat

4 slices American cheese

4 potato buns, toasted

2 pickles, very thinly sliced lengthwise on a mandoline

¼ head iceberg lettuce, finely shredded

Salt

Pepper

Summers with backyard burgers and potato salad are good summers. If you want incredible what's-in-this-burger burgers, you're going to have to get really good meat. Like find a farmer and drive to his farm and pick up some freshly ground beef that's got the perfect amount of fat. Budget for these burgers.

1. Whisk all the awesome sauce ingredients in a bowl and season with salt and pepper to taste. Cover and refrigerate for up to 3 days.

2. Fire up the grill or your stove to medium-high. Set a cast-iron griddle or steel griddle on top of the flames and wait for it to heat up.

3. Meanwhile, divide the meat into 4 portions and form gently into balls.

4. Once the griddle surface is hot, add a burger ball and smasssssh it down with a heavy-duty burger spatula or a pan. Give it a sprinkle of salt, then don't touch; wait 3–4 minutes, until the underside is crispy and browned. Flip, sprinkle the other side with salt, and leave it for about 2 more minutes, until that side is crispy and browned. At the last minute, add a slice of cheese. Transfer to a plate and tent loosely with foil.

5. Repeat with remaining burgers—however many fit on the griddle at a time.

6. Place on a burger bun and top with sauce, pickles, and lettuce. Enjoy!

Classic Potato Salad

Serves: 6

---

2 pounds red potatoes, skin on

2 tablespoons apple cider vinegar

1 small red onion, diced

2 stalks celery, diced

3 tablespoons fresh Italian parsley, chopped

2 scallions, chopped

2 pickles, diced

¾ cup mayonnaise

¼ cup sour cream

2 teaspoons Dijon or whole-grain mustard

Salt

Pepper

Bad potato salad is such a shame, because it can cause a lifetime of prejudice. Have a goopy mess of it on a flimsy plastic plate in eighth grade and you'll forever judge all potato salads because of it. Done right, it will make the best side dish you've had in a while. Cookouts aren't the same without a big bowl on a checkered tablecloth.

1. Add potatoes to a pot of salted water and bring to a boil. Reduce heat to a simmer and cook just until fork tender. You don't want them falling apart in the salad. Drain well.

2. Halve or quarter the potatoes, depending on size, and place them in a large bowl while still warm. Gently toss them with the apple cider vinegar. Set aside.

3. Add onion, celery, parsley, scallions, and pickles to the potatoes.

4. In a small bowl, mix the mayo, sour cream, mustard, 1 teaspoon salt, and 1 teaspoon pepper.

5. Pour the mayo mix into the large bowl and gently stir everything together. Taste—usually you'll need more acidity or salt. Let it rest for at least 15 minutes. Serve at room temperature or refrigerate until ready to eat.

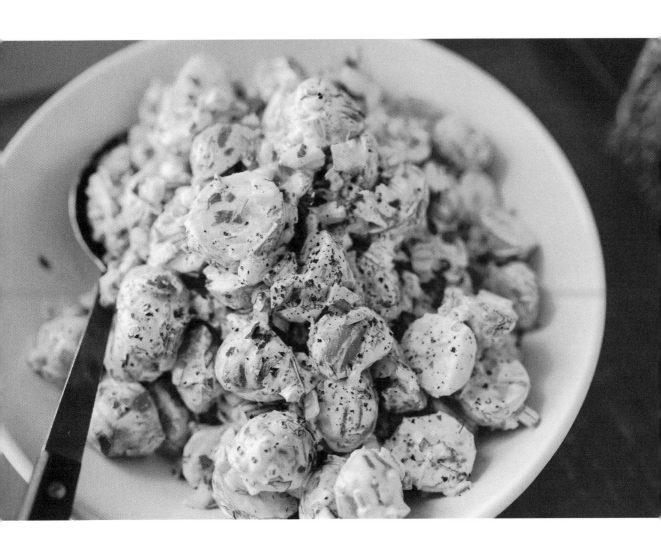

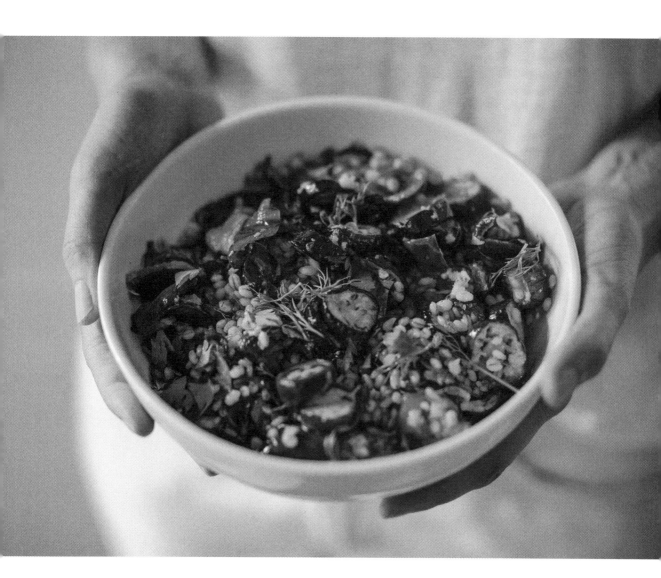

Quick-Marinated Eggplant & Poblanos with Herbed Barley

Serves: 4

_____

Eggplant and poblanos

1½ pounds eggplant; we love the slender Chinese or Japanese eggplants

4 poblano peppers

Grapeseed oil

Barley

1 cup pearl barley

3 cups water

Garlic-lemon marinade

6 cloves garlic, minced

½ cup extra-virgin olive oil

Juice of 1 lemon

½ bunch fresh dill, chopped

1 bunch fresh Italian parsley, chopped

Salt

Pepper

This is your summer potluck side dish. Take it everywhere or serve it at home with any and all grilled meat or fish. It tastes amazing at room temperature or right out of the fridge.

1. Preheat oven to 400°F.

2. Cut eggplant into ½-inch slices and chop poblanos into 1-inch pieces; lay them on a large sheet pan. Drizzle with oil and season with a few pinches of salt and pepper. Transfer to the oven and roast for 20–30 minutes, flipping veggies halfway through.

3. Add the barley, 1 teaspoon salt, and water to a pot; bring to a boil. Cook for 25–35 minutes or until barley is tender. Drain and set aside.

4. In a large bowl, whisk the garlic, olive oil, lemon juice, and ½ teaspoon each salt and pepper.

5. Add the roasted eggplant and poblanos to marinade. Stir well and let them sit for at least 30 minutes, then stir in the barley and chopped herbs. Taste and add more salt, lemon, or herbs if you'd like.

6. Cover and refrigerate for up to 2 days. The more it sits, the better it tastes, so make it a couple of hours before serving (although we've eaten it immediately and it's still delicious).

I Make You (Best) Lamb Taco

Serves: 4

Lamb

1 tablespoon extra-virgin olive oil

1 yellow onion, chopped

5 cloves garlic, minced

1 teaspoon salt, plus more to taste

½ teaspoon pepper

2 teaspoons paprika

2 teaspoons dried oregano

1 teaspoon ground cumin

½ teaspoon ground cinnamon

2½ teaspoons tomato paste

1 pound ground lamb

½ cup beer

Taco fixings

8 corn tortillas, charred or warmed over an open flame

1 English cucumber, diced

1 small red onion, thinly sliced

1 large tomato, diced

½ cup feta cheese, more to taste

¼ cup Greek yogurt

One of our favorite scenes in movie history is when the entire *My Big Fat Greek Wedding* family dramatically gasps at the thought of someone being vegetarian. Our entire childhood flashed before our eyes. So this is us, in our best Aunt Voula voice, telling you that if you love lamb, we'll make you this taco. And if you don't love lamb, that's okay, we'll still make you this taco. It's really that good.

1. Place oil in a large skillet and set over medium heat.

2. When hot, add the onion and sauté for about 4 minutes, until soft.

3. Add the garlic, salt, pepper, and spices and cook for another minute or so.

4. Stir in the tomato paste and cook 1–2 minutes, until it's combined with the onion mixture.

5. Add the lamb and raise heat to medium-high. Break up the meat into smaller bits with a spoon or spatula. When the lamb is no longer pink, pour in the beer, stirring occasionally until it's completely evaporated.

6. Now, in order to get the lamb gorgeous, with crispy bits here and there, you have to continue cooking another 10 minutes or so. Don't stir often—the bottom of the pan will get brown, but don't worry, pay no attention. Every couple of minutes, try to stir up those brown bits along with the lamb.

7. Serve lamb with charred tortillas, cucumber, red onion, tomato, feta, and yogurt.

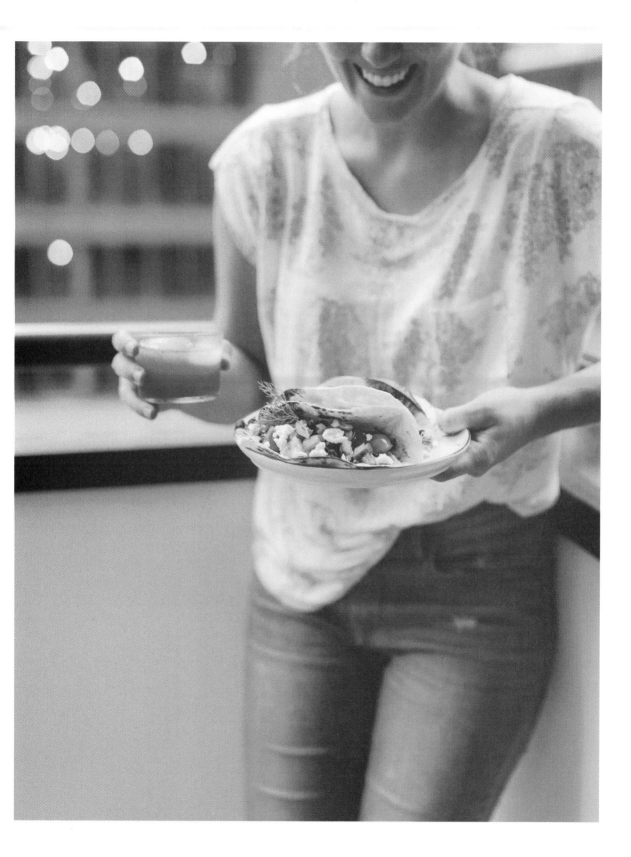

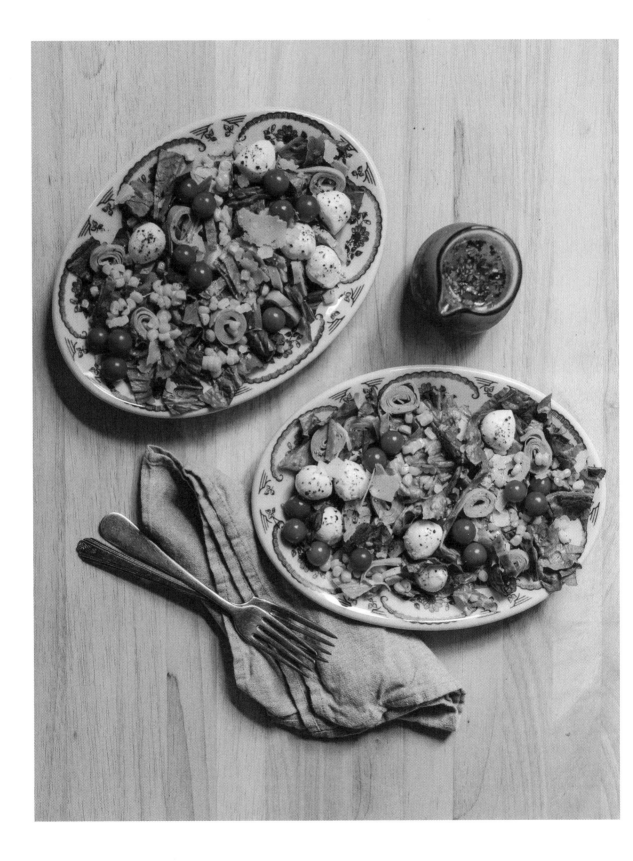

Brooklyn Pizzeria Summer Salad

Serves: 3–4

Vinaigrette

1 shallot, finely minced

2 cloves garlic,
finely minced or grated

½ cup red wine vinegar

2 teaspoons dried basil

2 teaspoons dried oregano

1 teaspoon maple syrup

¾ cup olive oil or other
neutral-tasting oil

Salad

¼ pound soppressata
and mortadella, or any
Italian deli meats

1 head romaine lettuce,
torn into 1-inch pieces

1 pint cherry tomatoes,
halved or whole if they're tiny

1 cup corn kernels, cooked,
from about 2 ears of corn

¾ cup mini fresh
mozzarella balls

½ cup Parmigiano-Reggiano,
shaved

Salt

Pepper

Eating this bursting-with-summer antipasto salad outside may instantly transport you to the back patio of a Brooklyn pizza joint. You're surrounded by colorful murals, wood-fired pizza, tattoos, and a view of the bridge.

Kitchen note: Some options for cooking corn: (1) Slice kernels off cob and sauté over medium heat in a little butter or oil for a few minutes. (2) Grill with the husks on, then slice off kernels. (3) Bring a large pot of water to boil, add cobs, cover pot, turn off heat, and let them cook for 10 minutes. Char a little on an open flame for some extra flavor and slice off kernels.

1. Shake vinaigrette ingredients in a jar with about ¾ teaspoon each salt and pepper, about 1 minute. It keeps in the fridge for up to a week.

2. Prep the deli meat. For the thinner, fragile varieties like mortadella and prosciutto, stack a few slices, roll up tightly, and slice into thin strips. For thicker varieties like salami, thinly slice or cube.

3. Divide remaining salad ingredients onto plates, top with deli meat, and let everyone drizzle on vinaigrette to their preference. Dig in.

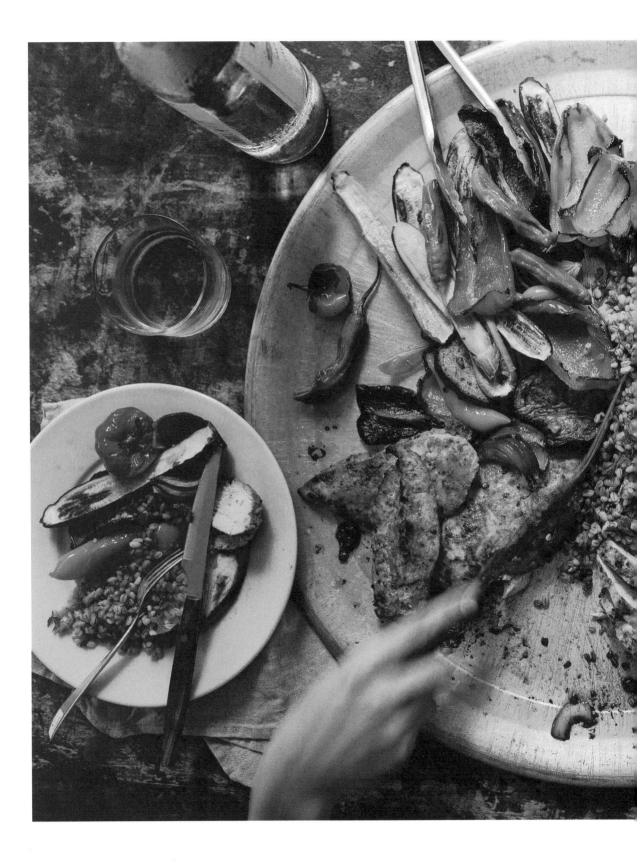

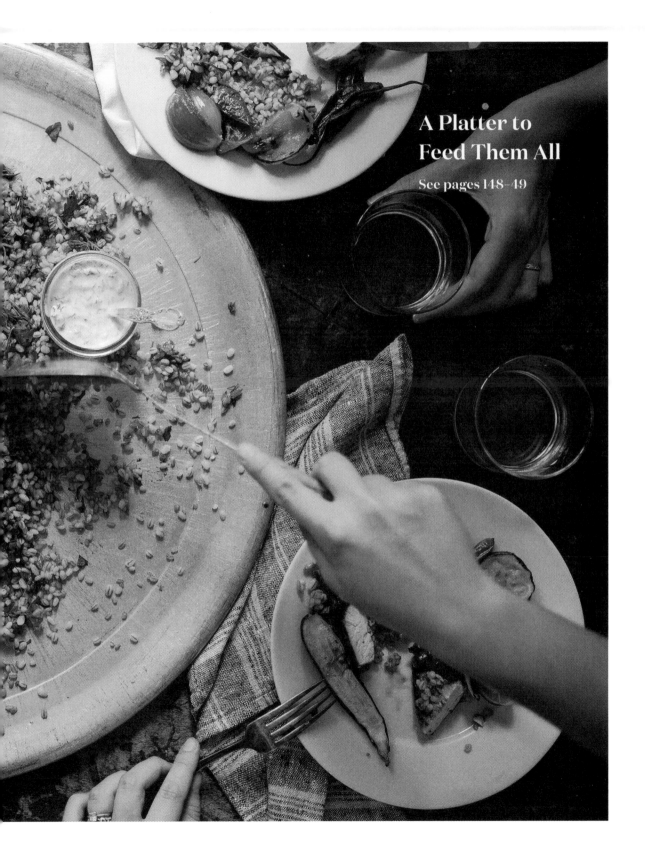

A Platter to
Feed Them All

See pages 148–49

A Platter to Feed Them All

Serves: 4–6

Spiced yogurt chicken

4 cloves garlic, minced

1½ teaspoons ground coriander

1½ teaspoons paprika

½ teaspoon turmeric

Juice of ½ lemon (you need about 1 tablespoon)

3 tablespoons extra-virgin olive oil

⅓ cup plain yogurt

1½ pounds boneless, skinless chicken breast

Barley

1½ cups barley

4 cups water

2 teaspoons extra-virgin olive oil

3 tablespoons chopped fresh herbs: parsley, dill, cilantro, whatever you have on hand

One thing that hasn't changed throughout centuries of humans eating together is the curious thrill we get when an oversize platter piled high with heaps of food gets ceremoniously plopped in the middle of a table. It's the culmination of all things festive and celebratory. This is why we gather—to eat lots of food with people we love (or at least kinda like).

The beauty here is that this is just seared meat, barley fragrant with all the herbs you have in your fridge, and a roasted assortment of all the vegetables you have in your fridge. You've probably even eaten something like this before but didn't know it because it was in three separate serving dishes. To get the dramatic oohs and aahs, make sure your platter is really big. Like hard-to-find-storage-for-it big. We snagged ours for a mere five bucks at a thrift store. (It's actually just a used pizza platter.) Get creative.

Kitchen note: You can let the chicken marinate several hours before grilling and even have all the veggies sliced and ready to go in the fridge. The barley can be served at room temperature. If you don't have an outdoor grill, cook chicken in a pan and roast the veggies at 425°F in 2 sheet pans.

1. In a bowl, whisk all the spiced yogurt chicken ingredients (except chicken) along with 1 teaspoon each salt and pepper.

2. Add chicken to the yogurt marinade, making sure it's coated on all sides. Cover and refrigerate at least 2 hours, up to overnight.

3. When ready to eat, heat up a grill to medium-high and cook chicken 3–4 minutes on each side until opaque throughout. Keep warm.

4. Bring the barley, water, and 1 teaspoon salt to a boil. Lower heat to a simmer and cook until tender, about 25–30 minutes. Drain, return to pot, and stir in oil and chopped herbs.

Grilled vegetables

2 heirloom bell peppers
(assorted colors), quartered
lengthwise

2 red onions, sliced into
large wedges

2 or 3 summer squashes
and/or zucchini, halved
lengthwise

I eggplant, sliced into
$^1/_3$-inch rounds

½ pound shishito peppers

2 tablespoons extra-virgin
olive oil

Salt

Pepper

5. Brush all the vegetables with a little oil and season with ½ tea-spoon each salt and pepper. Add them to the grill (next to the chicken if they fit). Grill until slightly charred and cooked through, 5–7 minutes per side.

6. Arrange the vegetables, chicken, and barley on a platter. Then make sure everyone's sitting; this platter needs an entrance.

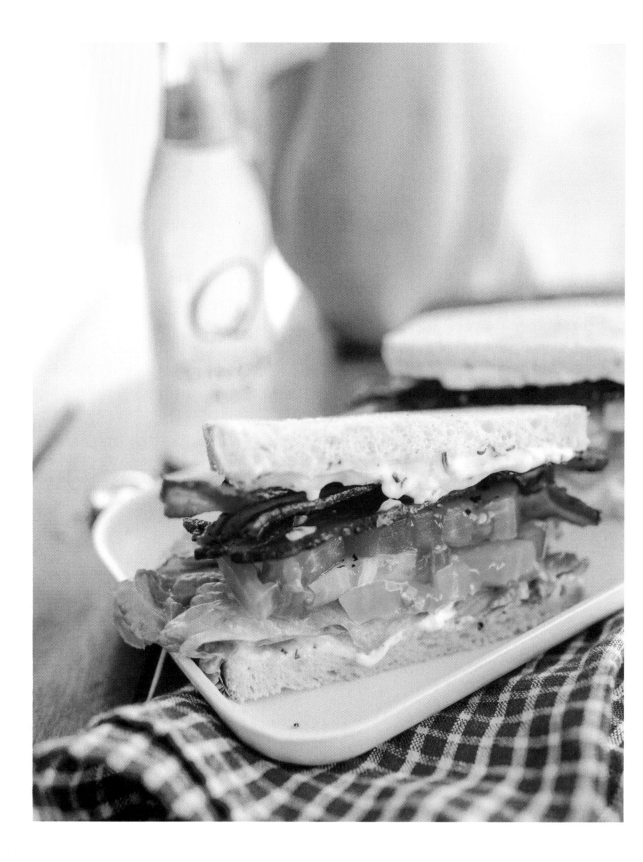

Classic B-L-Double-T with Rosemary Mayo

Serves: 4

_____

Rosemary mayo

½ cup mayonnaise

2 sprigs fresh rosemary, leaves removed from stem and very, very finely minced; add another sprig if you like rosemary

1 clove garlic, finely minced or grated

¼ lemon, just a squeeze

Sandwich

8 slices bacon

8 slices white bread

4 leaves romaine lettuce

2 really good large tomatoes, sliced into ¼-inch rounds

Salt

Pepper

Optional sandwich add-ins: 8 slices smoked turkey and 1 ripe avocado, thinly sliced

Optional, for serving: dill pickles and kettle chips

You might as well add this to your meal plan weekly during tomato season. And only during tomato season. Why settle for average when you know actual perfection is out there? And by *perfection* we mean heirloom tomatoes (the heaviest, most fragrant, bursting with juice); really good bread (not the kind you can squeeze into a ball in your hand); lettuce that's crisp and fresh (no sad lettuce!); thick bacon you can't afford to serve for breakfast (but make an exception for this sandwich). There's no "I" in "team"—everyone has a job to do.

1. In a small bowl, whisk together mayo ingredients with ¼ teaspoon salt and a crack of pepper. Add a tiny squeeze of lemon to brighten up the mayo. Refrigerate for up to several days if not using right away.

2. Heat a skillet over medium heat and add half the bacon; the skillet can be cold so the fat renders. Cook on each side for a few minutes, until browned and crisped. Transfer to a paper-towel-lined plate, pour the fat in your phat jar (see note), and cook the second batch. Alternatively, bake on a sheet pan in a 350°F oven for 15–20 minutes.

3. Toast the bread until golden, spread mayo on all slices, and divide bacon, lettuce, and tomatoes among the 4 sandwiches, sprinkling a little salt and pepper on each tomato round. Slice each sandwich in half diagonally and eat outside with a cold, fizzy drink.

_____

Note: We're bringing back that jar your grandma kept in her fridge. It made everything taste better. Starting your phat jar is really easy. Find a cute empty jar with a lid that's already in your pantry. Cook bacon, then pour the liquid gold into your jar. Keep in the fridge for up to a few months. Add it here and there to stews, soups, chilis, roasts, home fries, and anywhere you want to add a little extra depth and love.

Pappardelle de Francese

Serves: 4

---

1 tablespoon extra-virgin olive oil

3 tablespoons unsalted butter, divided

1¼–1½ pounds chicken drumsticks, at room temperature

1 head garlic, cloves peeled and finely minced

½ cup dry white wine, plus more if needed

2 medium carrots

2 large bell peppers or sweet peppers

2 medium zucchini or any type of summer squash

2–3 sprigs fresh summer savory, leaves picked, optional

8 ounces pappardelle pasta

6 tablespoons crème fraîche

¼ bunch fresh Italian parsley, finely chopped

Salt

Pepper

Parmigiano-Reggiano, optional, for serving

Herby microgreens, optional, for serving

If an Italian kitchen and a French kitchen had a baby, this would be it. It uses a bunch of stuff you don't ordinarily see in pasta: carrots, parsley, dark meat. Braising the meat boosts the dish's overall flavor and puts under-utilized cheap cuts of meat to work. The fine chop of the vegetables helps them cling beautifully to the pasta. And adding crème fraîche to pasta water yields a luxurious sauce without the heaviness. Tossed together with this light, summery sauce, it feels straight out of a fancy bistro, yet is super economical—channeling that *je ne sais quoi*.

1.   Set a braiser or a large, lidded sauté pan over medium-high heat. Swirl in oil and 2 tablespoons butter. Generously season drumsticks with salt and pepper and, once butter and oil sizzle, add meat. Don't move for 3–4 minutes, until gorgeously seared, then flip for another 2–3 minutes.

2.   Turn heat down to low and nudge chicken to the pan's edges, creating a well in the middle. Add garlic and stir for 30 seconds, then pour in the wine and scrape up all the brown bits. Add ¼ cup water, cover, and let chicken braise on low for 30–35 minutes, up to 45 minutes for larger drumsticks. The meat should be opaque and come apart easily with a fork. Transfer to a plate and shred.

3.   Meanwhile, bring a large pot of well-salted water to boil for the pasta. Then pour yourself a glass of wine and chop carrots, peppers, and zucchini or squash finely, in ¼-inch pieces.

4.   In the same pan in which you cooked the drumsticks, splash in a few more tablespoons of wine to deglaze and turn up heat to medium. Let wine reduce, then add in vegetables with a big pinch of salt and summer savory, if using. Stir occasionally for 5–7 minutes, until tender, then turn off heat.

5.   When vegetables go into the pan, that's your cue to drop the pasta into the boiling water. Cook 1–2 minutes shy of package directions. Use tongs to transfer directly to vegetable pan, reserving the pasta water.

6.   Now working quickly, ladle ½ cup pasta water into a measuring cup and whisk in crème fraîche until smooth.

7.   Pour into the pan and toss gently with pasta and vegetables. Turn heat to low and drop in the remaining tablespoon of butter to melt and coat the pasta as you toss. Simmer for a few more minutes so sauce thickens and pasta finishes cooking. If it looks like you need a little more sauce, splash in a couple of tablespoons of pasta water at a time.

8.   Taste for salt and pasta doneness, crack in a little more pepper, sprinkle in parsley. Remove from heat and serve right away with grated Parm and microgreens.

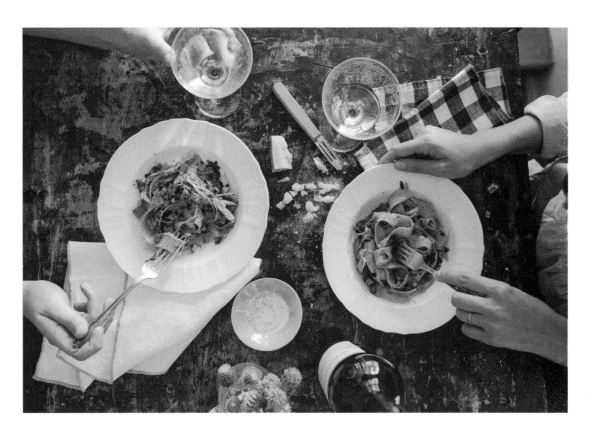

Southwestern Summer Salad with Jalapeño-Cilantro Ranch

Serves: 4

_____

Ranch

½ bunch fresh cilantro, plus more for garnish

¼ cup Greek yogurt or sour cream

¼ cup mayonnaise

2 garlic cloves, chopped

I lime, half juiced and half cut into wedges

½ jalapeño pepper, seeds removed, chopped

Salt

Pepper

Chicken

2 tablespoons extra-virgin olive oil

I½ tablespoons fajita seasoning

I pound boneless, skinless chicken breast, cut in half lengthwise

Salad

I yellow onion, diced

I cup fresh corn kernels, from 2 ears of corn

I head romaine lettuce, chopped

I bunch baby kale

I pint cherry tomatoes, halved

I small red bell pepper, diced

I 15-ounce can black beans, or I½ cups

2 corn or flour tortillas, for crispy tortilla matchsticks, optional

Grapeseed oil, or any neutral oil, optional

The perfect mix of detox and hearty—gorgeous colored vegetables, vibrant and creamy dressing, and crispy tortilla strips. Even our kids request this all summer long.

1. In a blender, puree the ranch ingredients with ¼ teaspoon each salt and pepper. Refrigerate for up to 3 days.

2. In a shallow bowl, mix 1 tablespoon oil with the fajita seasoning. If your seasoning mix doesn't have salt or pepper, add 1 teaspoon of salt and ½ teaspoon pepper as well. Add the chicken breasts and use your hands to massage the seasoning over each piece. Make sure they're coated well. Set aside on the counter.

3. Heat a large sauté pan over medium-high heat. Add the remaining tablespoon of oil and, when hot, add half the chicken breasts. Cook for 3 minutes or until the bottom gets slightly brown, then turn over and cook 2 more minutes until cooked through. Remove to a plate and cook the remaining chicken, adding more oil if needed.

4. In the same pan you cooked the chicken in, place the onion and corn. You'll see all the brown bits on the bottom of the pan release as the onion cooks. Stir a few times and cook for 3–4 minutes or until a little soft. Remove from heat and set aside while you assemble the salad.

5. In a shallow serving dish, mix the greens together. Now gently add all your veggies and toppings on top: the cherry tomatoes, bell pepper, black beans, and corn/onion mix.

6. Serve with the jalapeño-cilantro ranch on the side or drizzled over the salad, extra lime wedges, and these crispy tortillas below.

7. Halve the tortillas, then slice them into very thin strips (or thicker if you prefer, as on page 85). Pour enough oil into a small skillet to coat the bottom by ⅛ inch and set over medium-high heat. Once the hot oil shimmers, after about 2 minutes, test one matchstick. The oil should bubble all around it. Add half the strips in an even layer; they should be nearly submerged. Fry for about 2 minutes, flipping with tongs halfway through, until golden brown and crispy.

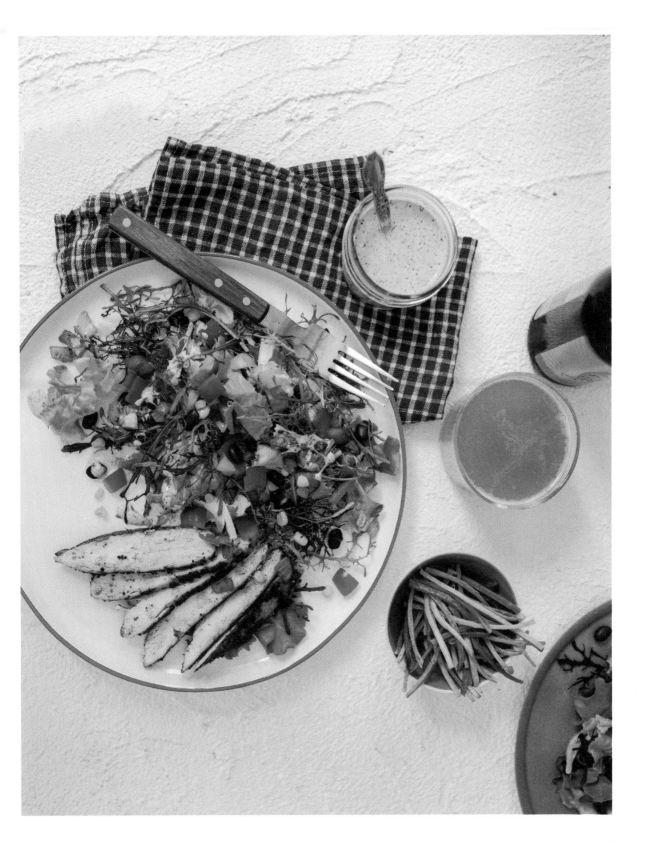

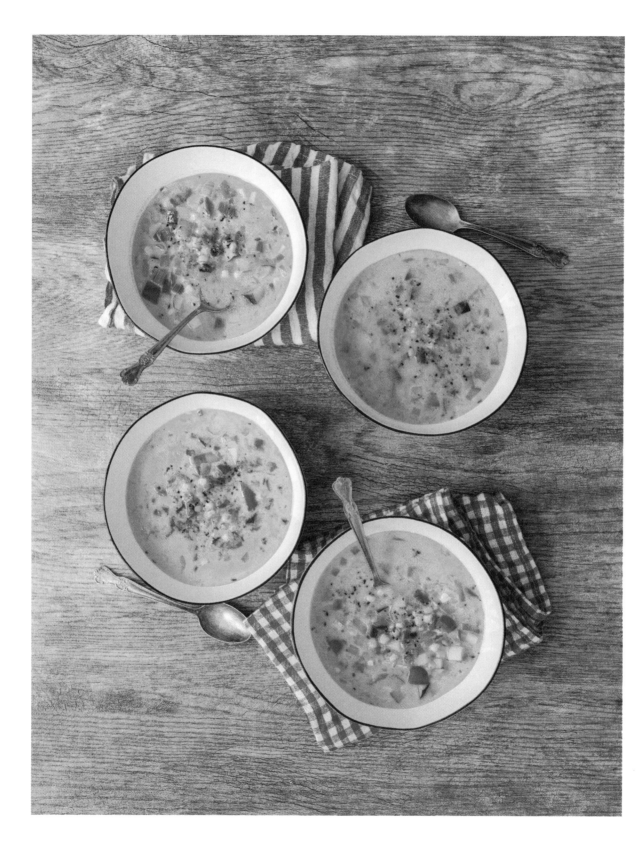

Market Corn Chowder with Summer Savory

Serves: 4–6

---

4 slices bacon, diced

2 stalks celery, finely chopped

1 large yellow onion, diced

1 small red bell pepper, seeded and diced

6 cloves garlic, minced

2 teaspoons paprika

3 sprigs fresh summer savory, leaves only, or fresh thyme

4 cups low-sodium chicken stock

2 medium red potatoes, skin on, diced

1½ cups fresh corn kernels, from 3 ears of corn

1 small to medium zucchini, diced

½ cup heavy cream

Salt

Pepper

We're firm believers that there's no such thing as "soup season." Soup's always on. Even in the late-August heat, we could all use a little warming soul food—when summer's got a month left and the school bus comes around again.

1. In a Dutch oven or a medium soup pot, cook the bacon over low heat to render the fat slowly, 7–10 minutes, stirring occasionally. Remove bacon bits with a slotted spoon once they're browned and crispy. Transfer to a paper-towel-lined plate and set aside.

2. Add the celery, onion, and bell pepper to the pot and raise the heat to medium. Cook for about 5 minutes, until veggies are softened.

3. Stir in the garlic, paprika, and summer savory leaves. Cook for another minute or so and pour in the chicken stock.

4. Add the potatoes and corn. Give everything a good stir and season with 1 teaspoon of salt and a few good cracks of pepper. Cover and simmer for 10 minutes.

5. Remove lid and add the zucchini. Continue simmering for 3–4 minutes, until potatoes are fully cooked and zucchini is tender but not mushy.

6. Pour in heavy cream and give the soup a taste. Add more salt if needed. Ladle into bowls and serve immediately with the bacon bits.

An Intro to Okra with Asian Marinated Flank Steak

Serves: 3–4

1 tablespoon sesame oil

3 tablespoons grapeseed oil, divided

¼ cup soy sauce

2 tablespoons rice wine vinegar

2 tablespoons brown sugar

8 cloves garlic, minced

2 teaspoons fresh ginger, grated

3 scallions, thinly sliced, divided

1 pound skirt or flank steak

1 cup uncooked brown rice

1 pound okra

Okra's one of those you-need-to-get-to-know-it vegetables. Its appearance can be a little intimidating, and it tends to get slimy. But it's pretty delicious and delightful if cooked quickly over high heat and sliced in ways to highlight its shape and seeds. And what vegetable isn't living its best life dressed in soy sauce and garlic?

1. In a measuring cup, whisk together the sesame oil, 1 tablespoon grapeseed oil, soy sauce, vinegar, brown sugar, garlic, ginger, and 2 of the scallions.

2. Take out a glass or ceramic dish that will fit the steak snugly, poke holes in the meat with the tines of a fork, place steak in the dish, and pour the marinade over, reserving 1–2 tablespoons for cooking the okra.

3. Refrigerate meat and reserved marinade at least 8 hours or overnight, then bring to room temperature 30–45 minutes before cooking.

4. When ready to eat, cook the rice like pasta—in a medium pot of salted boiling water, according to time on package instructions. Drain well, dump back in the pot, then cover so the remaining water is absorbed.

5. Remove the okra tips and tails, then slice into thin strips or rounds, or both, to mix it up.

6. Set a large skillet or cast-iron pan over medium-high heat. Drizzle in a tablespoon of oil and swirl to coat evenly. Cook the steak 3–5 minutes on each side, depending on thickness, until it's nicely seared and pink in the middle. Transfer to a cutting board or platter and let it rest for 5–10 minutes.

7. Set the same pan back over medium-high heat and swirl in another tablespoon of oil. Once it's hot, stir-fry the okra until browned in some parts. Remove from heat and pour in the reserved marinade, coating all the okra evenly.

8. Slice steak against the grain and serve with okra and rice. Sprinkle on remaining scallions and serve immediately.

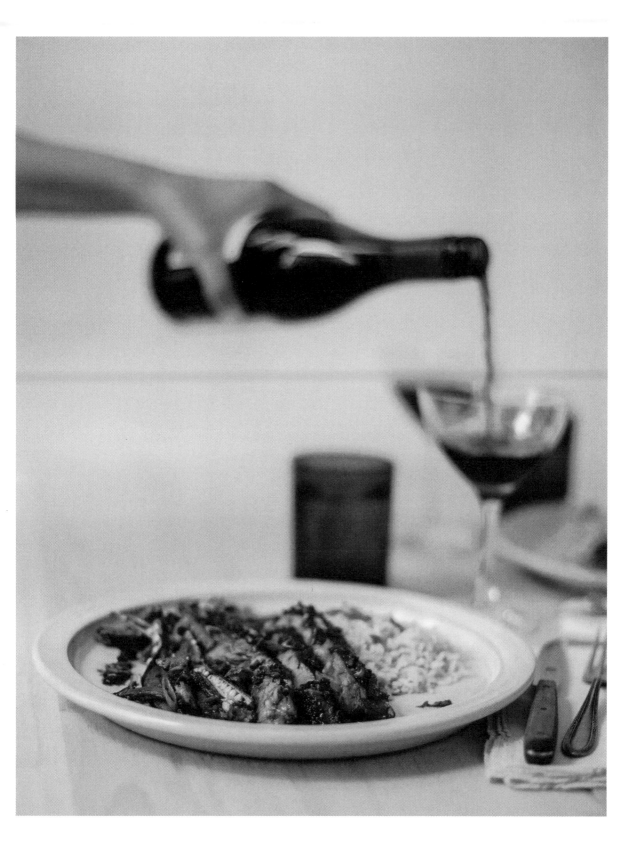

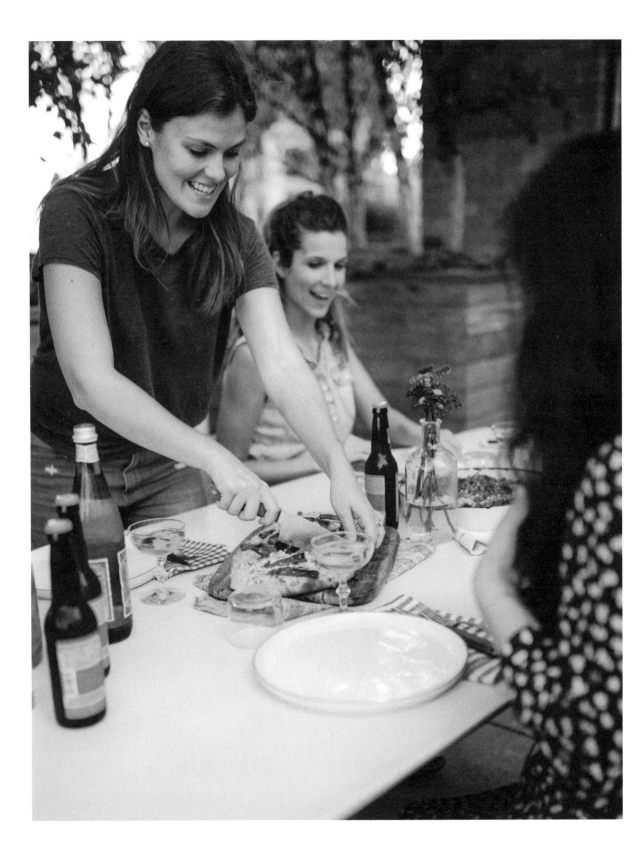

Rooftop Shishito & Corn Pizza with Garlic-Basil Oil

Serves: 4

———————

6 cloves garlic, minced

1 bunch fresh basil,
finely chopped

¼ cup extra-virgin
olive oil

¼ teaspoon salt

¼ teaspoon pepper

16-ounce ball of homemade
or store-bought pizza dough

2 tablespoons coarse
cornmeal

8 ounces low-moisture
mozzarella cheese, shredded

½ cup Parmesan cheese,
freshly grated

1 pint shishito peppers

1 cup fresh corn kernels,
from 2 ears of corn

We love our baking steel and how it produces pizza that rivals pizzeria pizza. In the summer, there's nowhere else you should be eating this corn- and shishito-pepper-topped pie but outside, preferably on a rooftop.

1. Preheat oven to 500°F and move the oven rack to the top position in the oven just below the broiler. Set a baking steel (we love ours from Baking Steel) on the rack and let it get hot for 45–60 minutes. If you don't want to use the broiler during the last minute of baking, put the steel anywhere in your oven.

2. Meanwhile, in a bowl, mix the garlic, basil, oil, salt, and pepper. Set aside.

3. Divide the pizza dough in half to make two pizzas. Use your hands to stretch each ball into a round or oval shape (just make sure it's thin).

4. On a pizza peel, spread 1 tablespoon of the cornmeal over it. Place the stretched pizza dough on top.

5. Brush the dough with half the garlic oil, leaving a 1-inch border all around.

6. Top with half the cheeses and then half the peppers and corn.

7. Transfer to the baking steel and bake for 5–7 minutes. (If you'd like a more charred top, just turn on the broiler for 1 minute.) But make sure to check after 30 seconds, because things go from charred to completely burned in a matter of seconds.

8. Prepare the second pizza while the first one is baking. Cut and serve immediately.

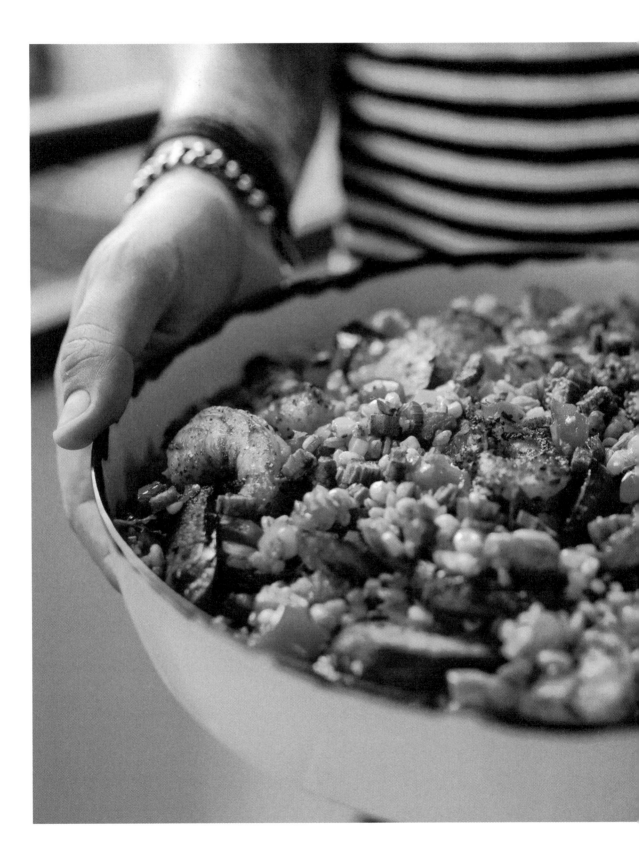

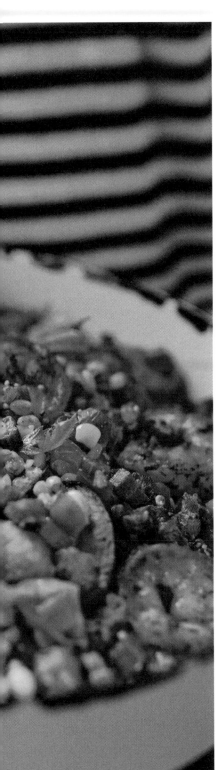

Cajun Potluck Platter with Warm Bacon-Jalapeño Vinaigrette

This is truly an impressive potluck-worthy production and a sure ticket to every summer gathering.

Serves: 4-6

Farro and vinaigrette

1 cup farro

1½ tablespoons bacon fat or unsalted butter

2 jalapeños, chopped

1 yellow onion, chopped

1 bunch scallions, thinly sliced

6 cloves garlic, minced

1 teaspoon Worcestershire sauce

1 teaspoon maple syrup

1 teaspoon dried basil

¼ teaspoon dried oregano

¼ teaspoon dried thyme

2½ tablespoons red wine vinegar

Vegetables

3 bell peppers, sliced into 1-inch pieces or smaller

1 pint cherry tomatoes, halved

2 cups fresh corn kernels, from 4 ears of corn

1 pint okra, thinly sliced into rounds or lengthwise strips

Shrimp and sausage

½ pound shrimp, peeled and deveined

1 teaspoon paprika

1 teaspoon garlic powder

½ teaspoon coriander

½ teaspoon chili powder

½ pound andouille sausage, fully cooked

1 cup mixed fresh herbs: Italian parsley, basil, and summer savory if you can find it

Grapeseed oil

Salt

Pepper

1. Cook farro like pasta; drain and set aside. For extra-good, toasted farro, slide it under the broiler on a sheet pan for another 8–10 minutes, stirring halfway through.

2. Grab a sauté pan for vinaigrette and set over medium heat. Swirl in bacon fat, wait for it to get hot, then scrape in jalapeños, onion, and

scallions with a pinch of salt. Sauté until soft, then add garlic and cook another minute. Add Worcestershire, maple syrup, dried herbs, vinegar, and ¼ cup oil with another generous pinch of salt and some cracks of pepper. Turn off heat and stir to combine.

3. Combine toasted farro and vinaigrette in the pan; set aside.

4. Preheat oven to 400°F.

5. On a sheet pan, toss bell peppers with a drizzle of oil and salt and pepper. Spread out and roast for 20 minutes or until charred in some parts. Remove sheet pan, nudge the peppers to one side, and add tomatoes and corn, tossing with a little oil and salt and pepper. Roast for another 10 minutes. Transfer to pan with farro.

6. Meanwhile, prep shrimp and sausage. In a small bowl, toss shrimp with a drizzle of oil, spices, some pepper, and ½ teaspoon salt. Arrange on the now empty sheet pan, leaving just a tiny bit of space between them.

7. Cut sausage into ¼-inch slices on the diagonal. Toss with a little oil in the same bowl you used for the shrimp and pile onto the sheet pan. It doesn't have to be spread out or it'll dry out.

8. In the space that's left, toss the okra with a little oil, salt, and pepper, then spread it out a bit. Turn on the broiler and slide the pan in for 5–7 minutes, turning halfway through, until shrimp is opaque, okra is charred, and sausage is browned.

9. Toss everything right on the sheet pan or on your biggest platter and serve. Toss everything with the fresh herbs, right on the sheet pan or on your biggest platter, and serve.

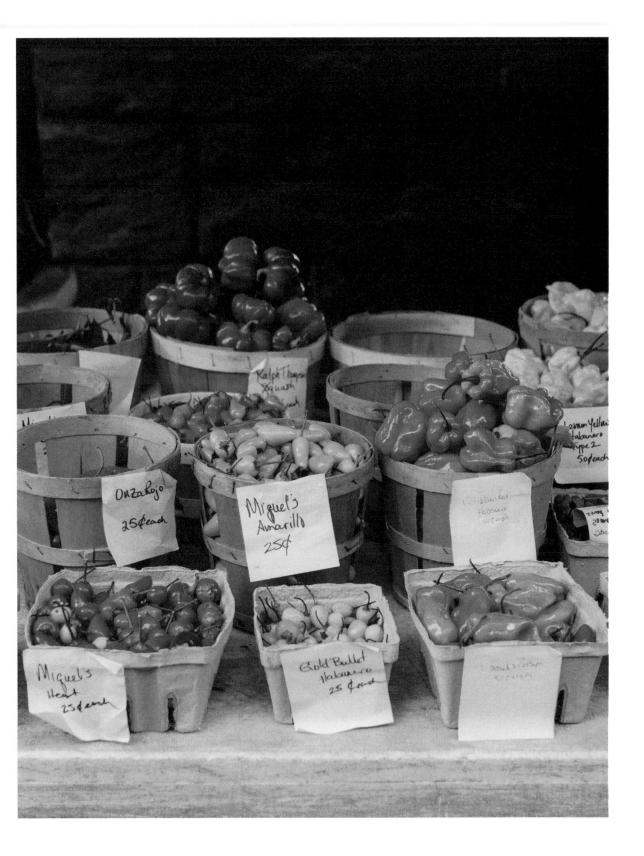

Thai Basil Chicken Wraps with Peanut Sauce & Cucumber-Carrot Slaw

Serves: 4

_____

Chicken

1 teaspoon ground coriander

1 teaspoon chili powder

1 teaspoon garlic powder

½ teaspoon turmeric

2-3 teaspoons grapeseed oil

2 bone-in chicken breasts (1½-2 pounds)

Peanut sauce

2 tablespoons peanut butter

2 tablespoons rice wine vinegar

4 teaspoons soy sauce

4 teaspoons sugar

2 cloves garlic, grated

2 teaspoons fresh ginger, grated

Salt

Pepper

I (Christine) once brought home a package of *skin-on, bone-in* chicken parts. Completely by accident, obviously. Panic ensued. *Gross. I have no idea what to do with these.* Turns out they're ten times more delicious, and not as scary as I imagined. You can roast them or sear-and-cover on the stovetop and let the flavor from the bone infuse the meat while it cooks. Then the bone comes off pretty easily in the end. And if a closet vegetarian like me who has to go to my happy place while handling raw meat can enjoy cooking and eating bone-in/skin-on, you can, too.

_____

Kitchen note: Thai basil can be kind of an herb unicorn in grocery stores, but if you ever stumble on it at the farmers' market, snatch it immediately. Use up the rest of the bunch in Don't-Get-Takeout Take-out (page 276) or anything else you dream up. If you must, substitute regular basil.

1. Preheat oven to 400°F.

2. In a small bowl, mix the spices for chicken with 1 teaspoon each salt and pepper. Coat the chicken lightly with oil, then rub/pat the spice mix all over.

3. Transfer to a small baking sheet or roasting dish and roast for 20–25 minutes, until the skin is slightly browned and the chicken is fully cooked. Remove from oven and let it rest. When you're ready to eat, pull the meat off the bones and shred or cut into larger-than-bite-size pieces.

4. While the chicken is in the oven, grab a small bowl. With a fork, mash in the peanut butter so it's not clumpy. Add in remaining peanut sauce ingredients, along with a pinch of salt, then whisk in 1 or 2 tablespoons of water. Adjust sauce thickness with a little more water if needed; it should be thick but slightly runny. Set aside.

Cucumber-carrot slaw

1 medium carrot, sliced into very thin matchsticks

1 medium cucumber, sliced into very thin matchsticks

1 jalapeño pepper, thinly sliced

2 tablespoons Thai basil, chopped, divided

1 tablespoon rice wine vinegar

For wraps

1 package gluten-free or flour tortillas

1 lime, sliced into wedges

5. Place sliced slaw vegetables and half the Thai basil in a medium bowl; toss with vinegar and a big pinch of salt and pepper. Set aside.

6. Using tongs, char tortillas over a stovetop flame. Let everyone pile in their own chicken and slaw and drizzle generously with peanut sauce. Garnish with black sesame seeds if you have them, remaining Thai basil, and a squeeze of lime. Roll 'em up!

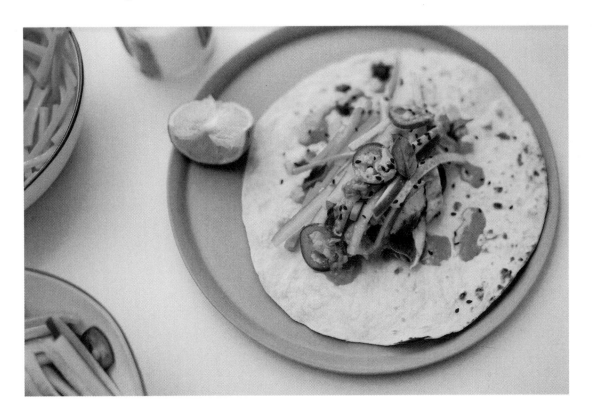

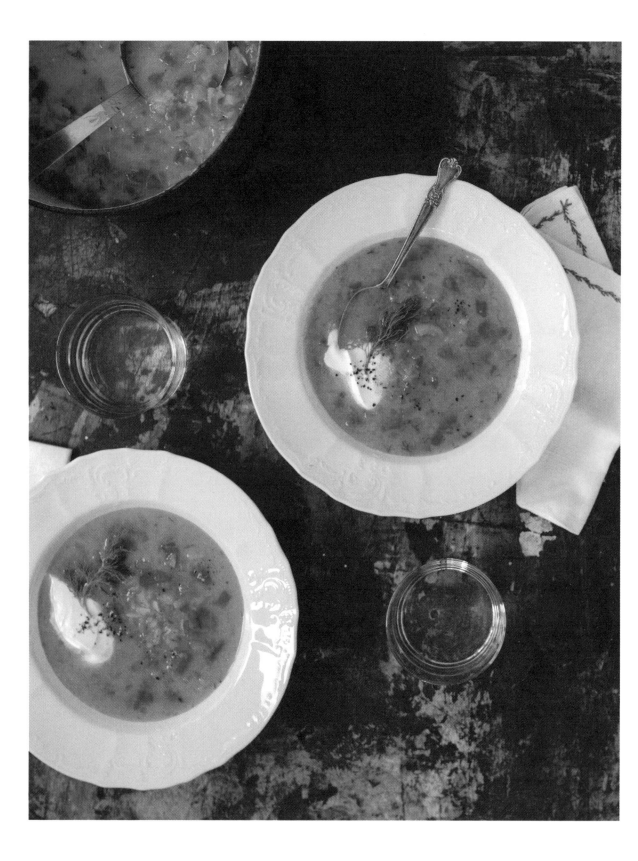

Transylvanian Herbed Squash & Tomato Soup

Serves: 4

I pound winter squash

Extra-virgin olive oil

I medium yellow onion, diced

I large red bell pepper, finely diced

I teaspoon paprika

4 cups water

I sprig fresh thyme, or a pinch of dried thyme

2 medium tomatoes, peeled and diced

I tablespoon fresh dill, chopped, plus more if you're into dill

Salt

Pepper

Optional for serving

Extra dill

Dollops of sour cream, crème fraîche, or yogurt

Crusty bread

In August, winter squash shows up at the market amid the peppers and tomatoes. Farmers are sad that people ignore them and wait for fall to finally buy them. So instead of avoiding eye contact with winter squash until September, embrace the transition with this late-summer soup, inspired by Grandma's kitchen and our Transylvanian roots. It's traditionally made with a roux, but we've eliminated the flour and milk for an equally delicious detox version, and the grated squash adds a really unique texture. Eez good.

1. Remove skin from squash with a sharp knife and scoop out the seeds. In a food processor fitted with the grating disk, grate the squash. If you don't feel like washing the food processor, you can also shred carefully by hand using a box grater. You need about 2 cups.

2. Meanwhile, heat a tablespoon of olive oil in a medium soup pot or Dutch oven. Sauté onion and pepper until soft, 7–10 minutes. Sprinkle in the paprika and stir.

3. Add squash, water, thyme, and tomatoes. Season with a teaspoon of salt and ½ teaspoon pepper. Bring to a low boil, then cover and simmer for 20 minutes. Taste for seasoning and adjust, then stir in dill.

4. Ladle into bowls and serve immediately with extra dill, sour cream, lots of cracked pepper, and crusty bread. If reheating leftovers, add a splash of water if the soup has thickened up.

Basil-Lemon Fish with a Sunny Sauté

Serves: 4

_____

Veggie sauté

2 tablespoons extra-virgin olive oil or butter

¼ pound green beans (cut into thirds)

1 cup fresh corn kernels, from 2 ears of corn

1 pint yellow cherry tomatoes, halved

Fish

4 sole fillets (or haddock or halibut), about 1 pound

1 teaspoon dried basil

½ teaspoon dried parsley

Zest of 1 lemon, and lemon cut into wedges for serving

½ teaspoon garlic powder

2 tablespoons unsalted butter

Salt

Pepper

This is one of the best ways to eat summer vegetables. Simple, fresh, and fast. No fancy sauce or elaborate chopping. Just a quick sauté in a bit of butter or olive oil to soften them. Bring home any vegetables that make you smile at the market—snap peas, shishito peppers, green tomatoes, summer squash, grape tomatoes, anything and everything. Yellow and green make such a cheery combination.

1. Add the olive oil to a large skillet over medium heat. When hot, add the green beans and sauté for 2 minutes, shaking the pan occasionally.

2. Add the corn to the green beans and cook for 3–4 minutes or until veggies are just tender, but not mushy. Season with ½ teaspoon each salt and pepper. Turn off heat and gently stir in tomatoes just to heat through. Set aside while you cook the fish.

3. In a small bowl, mix the basil, parsley, lemon zest, garlic powder, ½ teaspoon salt, and ¼ teaspoon black pepper.

4. Season both sides of the fish fillets with the mix.

5. Set a skillet (big enough to hold all the fish fillets at once) over medium-high heat for 1–2 minutes. Add in butter; once it foams, swirl to coat and add the fish. Make sure the skillet is hot or the fish will stick. Cook 1–2 minutes per side.

6. Serve the fish with the veggie sauté and lemon wedges.

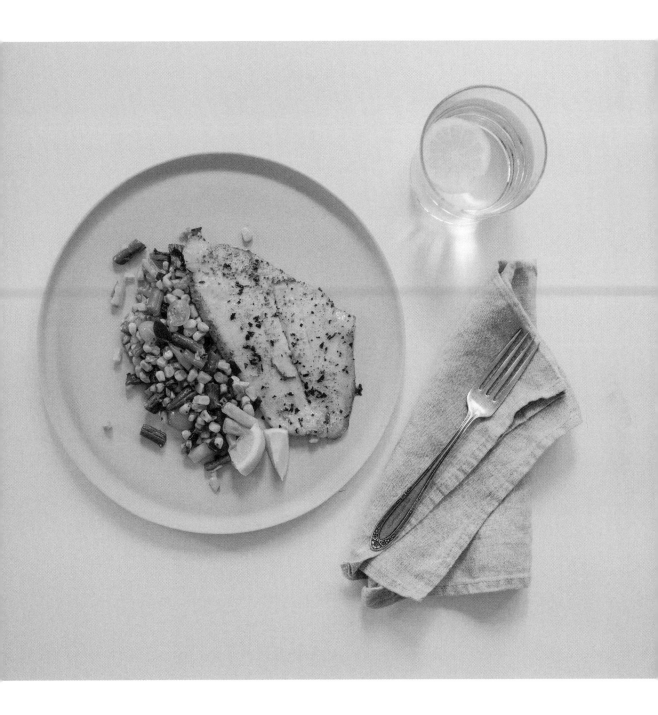

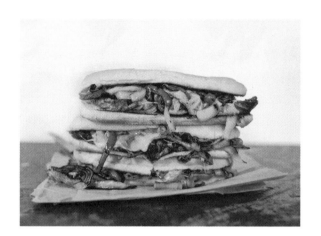

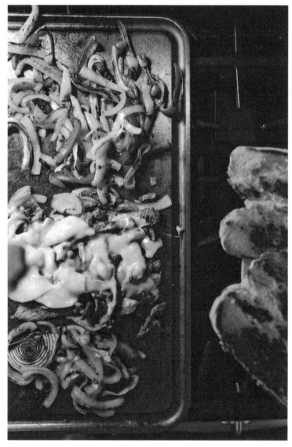

Philly Cheesesteaks with Heirloom Peppers

Serves: 4

_____

2 tablespoons extra-virgin olive oil

I pound heirloom peppers, in a mix of colors, sliced

2 medium white onions, sliced

3 cloves garlic, minced

I¼ pounds sirloin steak, very thinly sliced

²/₃ pound provolone, thinly sliced or shredded

2 tablespoons unsalted butter

4 hoagie rolls

Salt

Pepper

Our take on the legendary Philly cheesesteak: really good meat and *a lot* of bright, market heirloom peppers.

_____

Kitchen note: We used the baking steel for this and loved it, but if you don't have a massive, heavy block of steel lying around, a large skillet will get the job done perfectly fine.

1. Heat your baking steel on the stovetop over medium-high heat for at least 10 minutes. Add a drizzle of oil and then the peppers, with a sprinkle of salt; cook for about 4 minutes. Add the onions next to the peppers, season, and flip every few minutes, until soft and charred.

2. Stir in the garlic and cook an additional minute; transfer veggies to a bowl.

3. Drizzle extra oil onto the baking steel and then add the meat, seasoning with salt and pepper. Use a metal spatula to press it down so it can get some nice color. Stir a bit until no longer pink.

4. Add the veggies back in; mix well with the meat. Then, using the spatula, divide the meat-onion-pepper mix into 4 portions. Top each with cheese.

5. Meanwhile, melt some butter in another pan. Cut the rolls lengthwise and add 2 at a time, cut side down. Toast until golden brown. Remove to a plate.

6. Gently scoop up cheesesteaks into the rolls and serve immediately.

Almond Blender Pancakes

Serves: 4

½ cup kefir (kinda like buttermilk, but healthier–probiotic and lactose free)

2 large eggs, room temperature

1 teaspoon vanilla extract

1 cup almond flour

2 tablespoons ground flaxseed

1½ tablespoons coconut sugar

½ teaspoon baking powder

½ teaspoon baking soda

⅛ teaspoon salt

2 teaspoons coconut oil, for pan

1 pint seasonal fruit, cut up for serving

Butter, maple syrup, and/or whipped cream, for serving

Pancakes are one of the highest callings for spring and summer fruit. But sometimes your body needs a break from the heavy (but heavenly) buttermilk ones, with some lighter, wholesome ones. Throw all these good-for-you ingredients into a blender and you can even have them on a weekday morning if you got up with the sunrise. It's a year-round breakfast canvas for whatever fruit is in season. Winter: citrus. Spring: rhubarb and strawberries. Summer: berries and peaches. Fall: pear and apple compote.

1. Place all the pancake ingredients (kefir through salt) in a blender and give them a whir for about 10 seconds, just until well combined.

2. Let the batter rest for 10–15 minutes to thicken up.

3. Heat a griddle or nonstick skillet over low heat and brush with coconut oil. Once hot, pour in about 2 tablespoons of batter for each pancake—they'll be silver-dollar size. You can ladle the batter onto the pan or just eyeball it and pour directly from the blender.

4. After 2–3 minutes, when you see the top is kind of bubbly and set, check the underside to make sure they're golden brown, then flip for another 30 seconds–1 minute. Repeat with the remaining batter until all pancakes are cooked.

5. Serve with maple syrup, fruit, a pat of butter, and/or whipped cream.

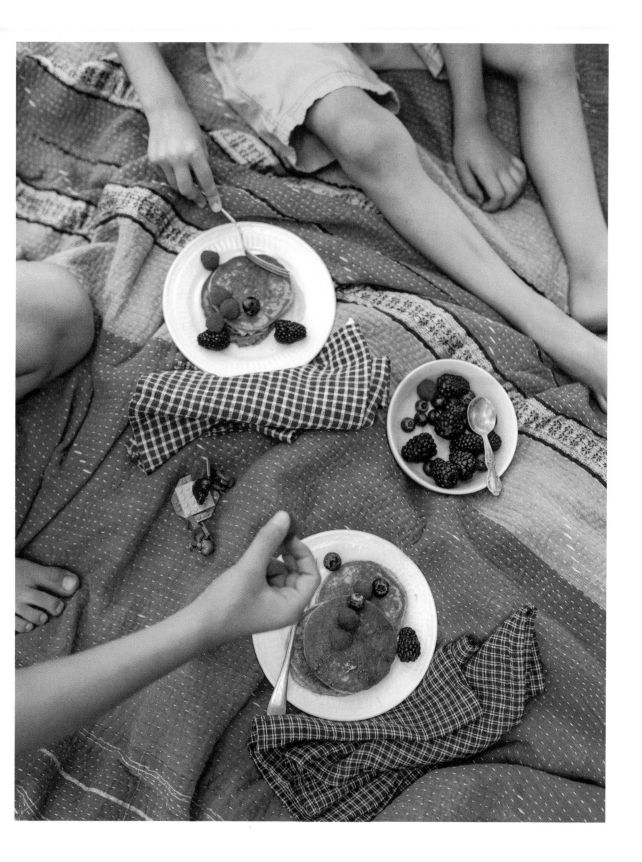

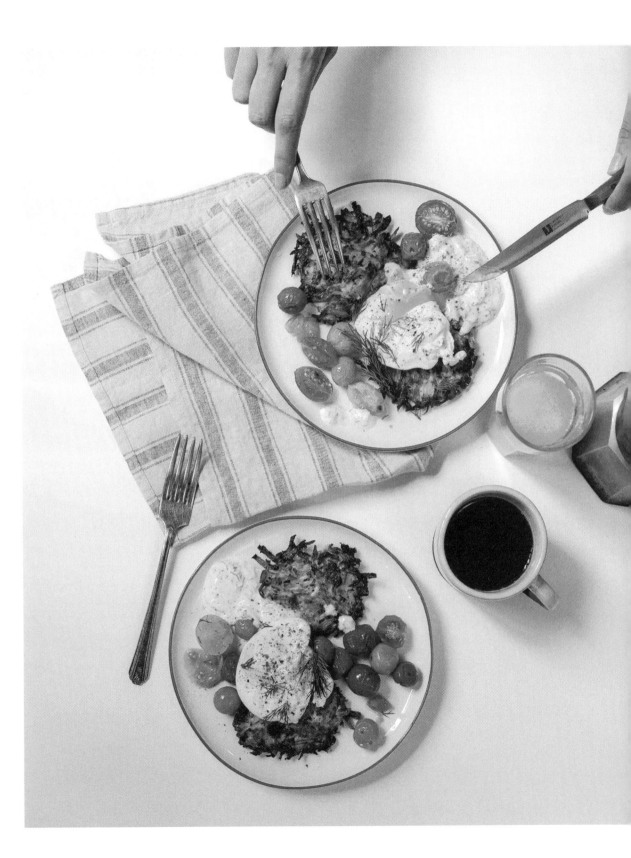

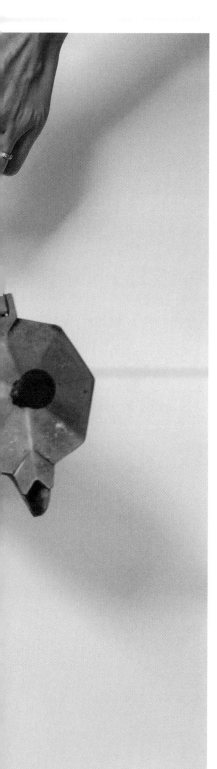

The Dilly Dally

Firmly decide to ignore your to-dos for a few hours and cook this. It should take almost as much time to eat as it took to make it. Let yourself dillydally. It might spark a new idea.

Serves: 3–4

Tzatziki

I small cucumber

½ cup Greek yogurt

2 cloves garlic, finely minced or grated

2 teaspoons lemon juice

I teaspoon extra-virgin olive oil

½ teaspoon white vinegar

2 tablespoons fresh dill, chopped

Tomatoes

I pint cherry tomatoes; halve any large ones

I tablespoon extra-virgin olive oil

Fritters

I½ pounds zucchini, yellow zucchini, or summer squash

I large egg

¼ cup all-purpose flour

2 tablespoons fresh dill, chopped

I tablespoon fresh Italian parsley, chopped

Neutral oil for cooking

Large eggs

3–4 large eggs, for poaching

Salt

Pepper

Extra dill and a few dashes of paprika for garnish

Kitchen note: Use the cucumber juice from tzatziki to make yourself a Green Gemini (page 186) later.

1. Tzatziki: Grate cucumber and squeeze out the liquid, one handful at a time. Transfer to a bowl with remaining tzatziki ingredients, ½ teaspoon salt, and a few cracks of pepper. Cover and refrigerate for up to 3 days.

2. Tomatoes: Preheat oven to 300°F.

3. Pile tomatoes onto a small sheet pan, drizzle on oil, sprinkle generously with salt, and slide into the oven for 30–35 minutes, until soft and juicy. Then turn the oven down to 175°F and keep warm until ready to eat.

4. Fritters: Grate squash with a box grater into a medium bowl. Grab another medium bowl and beat 1 egg.

5. Take handfuls of squash and squeeeeeze out as much liquid as you can, adding the squeezed squash to the egg bowl as you go.

6. Now sprinkle in flour, herbs, ½ teaspoon salt, and a few cracks of pepper; combine well with your hands.

7. Take about ¼ cup of the mixture, press it together with your hands so it adheres, and place mounds on a sheet pan.

8. Meanwhile, pour oil into a large skillet, enough to coat the bottom really well, and turn heat to medium-high.

9. Once oil is hot, use the spatula to gently transfer in 4 fritters, flattening well. Let them sizzle for about 3 minutes, until lightly browned and crispy; flip and cook the other side for about 2 minutes, until also lightly browned and crispy. Transfer to a towel-lined plate to absorb any residual oil and repeat 2 more times for remaining fritters. You should have about 12 total.

10. Then make some room for them next to the tomatoes to keep warm in the oven.

11. Eggs: Fill a medium pot with water. Bring to a boil, then turn the heat down so the water just barely simmers. The water should look shaky, but there shouldn't be bubbles.

12. Crack 1 egg into a tiny bowl or ramekin.

13. Now grab a spoon and stick it right in the middle of the water pot. Start swirling and swirling until it looks like a tornado. Have the egg ready to go in the other hand and drop it right into the eye of the storm.

14. It'll need 5 minutes to poach, on average. You can gently lift the egg out with a slotted spoon and prod with your finger to check whether the white is set. Transfer to a paper-towel-lined plate and repeat for the other eggs.

15. Assemble your plates: Place 3 fritters on each plate and nestle tomatoes next to them, along with a dollop of tzatziki. Top with a poached egg sprinkled with salt and pepper. Garnish with dill sprigs and dashes of paprika. Take your plate outside, along with a speaker playing cheerful café tunes. Slice into that gorgeous orangey-yellow yolk and you're on your way to a really great weekend.

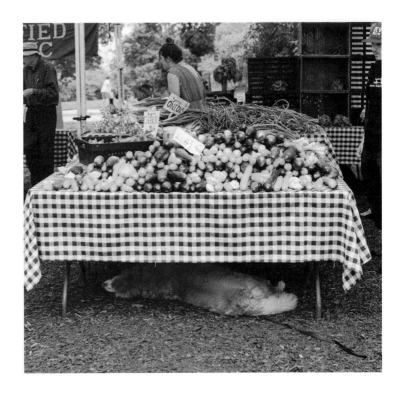

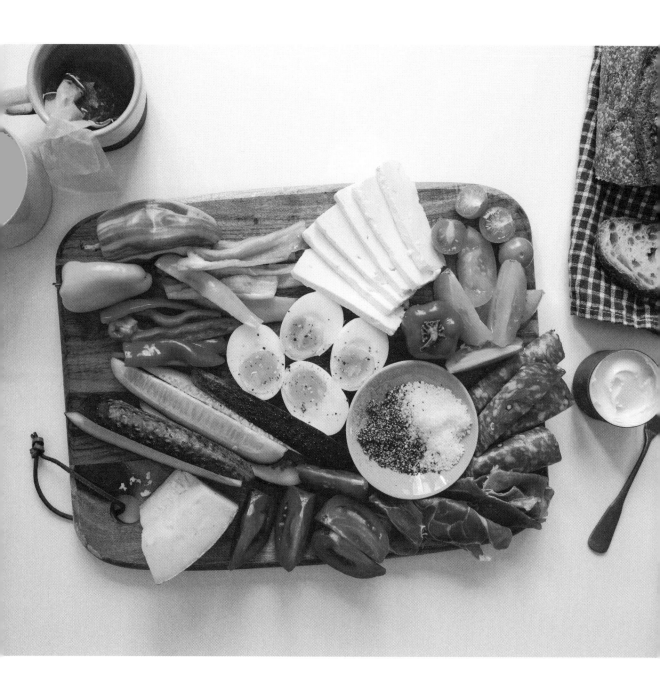

A Tale of a Countryside Breakfast Board

Serves: 4

_____

Vegetables

2 heirloom tomatoes, sliced into wedges, or I pint cherry tomatoes

2 small cucumbers, sliced lengthwise

4 snacking peppers, sliced into strips

Optional: I spring onion, thinly sliced

Everything else

4–6 large eggs

2 ounces feta cheese, sliced

2 ounces semi-hard, aged cheese, sliced

¼ pound salami or Serrano ham

I loaf whole-grain, heirloom-style bread from that stand at the market that sells out within the first hour

4 tablespoons salted butter, softened

Salt and pepper

This is the European secret to a long and happy life—starting the day with sliced, garden-fresh vegetables served, unapologetically, with old-school bread, butter, cheese, and charcuterie. We grew up on this breakfast. It's no-cook, no-stress, impressive, and as close to "raw" or "vegan" or "gluten-free" as you're allowed to get in Europe. Everyone lingers and grazes and the board gets replenished into the late morning. Brew big mugs of forest berry tea or Earl Grey to go round.

1. To make perfectly jammy, 7-minute eggs, fill a saucepan ¾ full with water. Set over high heat and bring to a boil. Once it's boiling, gently add eggs. Set a timer for 7 minutes. If you prefer them more cooked, go to 8 or 9 minutes, but not past that. Immediately remove eggs and run under cold water to stop the cooking process. Peel and slice in half; sprinkle with salt and pepper.

2. Channel your inner artist and arrange everything on a large platter or cutting board.

3. Serve with bread and butter and let everyone reach in and assemble their plates.

4. Sip your tea, eat slowly, and keep grazing throughout the morning.

French Farmhouse Skillet Hash with Sunny-Side-Up Eggs

Serves: 2

_____

Hash

1 tablespoon bacon fat, from your phat jar

½ small yellow onion, finely diced

1 bell pepper, chopped into ¼-inch pieces

1 very small eggplant, chopped into ¼-inch pieces

1 very small zucchini, chopped into ¼-inch pieces

Optional: 1 teaspoon thyme, summer savory, or parsley, finely minced

Eggs

½ tablespoon extra-virgin olive oil

2 large eggs

Salt

Pepper

Pinch of all-purpose seasoning

Optional, for serving: good, grainy buttered toast

Tiny Cubes, reporting for breakfast duty. Chop the night before and have an egg- and vegetable-packed plate the next morning. The sauté would make an amazing dinner side as well.

1. Set a large cast-iron or nonstick skillet over medium heat and swirl in the bacon fat.

2. Once it's hot, add onion and pepper. Leave undisturbed for 2–3 minutes, then stir in eggplant and zucchini with a generous pinch of salt and pepper. Stir occasionally for another 7–10 minutes, until vegetables are tender. Divide between 2 plates.

3. Drizzle olive oil into the same skillet and place it back on the stove over low heat. Crack in eggs and cover with a lid for 4–5 minutes, until whites are set and yolks quiver just a bit. Season with salt, pepper, and all-purpose seasoning and serve immediately with the hash and buttered toast.

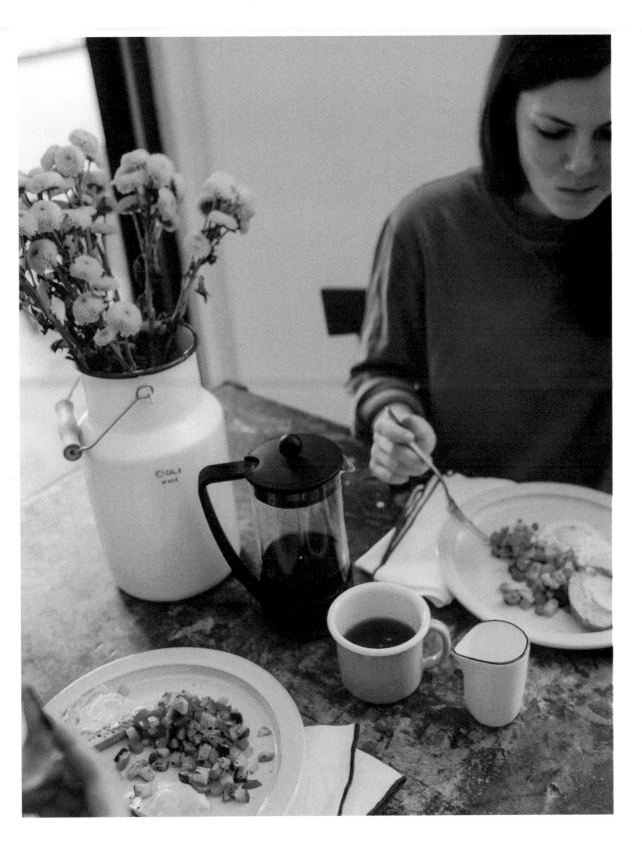

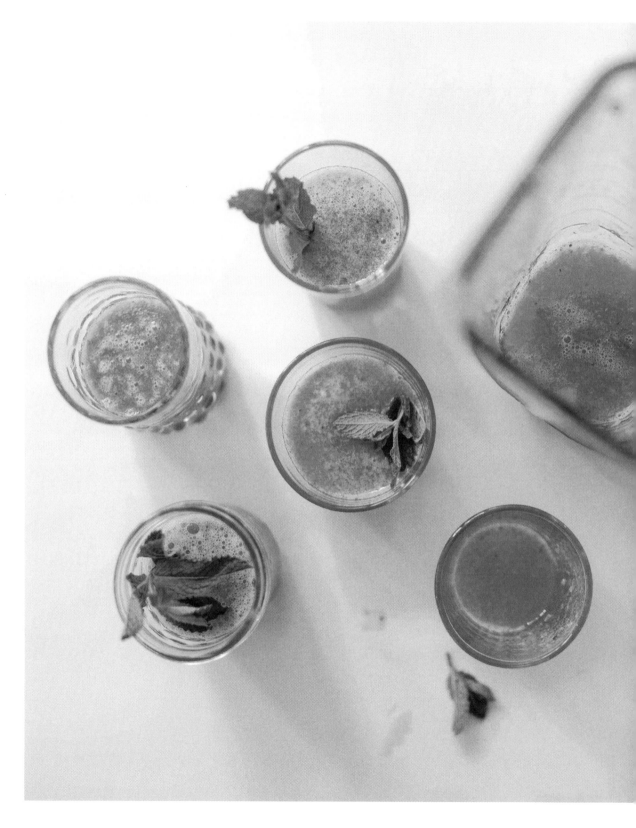

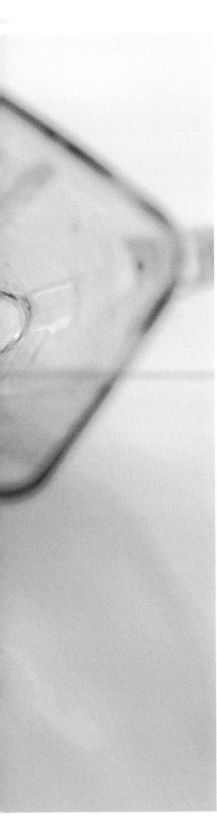

Melon Jubilees

We did a little research on melons and lost count of all the varieties! There are so many cute names, like moon and stars, little baby flower, yellow doll, but our favorite was jubilee. The definition is "a noisy celebration," and that's basically what summer is. A noisy, sticky, giggly celebration of sun and water and no school! So as you're sitting on your porch or in your backyard watching your kids run through the sprinkler, sip on an ice-cold Melon Jubilee to soak it all in.

Serves: 8

6 cups melon (I cantaloupe or I small watermelon, seeded and chopped)

Juice of I lime

2 cups water

Fresh mint or basil

1. Blend the melon, lime juice, and 1½ cups water until smooth. Give it a taste, and if it's too thick, add more water.

2. You can add a few leaves of mint or basil and give the blender another whir or serve them as garnish in a pitcher.

3. Chill and serve over ice.

Strawberry Swing Refresher

You can apply this blend-with-water-sugar-and-herbs concept to almost any fruit in your fridge that's blemished or about to turn.

I pound strawberries, hulled and roughly chopped

¼ cup sugar, or more to taste

4 cups water

Juice of ¼ lemon, just a squeeze

A small handful of mint or basil or tarragon

The Green Gemini

Serves: 2

---

2 cucumbers

10 fresh mint leaves

1 jalapeño, sliced

Juice of 3 limes

2 teaspoons maple syrup

Gin

Ice cubes

Just like the favorite Gemini in your life, this cocktail is cooling and spicy at the same time. It's really versatile and can be adapted to your mood and what you have in the fridge. No mint? Swap in basil or cilantro. Rum, vodka, or tequila can sub for gin, and if you love it even more spicy, use a serrano or bird's-eye chile instead of jalapeño.

1. Make the cucumber garnish first. Using a mandoline or a knife, thinly slice a cucumber lengthwise. You just need 2–4 pretty slices. The rest you'll juice.

2. Juice the cucumbers. If you don't have a juicer, you can do this in a high-powered blender and strain.

3. In a cocktail shaker, muddle 5 mint leaves and 2 slices of jalapeño. Add 2 ounces cucumber juice, 1 ounce lime juice, 1 teaspoon maple syrup, and 3 ounces gin. Put a few ice cubes on top, cover with the shaker lid, and give it a few good shakes.

4. Pour into an ice-filled glass of your choice and garnish with cucumber slices and jalapeño. Hand this off to your favorite person, then repeat steps to make your own.

Kitchen note: Yes, you could make a simple syrup, but sometimes you need a drink and have no patience for boiling water with sugar and then waiting for the syrup to cool. Enter maple syrup–better for you and does the job.

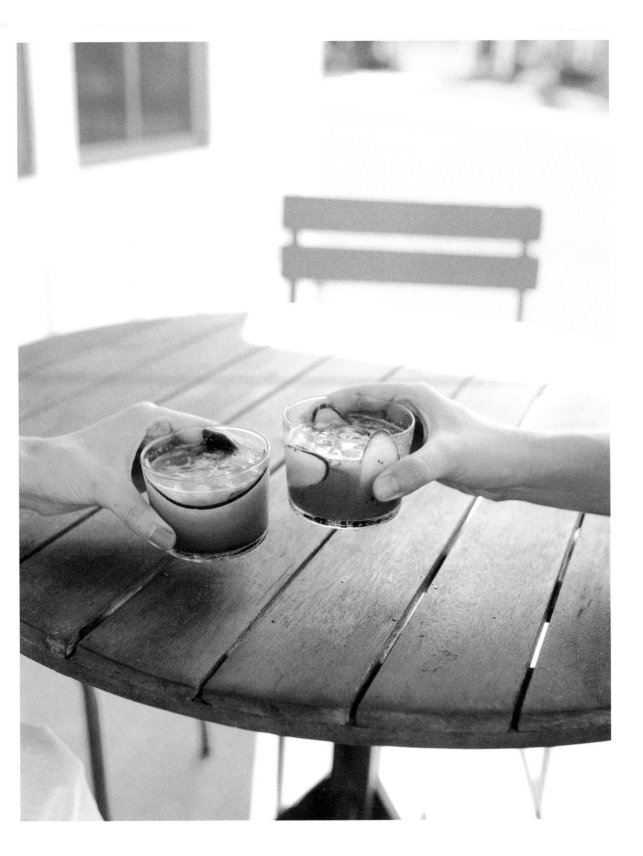

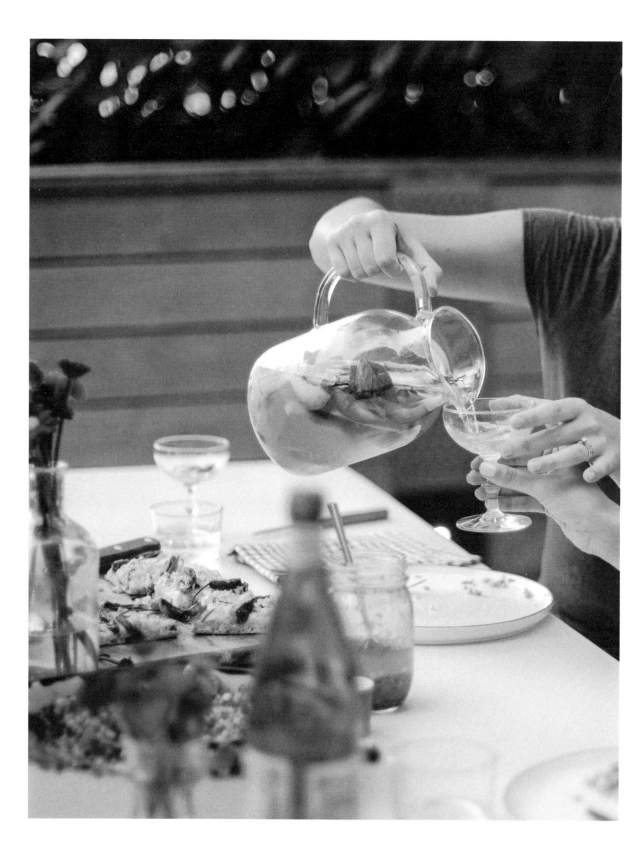

Summer Orchard Sangria with Elderflower & Basil

Serves: 4

_____

1 peach, very ripe, thinly sliced

1 nectarine, very ripe, thinly sliced

1 apricot, thinly sliced

2 plums, thinly sliced

1 cup fresh basil, mint, or lemon verbena

1 bottle white wine: Riesling or pinot grigio

1 cup St-Germain

Sparkling water, optional

At some point during that summer cookout you almost canceled, something magical happens. Everyone is eating seconds, laugh-crying, sharing stories, and then a sunbeam streams in at just the right angle through your sangria glass and makes it glow. And that is the moment. That's why you do this.

1. Place sliced fruit and basil in a medium pitcher that holds 60 ounces, give or take. Gently mash the fruit and basil to release their juices.

2. Pour the wine and St-Germain over the fruit and give everything a good stir. Refrigerate at least 6 hours, but ideally, make it the night before or early in the morning to serve in the evening. When ready to serve, pour sangria into glasses and top with sparkling water if desired.

Bakeshop Blackberry-Lavender Scones

Serves: 6

2½ cups all-purpose flour

½ cup sugar

2½ teaspoons baking powder

½ teaspoon baking soda

½ teaspoon salt

I tablespoon dried lavender

12 tablespoons unsalted butter, cold and sliced into tiny cubes

²/₃ cup cold buttermilk

2 large eggs: I for dough and I beaten with I teaspoon water for brushing

I tablespoon vanilla extract

1½ cups blackberries (halve any large ones), about I0 ounces

These scones can really help you keep to your weekly coffee shop budget. While they're baking and filling up your kitchen with the most incredible smell, whip up a latte for the full neighborhood bakeshop experience. Grab a pretty plate, play some music, and snag a comfy seat.

1. Preheat oven to 400°F and line a baking sheet with parchment.

2. In a medium bowl, combine the dry ingredients—flour, sugar, baking powder, baking soda, salt—and crumble in the lavender with your fingers.

3. Using a pastry cutter, cut in the cold cubed butter until it's the size of peas or smaller. Place the bowl in the freezer so the butter firms up again.

4. In a measuring cup, whisk together buttermilk, 1 egg, and vanilla.

5. Remove bowl from freezer and drizzle in the buttermilk mixture, stirring with a spatula until just combined, taking care not to overmix.

6. Gently fold in blackberries. Try to avoid over-smashing, but you do want some purple streaks in the dough.

7. Turn dough right onto the prepared baking sheet and gently flatten it into a 1-inch square/rectangle, pressing in any remaining dry flour bits from the bottom of the bowl. With a dough scraper or large knife, cut out 8 pieces. Slide in the freezer for 5–10 minutes so the dough firms up again just a bit.

8. Take them back out and brush each scone top with beaten egg. Slide in the oven for 15–20 minutes, until golden brown and craggly. Let scones rest for a few minutes; serve warm or at room temperature.

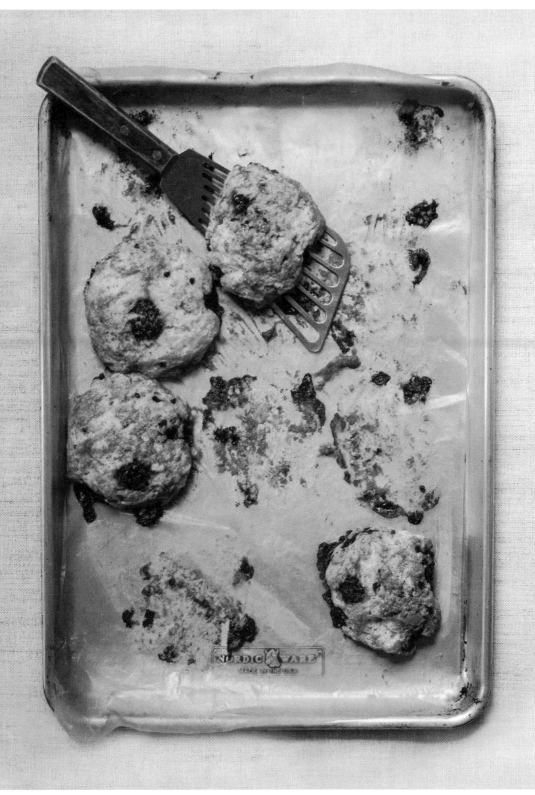

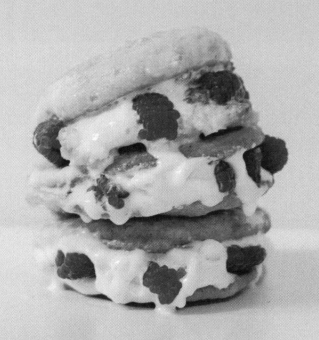

Corndoodle Ice Cream Sandwiches with Raspberries

Serves: 8

―――――――――

1 cup all-purpose flour

1 cup fine cornmeal

½ cup coarse cornmeal

½ teaspoon salt

½ teaspoon baking powder

2 teaspoons cornstarch

14 tablespoons unsalted butter, melted

1 cup sugar

1 large egg

1 cup corn kernels, raw

Vanilla ice cream

2 pints raspberries

There are ice cream sandwiches, and then there are corndoodle ice cream sandwiches. They're everything we love about summer in a handheld package. Make them ahead for a crowd, or enough to last you the week through the hottest of July days.

1. Mix together the flour, both cornmeals, salt, baking powder, and cornstarch in a bowl.

2. Place melted butter and sugar together in a large bowl, beat about 1 minute, then whisk in the egg until combined.

3. Stir the flour-cornmeal mixture into the large bowl; don't overmix. Fold in the corn kernels. Cover the bowl and transfer to the fridge for at least an hour or overnight.

4. When ready to bake, preheat the oven to 325°F and set dough on the counter to soften slightly.

5. Using an ice cream scoop, portion out dough to make 20–24 cookies. (Each should be about 2 tablespoons and form a 1½-inch ball.)

6. Using 2 small pieces of parchment and a small pan or heavy metal spatula, flatten each cookie ball between the parchment as you would a smash burger. You're aiming for ¼-inch thickness and just under a 3-inch diameter. They won't spread or rise too much.

7. Bake in 2 or 3 batches on a parchment-lined sheet pan for 13–15 minutes on the middle rack of the oven. You want the bottom to be just barely golden brown. Set aside to cool completely.

8. Meanwhile, take the ice cream from the freezer, let it soften for 5–10 minutes, and scoop into a bowl. Gently fold in the raspberries.

9. Assemble the sandwiches by scooping the ice cream onto one cookie and topping it with a second. It will be messy and the cookies will break a little; don't worry, just mold them back together. Wrap the sandwiches well in wax paper and transfer them to the freezer for at least 15–30 minutes or up to a week.

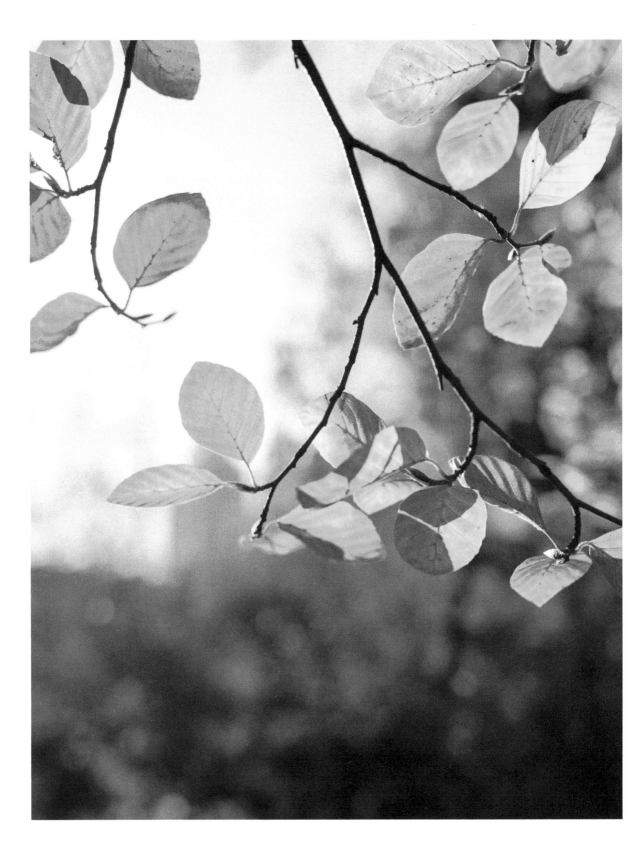

Autumn

NOTICE WHAT'S HAPPENING OUTSIDE (NATURE) . . .

You notice a single orange leaf on a tree full of vibrant green ones. Nature's cue that the season is shifting. Morning air is crisper, days are shorter. The pace picks up, with summer's leisure coming to a close. School supply lists, new outfits for the first days of school, summer Fridays ending at work, everything around us following the rhythm of the earth. It was fun, it was relaxing, but now we've got some things to get in order. Squirrels gather acorns as they sense winter is not very far away. They're planning, preserving, because soon things will wither and freeze while Mother Nature pushes the pause button.

. . . AND INSIDE (HUMAN NATURE)

There's a reflection of this in us, too—fall's energy moves us toward preparing and planning for the next thing. So listen to the promptings—plan, reflect, change, prepare, focus, align, shift, do whatever needs to be done. Be intentional about what kind of day you want. Break the day down and focus on each part—morning, noon, afternoon, evening. Get a routine on the books that will actually help you stick to habits.

HERE'S WHAT TO LOOK FORWARD TO:

The epic variety of apples at the farmers' market, flannel shirts, pumpkin everything, hot apple cider, first frost, pumpkin carving, apple pie, country drives to admire the leaves, renting a cabin in the woods, hayrides, festivals, a new notebook, Halloween, Thanksgiving, sweater weather, stews and soups.

Your Autumn Kitchen Plan

COOK 3X A WEEK:

Choose three dinners.

Add on breakfasts, something

sweet, and a drink, too, if you'd

like. Make a grocery list.

Remember to think in

cooking categories (page 34)

and add a new kitchen habit that

will help you stick to your

plan (pages 31–51).

After 4 weeks, mix and match

favorite recipes to cook the rest

of the season.

Week 1

Monday	Mini Greek Meatball & Orzo Tray with Eggplant, Peppers & Zucchini
Tuesday	Cumin-Oregano Squash & Bell Pepper Quesadillas
Wednesday	Goodbye Summer Golden Tomato Soup with Grilled Cheese
Thursday	Sheet Pan Miso-Glazed Fish with Broccoli & Coconut Rice
Friday	Chicken Tomatillo Chili with White Beans & Poblanos

Week 2

Monday	Crazy Cajun Chicken Pasta with Peppers & Pecorino Cream Sauce
Tuesday	Bam Bam Street Tacos with Herbs & Raita
Wednesday	Greens & Grain Bowl with Rosemary Roasted Garlic Dressing
Thursday	A Classic (Not Cafeteria) Meatloaf Dinner
Friday	Oven BBQ Sandwiches with Celeriac Caper Slaw & Sweet Potato Wedges

Week 3

Monday	Fettuccine Squash Fredo
Tuesday	Chile Chili
Wednesday	Broccoli & Parmesan Soup with Garlic-Kissed Bread
Thursday	Our Most Favorite Chicken Tikka Masala
Friday	Banh Mi-ish Burgers with Jalapeño-Cabbage Slaw

Week 4

Monday	I Can't Believe It's Not Spaghetti! with Tiny Basil Meatballs & Garlic Bread
Tuesday	Flannel Root Veggie Tacos with Chipotle Crema & Cilantro
Wednesday	First Squash Soup Greens with Amazing Apple Cider Vinaigrette
Thursday	Pork Medallions with Creamy Rosemary Pan Sauce & Roasted Fall Veggies
Friday	The Lumberjack Pizza with Brussels Sprouts & Bacon

Breakfasts, Drinks, Something Sweet

Breakfast	Neighborhood Café Frittata Sandwich with Early-Autumn Fruit
Breakfast	One-Bowl Banana Pumpkin Pancakes
Breakfast	Fall Scramble with Market Mushrooms & Aged Cheese
Breakfast	Huckle's Multigrain Harvest Muffins
Breakfast	Apple-Walnut Breakfast Crisp
Happy Hour	Apple-Picking Shrub (and a Cocktail)
Happy Hour	Pear Pitcher Margaritas with Chile-Lime Rims
Sweet	Pear Galette with So Much Hazelnut Crumble

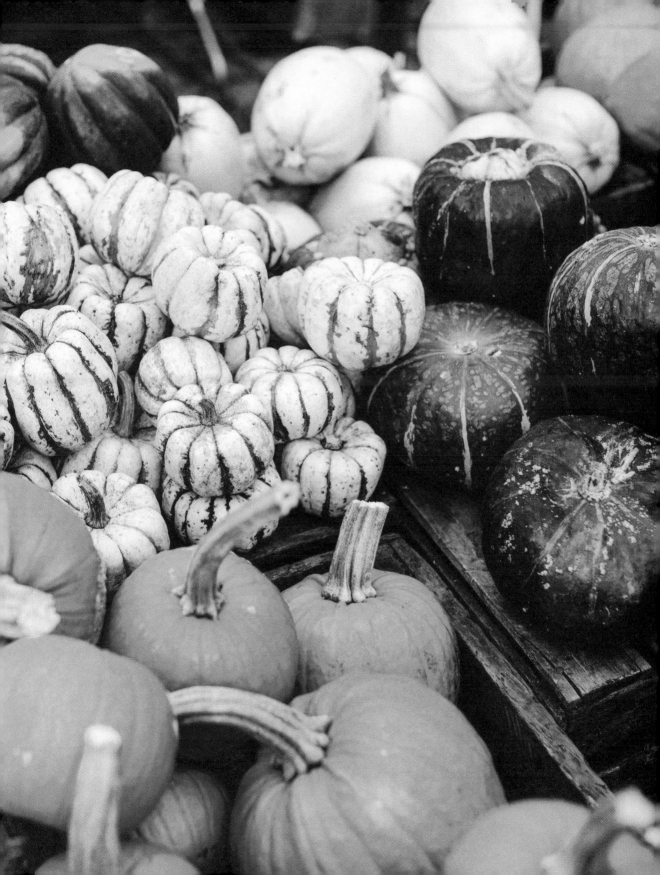

Mini Greek Meatball & Orzo Tray
with Eggplant, Peppers & Zucchini

Serves: 4

_____

Meatballs

I pound ground turkey

3 large cloves garlic, minced

⅓ cup white onion, minced

1½ teaspoons dried oregano

I teaspoon dried basil
or dried mint

I large egg, beaten

I cup panko breadcrumbs

Dill-jalapeño-feta sauce

6 ounces feta cheese

½ jalapeño pepper, seeded

I clove garlic, chopped

½ cup pickle brine or
pickled jalapeño brine

½ bunch fresh dill,
fronds and tender stems

Orzo and vegetables

I cup orzo

3 bell peppers, sliced into
I-inch squares

3–4 Japanese eggplants,
sliced into ¼-inch thick rounds

2 medium zucchini, sliced into
¼-inch rounds

Grapeseed oil

Salt

Pepper

Another fun, all-on-one-platter dinner. Eggplants, zucchini, and peppers are often available at the market even into November, so fall is the time to roast and roast some more. In the presence of meatballs and pasta, kids are less apprehensive about all the vegetables, and they might even venture to eat their entire bowl. A crowd-pleaser, for sure, and it's delicious as leftovers.

1.   Meatballs: In a large bowl, combine meatball ingredients with 1 teaspoon each salt and pepper, mixing really well with your hands; set bowl aside so meat reaches room temperature and flavors meld, about 30 minutes.

2.   Sauce: Toss feta, jalapeño, garlic, and half of the pickle brine in a blender and pulse until smooth and combined. Add the rest of the pickle brine if needed to adjust the consistency. Add the dill and pulse a few times, until combined but with little flecks of dill.

3.   Vegetables: Preheat oven to 425°F.

4.   All the vegetables should be about the same thickness and size for even cooking. Divide vegetables between 2 baking sheets, pile them in the middle, and drizzle a tablespoon of oil on each. Toss each pile well with a heaping ¼ teaspoon each of salt and pepper and spread them out. Slide into the oven for 30–40 minutes and bake until browned and tender, tossing halfway through. Keep warm in the oven at 175°F.

5.   Orzo: While veggies are roasting, cook orzo according to package directions. Drain and set aside in a bowl until ready to eat, tossing with a drizzle of oil, if you like, and any extra parsley or dill you have in the fridge.

6.   Back to meatballs: Start forming the meat mixture into tiny balls, less than an inch in diameter, and set them on a large plate. You should have about 40 total.

7. Heat a thin layer of oil in a large cast-iron skillet or sauté pan over medium-high heat. Add half the meatballs, and wait a minute or two until they sear nicely on one side. Shake the pan or turn meatballs with tongs every 2 minutes until cooked through, 5–7 minutes total. Veggies should be done cooking by now; make some room and transfer meatballs to the sheet pan to keep warm in the oven. Repeat with second batch.

8. Serve up everything in the warm sheet pan, letting everyone dig in and help themselves to big scoops of sauce and orzo, too.

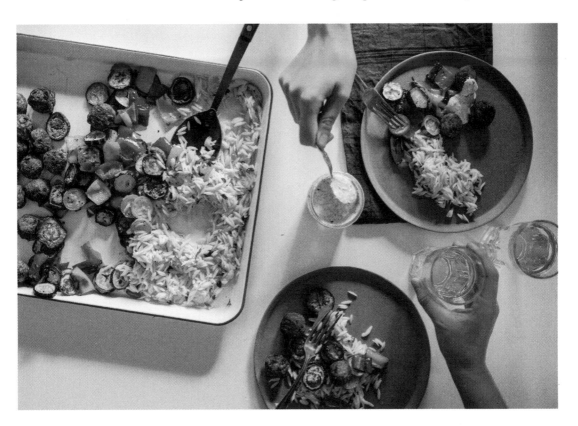

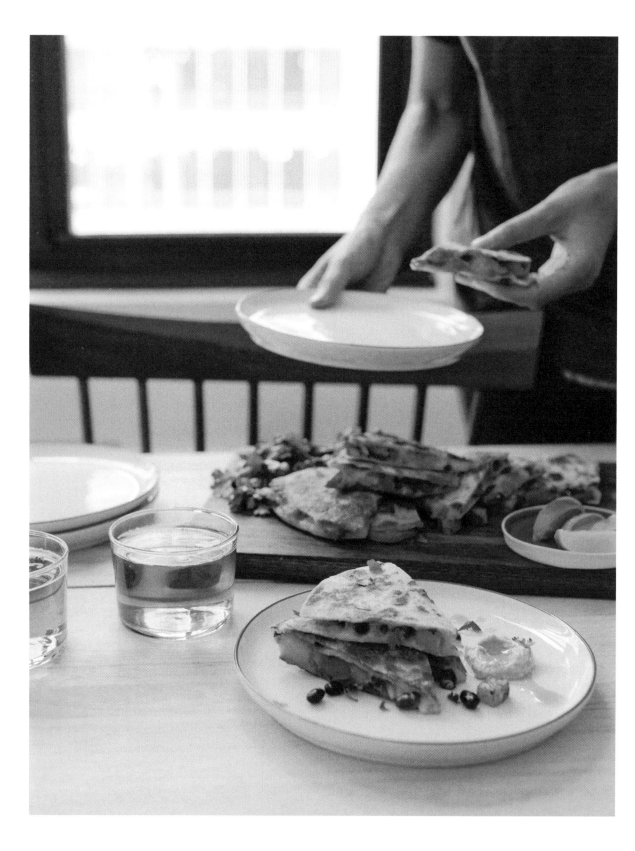

Cumin-Oregano Squash & Bell Pepper Quesadillas

Serves: 4

---

1 small butternut squash, peeled and cut into ½-inch cubes

1 large yellow onion, sliced thick

1 red bell pepper, sliced

1 tablespoon grapeseed oil

1 teaspoon chili powder

½ teaspoon ground cumin

Salt

Pepper

2 tablespoons unsalted butter, cut into 4 small pieces

8 flour tortillas

2 cups Monterey Jack or cheddar cheese, shredded

¾ cup canned or cooked black beans (about half a 15-ounce can)

¼ cup fresh cilantro, chopped

Sour cream, guacamole, and salsa, for serving

The quesadilla to make for people who think they'll never like a veggie quesadilla. It's the best back-to-school dinner—and the table's the best place to talk about new classmates, schedules, locker combinations, tryouts, and teachers.

1. Preheat oven to 400°F.

2. On a large sheet pan, toss the butternut squash, onion, and bell pepper with the oil, chili powder, cumin, and ½ teaspoon each of salt and pepper. Transfer to the oven and roast for 30 minutes or until veggies are soft and golden brown, giving the pan a shake halfway through. Remove from oven and set aside.

3. In a medium sauté pan, melt one butter piece over medium heat.

4. Once the butter is melted, lay 1 tortilla in the pan and add a thin layer of cheese, then scatter ¼ of the roasted veggies and black beans on top. Sprinkle on some cilantro and then another thin layer of cheese. Top with another tortilla and press down. When the cheese has melted on the bottom tortilla (about 1–2 minutes), gently flip and cook another 2 minutes or until the tortilla is golden brown and the cheese is melted.

5. Slide quesadilla onto a cutting board and tent with foil to keep warm. Repeat steps to make remaining quesadillas, wiping out skillet in between if needed.

6. Quarter quesadillas all with a large knife and serve with sour cream, guacamole, and salsa.

Goodbye Summer Golden Tomato Soup with Grilled Cheese

Serves: 4

_____

Soup

2 pounds golden plum tomatoes or regular red plum tomatoes

1 large yellow onion, sliced into thick wedges

6 cloves garlic, skin left on

1 tablespoon grapeseed oil

¼ bunch fresh basil

2 cups water, up to 2½ cups to adjust consistency if needed

3 tablespoons unsalted butter

Salt

Pepper

Sandwiches

Unsalted butter, softened

8 slices rustic sourdough, crusty whole wheat–any bread that would make a French person proud

1½ cups aged cheddar, thinly sliced or shredded, more if needed depending on your bread-slice size

Really, really good tomatoes from the market that are heavy and smell like tomatoes are essential for this recipe. It's summer-meets-autumn golden hour in a bowl. Remembering the flavor will carry you through until next tomato season.

1. Preheat oven to 400°F.

2. Halve tomatoes and toss them gently, along with onion and garlic, in a little oil on a sheet pan. Season with ½ teaspoon each salt and pepper; transfer to the oven. Roast for 25–30 minutes or until everything is soft.

3. Peel and squeeze out the garlic, adding it to a soup pot with the tomatoes, onion, basil, and half the water; puree using an immersion blender (or do this in a blender) until smooth. Gradually add the remaining water, using more if needed to adjust the consistency to your liking.

4. Warm the soup slightly over medium heat.

5. The soup may taste slightly acidic, depending on your tomatoes; adding a pinch of sugar will fix it.

6. Finally, to make the soup velvety, swirl in butter. Once it's melted, taste the soup one last time, adding more water, salt, or basil if you like.

7. For sandwiches, heat a griddle or large skillet over medium heat.

8. Butter one side of each bread slice. Divide cheese among the sandwiches, keeping the buttered sides on the outside of the sandwich.

9. When the griddle is hot, gently transfer the sandwiches and cook 3–4 minutes per side. Press them down with the back of a metal spatula or put a heavy pot on top (this gives you the panini effect).

10. Cut each sandwich in half, ladle soup into bowls, and get to dunking.

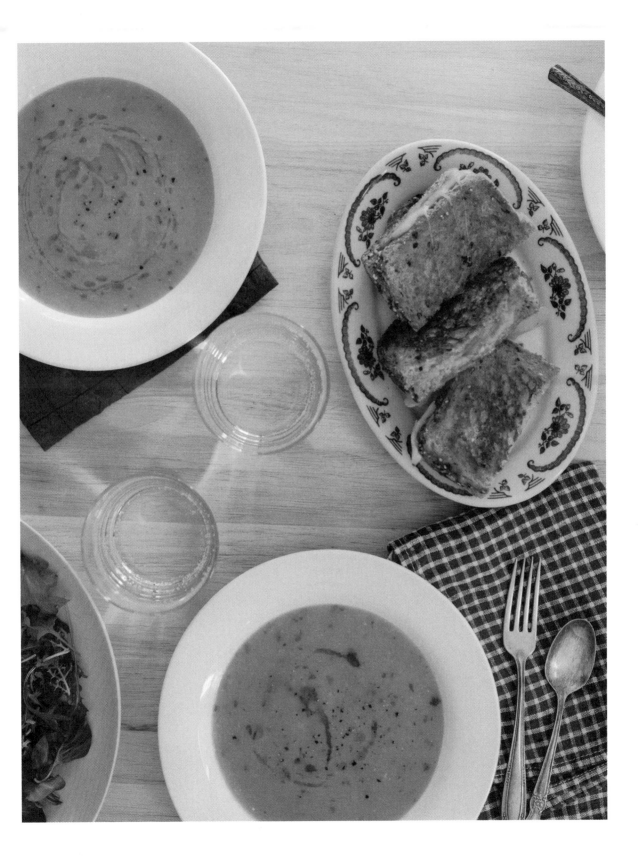

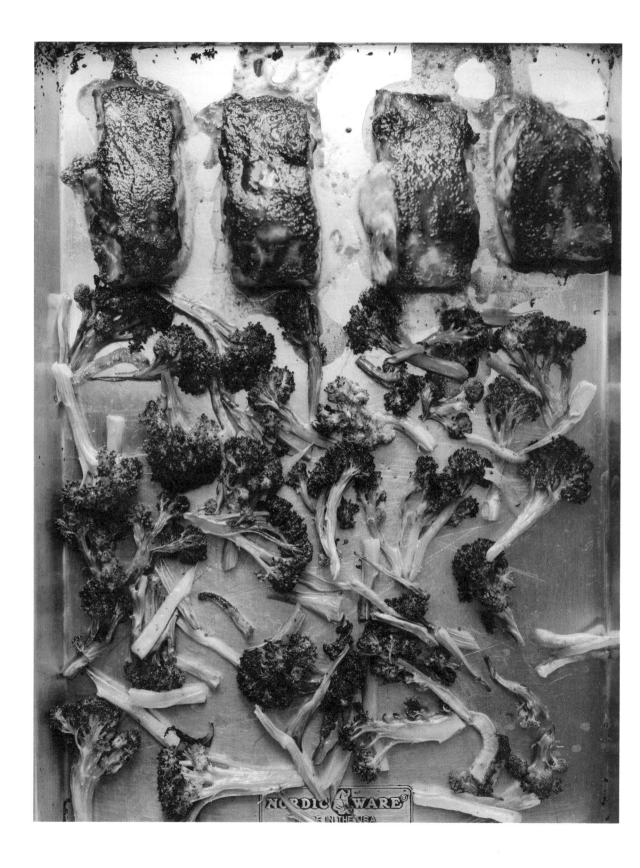

Sheet Pan Miso-Glazed Fish
with Broccoli & Coconut Rice

Serves: 4

_____

Miso-glazed fish

⅓ cup miso paste; red
or white is fine (red has
a stronger taste, white
is milder)

⅓ cup mirin

3 tablespoons maple syrup
or brown sugar

I teaspoon sesame oil

4 salmon, sea bass, cod,
or halibut fillets,
I¼–I½ pounds

Coconut rice

I cup jasmine rice

2 cups coconut milk

Broccoli

I head broccoli, florets
removed and stem peeled
and chopped into
French-fry shapes

I tablespoon grapeseed oil

Black sesame seeds,
optional, for garnish

Salt

Pepper

There's a miso-glazed cod at our favorite Japanese place that we fight over. The kind that tastes so good you assume it's got a lengthy list of ingredients and is too intimidating to attempt at home. Turns out that the ingredients for the glaze are pretty minimal and ones you might already have in your pantry.

1. In a shallow bowl, whisk the miso glaze ingredients together. Add the fish and coat all over with the marinade. Leave at room temperature for 30 minutes or refrigerate overnight.

2. Rinse the rice under cold water a few times and drain well (this prevents gloopiness, but it's not essential).

3. In a medium saucepan, combine the coconut milk, ¼ teaspoon salt, and rice; bring to a boil. Cover, reduce heat to a simmer, and cook for 15–20 minutes, until the coconut milk is just absorbed.

4. Remove from heat and let stand for 5 minutes, and then fluff with a fork.

5. For fish and broccoli, preheat oven to 400°F.

6. On a sheet pan, toss the broccoli with oil and ½ teaspoon each salt and pepper. Transfer to the oven and roast for 7 minutes.

7. Move broccoli to one side and add the fish fillets to the sheet pan. Transfer back to the oven and bake for 12–15 minutes. Use a pastry brush to brush on extra marinade if you notice the fish looks a bit dry. The marinade may start to burn around the fish because of the sugar—that's okay, brush on more and let it finish cooking. If you like the fish a bit more charred, broil for 30 seconds at the end.

8. Garnish with the black sesame seeds, if using, and serve with broccoli and rice.

Chicken Tomatillo Chili with White Beans & Poblanos

Serves: 6

---

4 skin-on, bone-in chicken thighs, about 2½ pounds

1 tablespoon bacon fat (see page 151)

2 large yellow onions, chopped

3-4 poblano peppers, chopped

8 cloves garlic, minced

1 tablespoon ground coriander

1 tablespoon ground cumin

1 tablespoon dried oregano

12-ounce bottle of beer

2 pounds tomatillos, husks removed and washed well to remove sticky residue, cut in half or quartered

1 bunch fresh cilantro, chopped

Salt

Pepper

For serving

Fresh cilantro, chopped

Sour cream

Lime wedges

Tortilla chips

This chili is so good, you'll wonder why you only made "red" chili before. It's even better the next day, so if you're hosting a dinner party, it's basically stress-free.

1. Preheat oven to 325°F.

2. Pat chicken thighs dry with a paper towel and season generously with salt and pepper.

3. Heat a Dutch oven over medium-high heat. Once it's hot, add bacon fat.

4. When the bacon fat is melted, nestle in the chicken thighs, skin side down, in the pot. Let them sear for 2–3 minutes (don't move them). Turn over and cook another 2 minutes. Transfer to a plate and set aside.

5. Add onions and poblanos to the Dutch oven and sauté until soft, 5–7 minutes total.

6. Add garlic, coriander, cumin, oregano, and 1 teaspoon each salt and black pepper; cook another minute.

7. Pour in beer and add tomatillos. Give everything a good stir. Set the chicken thighs back in, cover with a tight-fitting lid, and transfer to the oven to cook for 3 hours.

8. Remove from the oven and take out the chicken. Shred or cut the meat in large chunks, discarding the skin. Set aside.

9. Add chopped cilantro to the pot and, using an immersion blender, puree the chili until just slightly chunky.

10. Stir the shredded chicken back into the pot and serve immediately with your favorite garnishes.

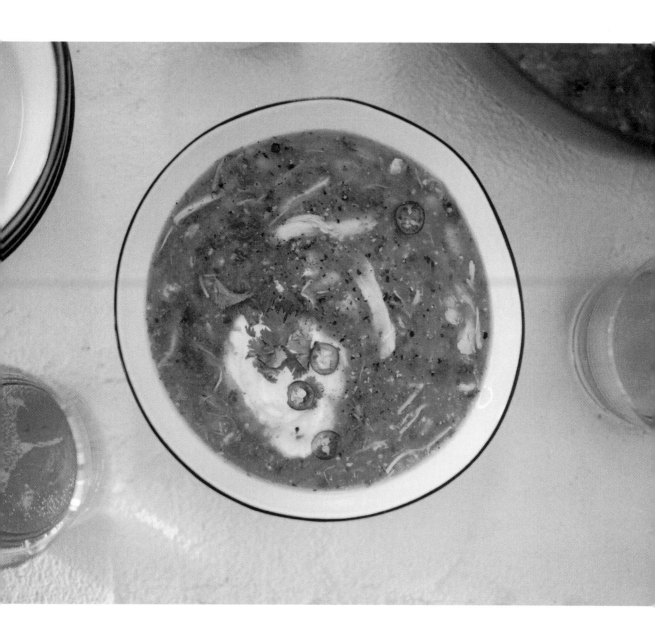

Crazy Cajun Chicken Pasta with Peppers & Pecorino Cream Sauce

Serves: 6

——————

1 pound short tubular pasta, like mezzi rigatoni or penne

4 tablespoons extra-virgin olive oil, divided

Juice of ½ lemon

2½ teaspoons paprika

1 teaspoon ground coriander

1 teaspoon chili powder

3 boneless, skinless chicken breasts, 1¼ pounds, halved horizontally through the middle so you have 6 total cutlets

2 bell peppers, any color, sliced

1 red onion, sliced

2 tablespoons unsalted butter

6 cloves garlic, minced

½ cup dry white wine

1½ cups heavy cream

⅓ bunch fresh Italian parsley, chopped

½ cup Pecorino Romano or Parmesan cheese, grated, plus more to taste

Salt

Pepper

The pasta that got our pepper haters to go from loathing peppers to *almost* liking them. Progress! Sometimes a single recipe will open the door to tasting a food (usually a vegetable) someone "hates." Adding pasta and heavy cream helps . . .

1. Pasta: Bring a large pot of salted water to a boil. Add penne and cook according to package instructions. Drain and return to pot. Set aside.

2. Chicken: Meanwhile, in a shallow bowl, whisk 2 tablespoons olive oil, lemon juice, spices, and ½ teaspoon each salt and pepper.

3. Using a meat mallet, flatten the chicken breast halves to an even thickness. In a shallow glass or ceramic dish, coat well with the marinade and let stand for 10 minutes (or up to an hour in the fridge).

4. Set a large sauté pan over medium-high heat. Add 1 tablespoon oil and once hot, add half the chicken breasts, without touching. Sear for about 3 minutes or until a nice brown crust forms, then turn cutlets over and cook an additional 2–3 minutes until chicken is opaque throughout. Transfer to a plate and repeat with the remaining chicken, adding another tablespoon of oil if needed. Set aside.

5. Veggies: In the same pan (full of brown bits and all kinds of goodness), cook the sliced peppers and onion. Sprinkle in a little salt so the veggies release their juices and cook for 5–7 minutes. Don't stir too often. Turn off heat and set aside.

6. Sauce: Heat a medium saucepan over medium heat and add the butter. When melted, stir in garlic and cook for 3 minutes, being careful not to burn it. Pour in wine and simmer for 4 minutes. Add heavy cream and ¼ teaspoon each salt and pepper. Lower heat to medium-low and simmer for 10 minutes.

7. Remove the sauce from heat; stir in parsley and cheese. Taste-test and adjust salt and pepper if necessary.

8. Pour the sauce over the pasta, add the peppers and onions, and stir well. Transfer to a serving platter.

9. Slice the chicken and arrange atop the pasta.

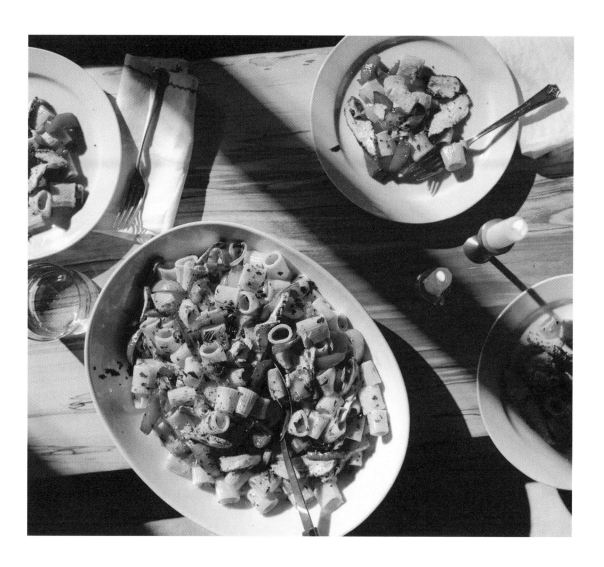

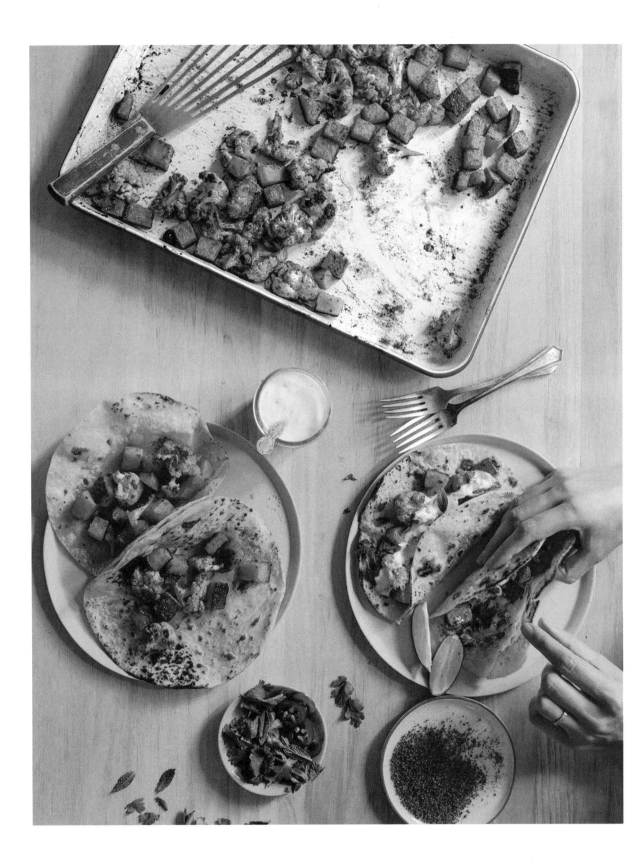

Bam Bam Street Tacos with Herbs & Raita

Serves: 4

Vegetables

1 small or medium butternut squash, peeled, seeds removed, chopped into ½-inch cubes

1 large head cauliflower, broken into 1-inch florets

2 tablespoons grapeseed oil

1 teaspoon curry powder

1 teaspoon garam masala

1 teaspoon paprika

1 teaspoon ground coriander

1 teaspoon turmeric

½ teaspoon smoked paprika

Garlicky yogurt sauce

1 cup yogurt

2 cloves garlic, minced

1 teaspoon white wine vinegar

1 teaspoon extra-virgin olive oil

Taco assembly

8 flour tortillas, charred on an open flame

¼ cup fresh mint, chopped

¼ cup fresh cilantro, chopped

Salt

Pepper

Almost as breezy as waiting in a food truck line for your favorite vegetarian tacos.

Kitchen note: If it's a nice day, grill the vegetables outside at the same temperature in a grill pan and warm the tortillas directly on the grates.

1. Preheat oven to 425°F.

2. Toss squash and cauliflower with grapeseed oil, 1 teaspoon salt, a few cracks of pepper, and all the spices. Spread out on a sheet pan. Roast for 30–40 minutes, until soft and slightly charred, tossing halfway through.

3. Meanwhile, whisk together sauce ingredients with a pinch of salt and pepper.

4. To serve, spoon vegetables down the center of a tortilla, drizzle generously with yogurt sauce, and sprinkle on herbs.

Greens & Grain Bowl with Rosemary Roasted Garlic Dressing

Serves: 4

_____

Vegetables and grain

3 bell peppers, cored and sliced into 1-inch squares

1 medium eggplant, cut into slices just shy of ¼-inch thick

1 large head cauliflower, cored and sliced into florets

2 tablespoons grapeseed oil

1 cup farro, or any other nutty, chewy grain

2 cups delicate, lacy greens such as frisée or Russian kale

Dressing

1 massive head garlic

1 tablespoon champagne vinegar

Juice of ¼ lemon, about 1 tablespoon

2 sprigs fresh rosemary, leaves removed from stems and minced very, very finely

¼ cup extra-virgin olive oil

Salt

Pepper

One of our go-to mix-and-match lunches to avoid the turkey sandwich repeat. A dressing that goes with anything—try zucchini, corn, and burst tomatoes in the summer, charred asparagus and green beans in the spring, caramelized squash and root vegetables in the winter. Or be adventurous with any greens, grains, or vegetables you're curious to try.

1. Preheat oven to 400°F. Divide peppers, eggplant, and cauliflower between 2 sheet pans. Toss each with 1 tablespoon grapeseed oil, ½ teaspoon salt, and ½ teaspoon pepper. Peel the garlic cloves for the dressing, wrap securely in parchment, and set on one of the sheet pans. Roast for 35–40 minutes, flipping halfway through, until vegetables are browned and tender and the garlic is soft.

2. Place farro in a small pot and cover with water by a few inches. Bring to a boil, reduce heat, then simmer according to the time on package instructions. Check for doneness, then drain and let the water evaporate for as long as you can so you don't have soggy grains. Sometimes we make this in the morning and just leave it on the stove uncovered till dinner.

3. In a small bowl, smash all the roasted garlic with a fork until you have a paste. Add in vinegar, lemon juice, rosemary, and ½ teaspoon each salt and pepper. Slowly drizzle in the olive oil, whisking constantly with the same fork. Adjust anything to taste.

4. Grab a large serving platter and place all the grain and greens at the bottom, all the veggies on top. Drizzle with half the dressing and reserve some to serve on the side.

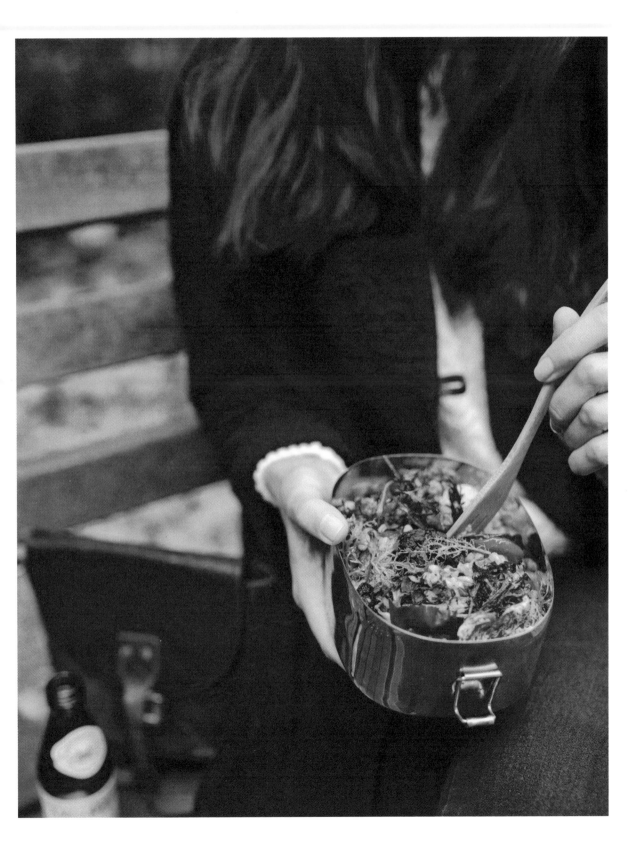

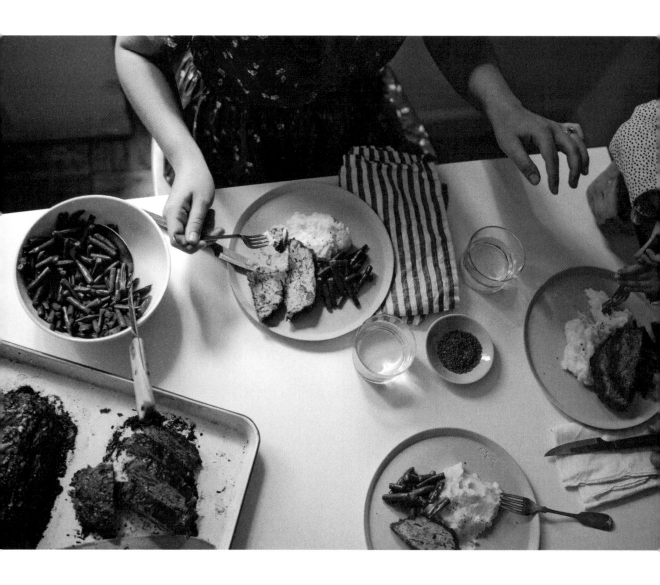

A Classic (Not Cafeteria) Meatloaf Dinner

Serves: 6–8

———————

3 tablespoons unsalted butter, plus a bit more for the pan

1 red or yellow bell pepper, diced

1 large yellow or red onion, diced

2 carrots, peeled and finely diced

3 stalks celery, diced

2 teaspoons paprika

1/8 teaspoon ground nutmeg

2 tablespoons Worcestershire sauce, divided

6 cloves garlic, minced

1/4 cup fresh Italian parsley, chopped

1/3 cup ketchup

1 tablespoon honey or maple syrup

2 pounds ground turkey

2 large eggs, beaten

1/2 cup panko breadcrumbs, up to 3/4 cup if needed

1/3 cup hot water

Grapeseed oil, for brushing sheet pan

Salt

Pepper

If you like to say you're not a meatloaf fan, you've probably had at least one person respond with "That's because you haven't had mine," and you have to explain that you've had plenty and you just don't like it. So we won't do that here. Make this for other people, at least—they'll love it. But taste a tiny bite to see if you've changed your mind.

———————

Kitchen note: Leftovers make some seriously epic sandwiches the next day. You can broil them open-faced on good bread, with cheese and some red onion, or make a cold sandwich with a little mayo and greens on a fresh baguette.

1. Preheat oven to 400°F.

2. Heat a large sauté pan over medium-high heat and swirl in butter.

3. Add the diced bell pepper, onion, carrots, and celery. Sauté for 3 minutes. Stir in paprika, 1/2 teaspoon each salt and pepper, nutmeg, and 1 tablespoon Worcestershire sauce; cook for an additional minute. Turn off the heat, give everything a good stir, and add the garlic and parsley. Leave on the stove to cool slightly.

4. Meanwhile, in a cup, mix the ketchup, honey or maple syrup, and remaining tablespoon of Worcestershire sauce. Set aside.

5. In a large bowl, mix turkey with 1 teaspoon salt and 1/2 teaspoon pepper, eggs, panko, and hot water. If mixture is not stiff or moldable enough, add more panko.

6. Add the sautéed vegetables to the turkey and mix well.

7. Brush some oil on a sheet pan. Divide the meat mixture in half and shape each half into a loaf. Brush the ketchup mixture all over.

8. Transfer meatloaf to the oven and cook for 40–45 minutes until the ketchup glaze has caramelized and the meatloaves feel firm to the touch. Remove from oven and let rest for at least 5 minutes before slicing.

Creamy Mashed Potatoes

Serves: 4

———————

2 pounds russet or Yukon Gold potatoes, peeled and cut into 1-inch cubes

1¼ cups whole milk, warmed

8 tablespoons unsalted butter, cut into pieces

2 teaspoons salt, divided, plus more if needed

¼ teaspoon pepper

1. Put potatoes and 1 teaspoon salt in a large pot. Pour in enough water to just cover them by an inch. Bring to a simmer and cook until potatoes are fork-tender, about twenty minutes.

2. Drain potatoes and return to same pot, set over low heat. (This helps evaporate remaining water.) Mash potatoes until mostly smooth. For extra-creamy mashed potatoes, use a handheld mixer to whip them.

3. Add half of the milk, ¾ teaspoon salt, and ¼ teaspoon pepper and continue mixing. Add the butter and more milk or salt if needed. Serve immediately.

Simple Skillet Green Beans

Serves: 4

———————

1 tablespoon unsalted butter or extra-virgin olive oil

1 pound green beans, trimmed and chopped into bite-size pieces

½ cup low-sodium vegetable or chicken stock, or more if needed

¼ teaspoon salt, plus more to taste

¼ teaspoon pepper

1. Heat oil or butter in a large skillet over medium heat and add the green beans. Give them a stir and arrange them with your wooden spoon so they're in one layer. Don't move them for a minute or two, so they char just a tiny bit. Stir for another couple of minutes.

2. Turn off heat (so stock doesn't scorch). Pour in stock, then add salt and pepper. Turn heat back on to low; partially cover the skillet and simmer for 7–10 minutes. Check at the 7-minute mark, then every minute until your beans are the way you like 'em.

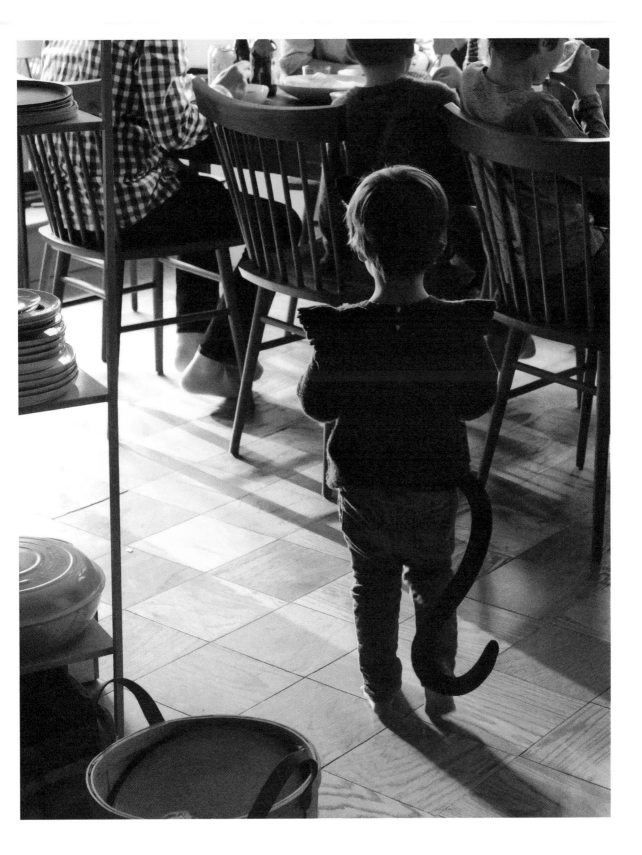

Oven BBQ Sandwiches with Celeriac Caper Slaw & Sweet Potato Wedges

Serves: 6

_____

Barbecue sandwiches

1 tablespoon grapeseed or canola oil

2½–3 pounds bone-in skinless chicken thighs, at room temperature

1 bottle barbecue sauce

8 brioche buns

Slaw

1 medium-size celeriac (celery root), peeled

Juice of ½ lemon

1 tablespoon pickle brine, plus more to taste

2 teaspoons Dijon mustard

2 tablespoons extra-virgin olive oil

¼ cup pickles, minced

2 tablespoons capers

¼ cup fresh chives, chopped

¼ cup fresh Italian parsley, chopped

If there ever were such a thing as a farmers' market barbecue joint, this would probably be what they'd serve. Set out a bunch of cold beers and colas and let everyone pile their plates high.

_____

Kitchen note: Meet celeriac (also called celery root), one of our favorite root vegetables. It tastes like celery in a starchier form, and you can eat it raw, roasted, or braised. You'll need a knife to peel it–this is not a job for your peeler. Cut away the dirt-filled knobs until you reach the smooth inside.

1. Barbecue: Preheat oven to 325°F.

2. Heat a tablespoon of oil in a Dutch oven over medium-high heat. Generously salt and pepper chicken thighs.

3. In batches, sear chicken for 3–4 minutes on each side until crisp and golden brown.

4. Nestle all the meat in the Dutch oven and pour barbecue sauce over. The amount of barbecue sauce is flexible here—you just want enough to almost cover the chicken. The fat will release from the chicken to contribute to the braising liquid, too.

5. Cook for about 1½ hours in the oven, until chicken pulls apart very easily. If it doesn't, give it another 30 minutes. Using 2 forks or your fingers, pull apart on a plate, discarding bones or anything mysterious. Then add back to pot, tossing with the sauce.

6. Slaw: Slice the peeled celeriac into very thin noodle-like strips using a mandoline. Place into a medium bowl, squeeze in lemon juice, sprinkle with a pinch of salt, and toss to prevent oxidation while you prepare the dressing.

7. In a small bowl or measuring cup, whisk together pickle brine, mustard, oil, and ½ teaspoon each salt and pepper.

Wedges

2 pounds sweet potatoes, scrubbed or peeled and completely dry, sliced into ⅓-inch wedges

2 tablespoons grapeseed or canola oil

2 teaspoons paprika

¼ teaspoon cayenne pepper, optional

Salt

Pepper

8. Toss celeriac with dressing and gently mix in the pickles, capers, chives, and parsley. Taste for acidity and seasoning.

9. Fries: Preheat oven to 425°F.

10. In a bowl, toss sweet potato wedges with oil, paprika, cayenne if desired, 1 teaspoon salt, and ½ teaspoon pepper. Spread them out evenly on 2 baking sheets, leaving a ½-inch space between each so they crisp, not steam.

11. Roast for 15 minutes, flip with a metal spatula, then slide back in the oven for about 10 more minutes until they're browned and puffy.

12. Sandwiches: Heap barbecued chicken onto buns with extra sauce if you'd like. Slaw can go in the sandwich, too, or on the side. Serve with sweet potato wedges straight out of the oven.

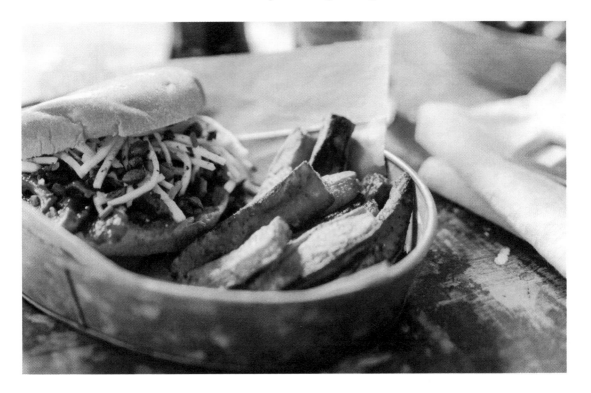

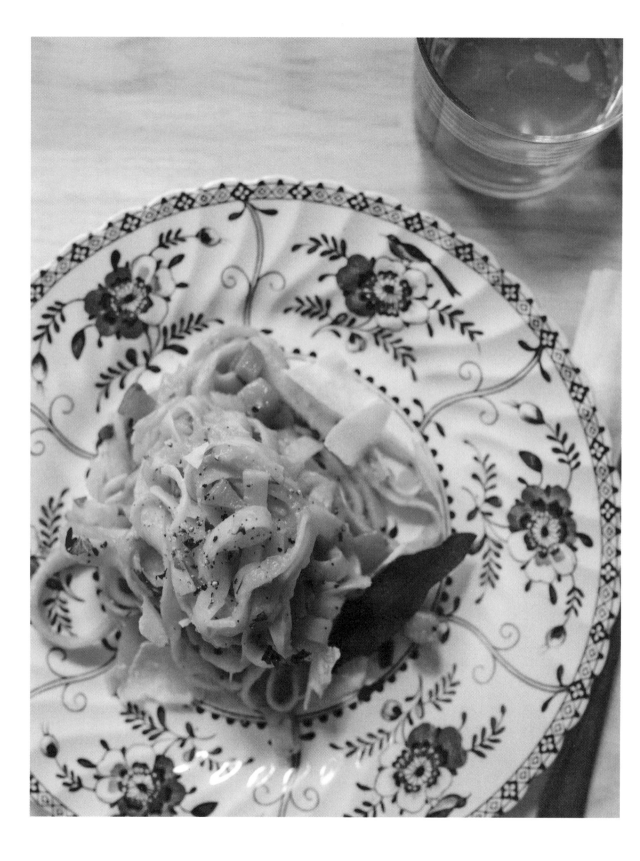

Fettuccine Squash Fredo

Serves: 4

---

1 butternut squash, about
2 pounds, peeled and cut into
½-inch cubes

1 yellow onion,
cut into 6 wedges

9 cloves garlic,
skin left on

2 tablespoons extra-virgin
olive oil

½ pound fettuccine

Salt

Pepper

Optional, but highly recommended for serving

1 bunch fresh sage leaves

⅓ cup grapeseed oil,
or another neutral oil

Parmigiano-Reggiano,
shaved

This is one of those genius five-ingredient, five-dollar sheet pan dinners that tastes of something else entirely. Dressed up with crispy sage and shaved Parm, it's perfect for a grown-up pasta party.

1. Preheat oven to 375°F and bring a pot of salted water to a boil.

2. On a sheet pan, toss the squash, onion, and garlic with oil and ½ teaspoon each salt and pepper. If you've got more than 2 pounds of squash, cube it up even tinier, to roast as garnish. Roast for 30–35 minutes or until squash is tender. Toss halfway through.

3. Meanwhile, add pasta to the boiling water and cook until al dente. Drain in a colander, reserving 1 cup of pasta water.

4. If you want to get fancy (recommended), make crispy sage: Grab a small skillet and set it over medium-high heat. Add a ¼-inch layer of grapeseed oil and, once it's hot, test one sage leaf. The oil should bubble around it. Fry all the sage leaves in one layer for 15–30 seconds, flipping with tongs. Don't let the leaves brown. Transfer to a paper-towel-lined plate and repeat with the remaining leaves. They'll crisp up as they rest.

5. Remove sheet pan from the oven, peel the garlic, and add everything to a blender, along with ½ cup of reserved pasta water. Puree until smooth. Adjust consistency with more pasta water if needed. Add more salt and pepper if needed.

6. Toss sauce with fettuccine in a big, warm pasta bowl. (An easy way to warm plates or bowls is to slide them into a just-turned-off oven.)

7. Arrange crispy sage, Parm, and extra cubed squash on top; serve right away.

Chile Chili

Serves: 6

---

3 dried ancho chiles

3 dried New Mexico chiles

1 tablespoon bacon fat
or extra-virgin olive oil

1 large yellow onion, diced

7 cloves garlic, minced

1 bay leaf

2 teaspoons ground coriander

2 teaspoons dried oregano

1 tablespoon ground cumin

2 pounds ground beef

1 bottle beer

1 28-ounce can diced
or crushed tomatoes

1½ teaspoons salt

¾ teaspoon pepper

1 cup water, plus more
for the chiles

1 15-ounce can black beans,
drained and rinsed

1 15-ounce can kidney beans,
drained and rinsed

Toppings: Sour cream, shredded
cheese, cilantro, red onion, lime,
avocado, hot sauce, tortilla chips

A big pot of chili—the ultimate comfort food. Perfect for Halloween, game nights with friends, after an afternoon spent jumping in leaves.

Kitchen note: Dried chiles give chili this depth, not to mention gorgeous color that you can't get from a tablespoon of powder. The extra work is just pouring some boiling water over the chiles and then putting them in a blender. These here are mild(ish), but feel free to play around with some hotter varieties like cascabel, pasilla, or arbol. And if you're making this in early fall add some fresh peppers (chopped) along with the onions.

1. Break off the tops of the chiles and remove most of the seeds by tapping on the counter upside down or using your fingers. Place them in a bowl and pour boiling water to cover. Top with any pot lid or plastic wrap; allow to rehydrate for 20 minutes.

2. Meanwhile, heat a Dutch oven over medium-high heat.

3. Swirl in bacon fat and, once it's melted, add onion. Stir occasionally for 5 minutes, then add garlic, bay leaf, and spices; cook another minute.

4. Add meat and cook until no longer pink, breaking it up with the spoon, about 5 minutes.

5. Pour in beer and tomatoes with salt and pepper, stir well, and lower heat to simmer.

6. Place the chiles in a blender along with 1 cup of the soaking liquid. Puree until smooth. Then add chile paste to the Dutch oven, plus 1 cup water (or stock if you have any you want to use up). Simmer for 2 hours, partially covered, stirring occasionally.

7. Add beans and simmer for another 30 minutes to an hour. If chili is too thick, you can add a little more water or stock.

8. Turn off heat and let the chili rest for 5 minutes. Serve with your favorite fixings.

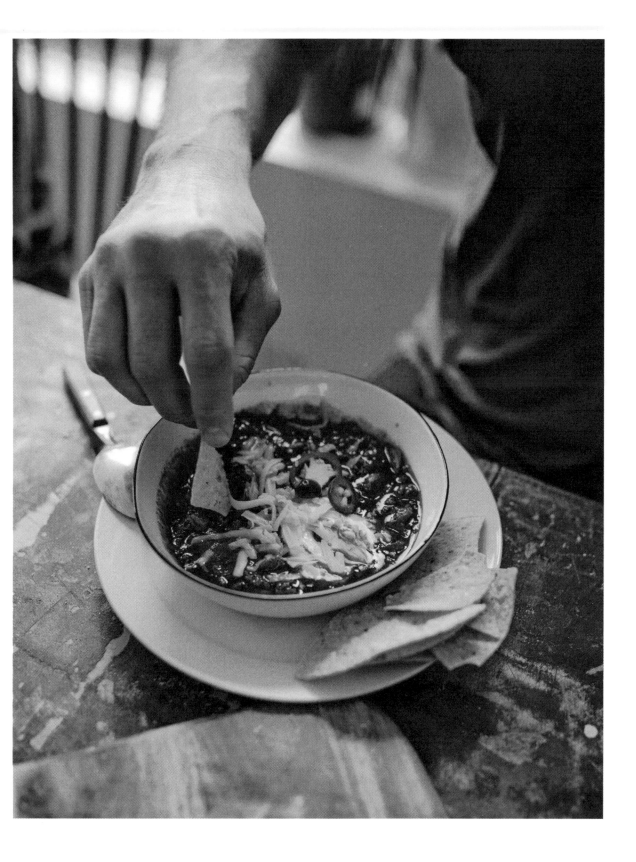

Broccoli & Parmesan Soup with Garlic-Kissed Bread

Serves: 4

———————

Soup

2 tablespoons extra-virgin olive oil

I yellow onion, chopped

I large leek, chopped, washed really well in a bowl of water

6 cloves garlic, minced

¼ teaspoon red pepper flakes

I teaspoon paprika

I teaspoon lemon pepper

I bay leaf

½ cup dry white wine

4 cups low-sodium chicken or vegetable broth

2 cups water

½ teaspoon soy sauce

¾ pound broccoli (I large head)

3 medium-small carrots, grated

I cup Parmesan cheese, grated

½ cup heavy cream, up to I cup

Garlic-kissed bread

8 slices really good crusty bread

Extra-virgin olive oil, for brushing

2 large cloves garlic

Salt

Pepper

The ideal soup for crispy-bread dunking—not fully pureed, not too chunky, just right. Truth be told, you may find yourself forgetting you have a spoon. We've often finished an entire bowl of soup with just the bread.

1. Swirl oil in a large soup pot over medium heat.

2. Add chopped onion and leek; stir for about 5–7 minutes, until soft.

3. Stir in minced garlic, spices, bay leaf, and ½ teaspoon salt and cook until fragrant, about 30 seconds.

4. Pour in wine and reduce for 2–3 minutes. Now add in broth, water, and soy sauce.

5. Let soup come to a low boil, then simmer on low. Meanwhile, prep broccoli and carrots.

6. Remove the broccoli florets and roughly chop. Using a knife, peel the outer layer of the remaining stem. Chop stem finely and add it to the simmering soup along with ¼ teaspoon more salt and a few cracks of pepper. After 10 minutes, add the florets and grated carrot. Let everything simmer for 7–10 more minutes, partially covered, until broccoli is tender but not overcooked.

7. Add the cheese and cream, stirring well.

8. Remove bay leaf and puree the soup just partially with an immersion blender so it stays chunky.

9. Taste the soup and adjust the salt and pepper if needed. Keep warm.

10. Heat a griddle or sauté pan over medium heat and brush both sides of bread slices with olive oil.

11. When pan is hot, add bread slices in single layer. Toast for 1–2 minutes on each side or until the bread reaches golden-brown, crusty perfection.

12. Rub a garlic clove on both sides of the bread and sprinkle a little salt on top. Serve immediately with the soup.

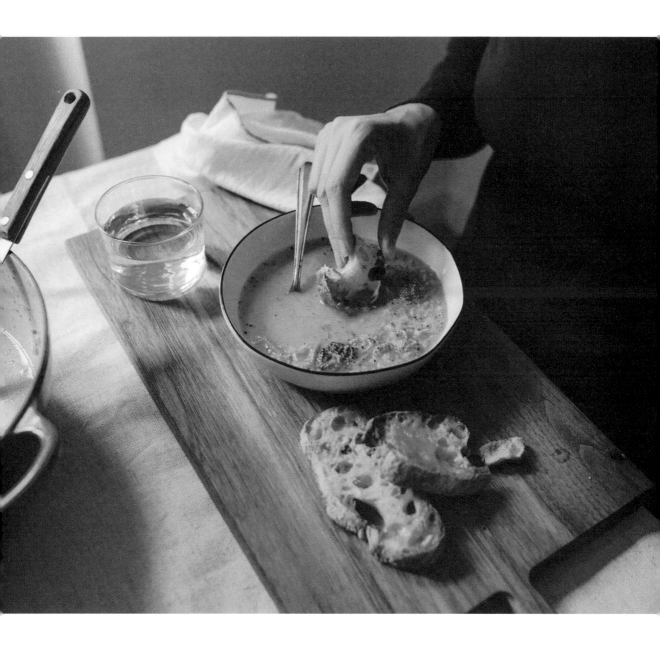

Our Most Favorite Chicken Tikka Masala

Serves: 4–6

¼ cup Greek yogurt

2 teaspoons paprika

1 teaspoon ground coriander

10 cloves garlic

3 tablespoons grapeseed oil

2-inch piece fresh ginger, peeled and minced

Salt

Pepper

3 boneless chicken breasts, cut into 1-inch cubes

1 large yellow onion, chopped

4 large plum tomatoes, chopped

½ teaspoon coconut sugar

1 teaspoon garam masala

½ teaspoon ground cumin

¼ teaspoon ground cinnamon

⅓ cup heavy cream, plus more if needed

3 tablespoons unsalted butter

2 tablespoons water

Juice of 1 lime

1 cup basmati rice

¼ teaspoon ground turmeric

¼ bunch fresh cilantro, chopped, for garnish

Raita, follow Tzatziki recipe on page 177, swapping dill with cilantro and/or mint

Store-bought naan

Pretty much the most popular dish at any Indian restaurant. Ugly, bursting ripe tomatoes (called *seconds* by farmers) are the secret ingredient here and they cost less. Not using canned tomatoes results in a delicate, velvety sauce you'll want to eat like soup.

1. In a medium bowl, whisk together yogurt, 1 teaspoon paprika, ½ teaspoon coriander, 4 minced garlic cloves, 1 tablespoon oil, 1 teaspoon of the ginger, 1 teaspoon salt, and ½ teaspoon black pepper. Coat chicken breasts with marinade. Cover and refrigerate overnight, or at least 25 minutes at room temperature.

2. Meanwhile, heat a sauté pan over medium-high heat. Add 2 tablespoons of oil and onion, remaining 6 cloves of minced garlic, and remaining ginger. Sauté for about 5 minutes or until onion begins to soften.

3. Stir in tomatoes and cover pan with a lid. Lower heat to medium and simmer until the tomatoes soften a bit, about 6 minutes. Uncover and stir occasionally, mashing the tomatoes.

4. Turn broiler to high. Arrange chicken cubes on a sheet pan without overcrowding. Broil for about 7 minutes until charred and opaque throughout. Set aside.

5. To the tomatoes add 1 teaspoon paprika, ½ teaspoon coriander, coconut sugar, garam masala, cumin, cinnamon, and 1 teaspoon each salt and pepper. Simmer for 5 more minutes.

6. Using an immersion blender, puree until smooth (or do this in a blender). Stir in heavy cream, butter, water, and lime juice, simmering for 3 more minutes. Taste and adjust seasoning if needed, then toss chicken with the sauce.

7. To make turmeric herbed rice, cook according to package directions, adding turmeric to the water. Fluff with a fork and keep warm. Mince a handful of parsley, cilantro, or mint and stir in.

8. Garnish chicken tikka masala with cilantro and serve with raita and rice. And naan; always naan.

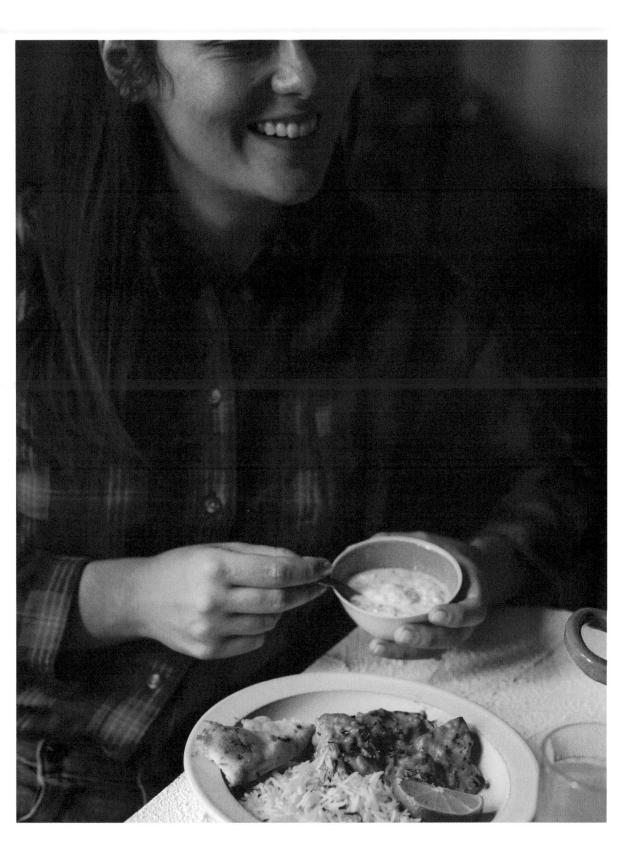

Banh Mi–ish Burgers with Jalapeño-Cabbage Slaw

Serves: 4

Burgers

1 pound ground turkey

1 carrot, shredded

2 scallions, finely chopped

2 tablespoons red onion, finely diced

3 cloves garlic, minced

1 tablespoon ginger, minced

1 tablespoon fresh cilantro, finely chopped

1 tablespoon fresh Italian parsley, finely chopped

1 tablespoon soy sauce

½ teaspoon sesame oil

2 tablespoons creamy peanut butter (the good stuff)

Grapeseed oil, for pan

4 hamburger buns or 6 flour tortillas

Sriracha mayo

¼ cup mayonnaise

2 tablespoons Greek yogurt (plain yogurt will work, too)

1 teaspoon lemon juice

1-2 tablespoons Sriracha; adjust to your taste

Ground meat is a great canvas for any and all flavors. Whatever cuisine/flavors you love, turn them into a burger. Thai, Mexican, French, Greek, Moroccan—you name it, you can make it. We're going Vietnamese-slash-Thai here.

1. In a bowl, mix all burger ingredients (turkey through peanut butter) with ¼ teaspoon each salt and pepper. Refrigerate while you prep the sauce and slaw.

2. Whisk Sriracha mayo ingredients in a small bowl with ¼ teaspoon each salt and pepper. Refrigerate for up to 3 days.

3. In a medium bowl, whisk together dressing ingredients (vinegar through fish sauce). Add cabbage, jalapeños, and cilantro with a pinch of salt and pepper; mix well to combine.

4. Take burger mix out of the fridge and form into patties. If using buns, shape into 4 round patties. If using tortillas, shape into 6 elongated patties.

5. Heat a large pan thinly coated with oil over medium (more toward medium-high) heat. Cook the burgers for 4-5 minutes per side until cooked through and nicely browned.

6. When ready to serve, spread mayo onto buns or tortillas; top with burger and slaw.

Jalapeño-cabbage slaw

1 tablespoon rice wine vinegar

Juice of 1 lime

2 tablespoons extra-virgin olive oil or grapeseed oil

1 teaspoon maple syrup or honey

1 teaspoon fish sauce

½ red cabbage

1–2 jalapeños, depending on how spicy you like it, sliced

½ bunch fresh cilantro, chopped

Salt

Pepper

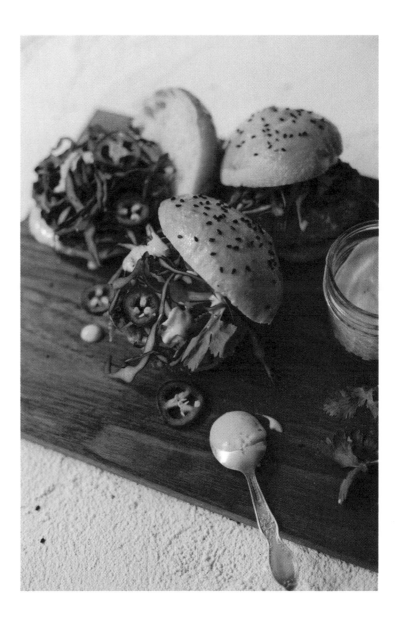

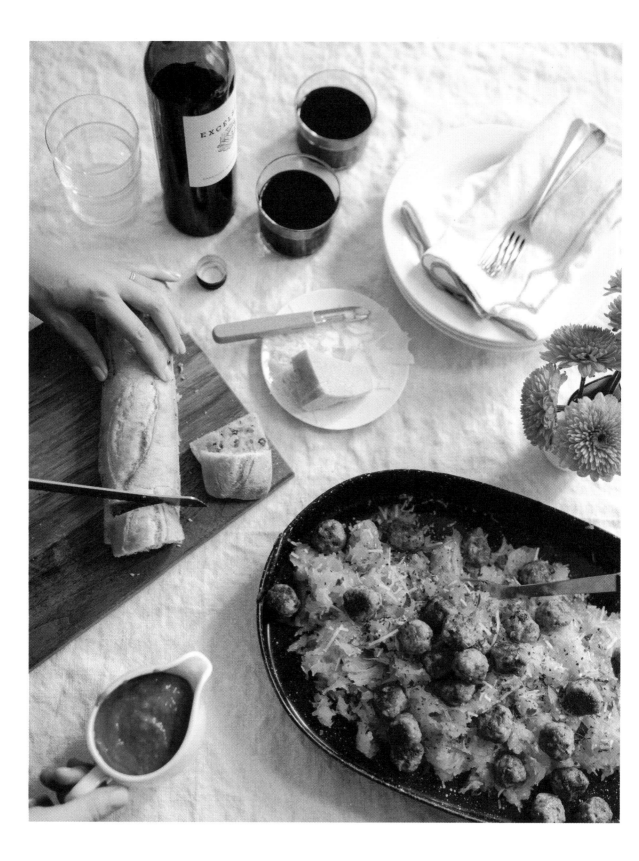

I Can't Believe It's Not Spaghetti! with Tiny Basil Meatballs & Garlic Bread

Serves: 5

_____

Squash

2½-pound spaghetti squash

1 tablespoon extra-virgin olive oil

¼ bunch fresh Italian parsley, minced

Meatballs

1 large egg, beaten

1 pound ground turkey

⅓ cup white onion, very finely minced

3 cloves garlic, minced

1 cup panko breadcrumbs

1 teaspoon dried oregano

1 teaspoon dried basil

2 tablespoons extra-virgin olive oil

Tomato sauce

2 tablespoons extra-virgin olive oil

5 cloves garlic, minced

¼ teaspoon crushed red pepper

2 tablespoons tomato paste

28-ounce can crushed tomatoes

1 teaspoon dried oregano

1 teaspoon dried basil

2 tablespoons unsalted butter

Salt

Pepper

Parmigiano-Reggiano, for serving

A gluten-free-ish feast any Italian grandma would approve of. We love piling everything onto the sheet pan (for fewer dishes on weeknights) or a pretty platter (for Sunday supper) and setting it right in the middle of the table, with great fanfare and lots of Parm. Everyone digs in, family-style.

1. Squash: Preheat oven to 400°F.

2. Slice the spaghetti squash in half lengthwise with a very sharp knife; scoop and discard the seeds. Drizzle a tablespoon of oil on the flesh and sprinkle generously with salt and pepper. Roast cut-side down on a sheet pan for 45–55 minutes, until very tender. When squash is cool enough to handle, scrape out the flesh onto the sheet pan, toss with minced parsley, and keep warm in the oven.

3. Meatballs, part 1: In a large bowl, mix meatball ingredients (sans oil) with 1 teaspoon salt and ½ teaspoon pepper. Refrigerate for up to a day, until ready to roll.

4. Sauce: Place a sauté pan over medium heat and drizzle in olive oil. Once hot, add the garlic and stir occasionally for 30 seconds, until fragrant. Stir in crushed red pepper, tomato paste, crushed tomatoes, dried herbs, and ½ teaspoon each salt and pepper. Simmer for 30 minutes, then swirl in butter until melted. Taste and add more salt if needed and/or mellow out acidity with a few pinches of sugar.

5. Meatballs, part 2: Start forming the meat mixture into tiny balls, less than an inch in diameter, and set them on a large plate. You should have about 40 total.

6. Heat a thin layer of oil in a large sauté pan over medium-high heat. Add half the meatballs, and wait a minute or two until they sear nicely on one side. Shake the pan or turn meatballs with tongs every 2 minutes until cooked through, 5–7 minutes total. Transfer to the warm sheet pan in the oven with the spaghetti squash and repeat with the second batch.

Garlic bread
(optional, but not really)

8 tablespoons unsalted butter, at room temperature

5 cloves garlic, minced

1 baguette or ciabatta, cut in half lengthwise

7. Garlic bread: Mix the butter, garlic, and ½ teaspoon each salt and pepper in a small bowl. Spread inside both halves of the bread. Wrap lightly in foil and bake at 375°F for 15–20 minutes (take out warm squash and meatball sheet pan).

8. Serve: Let everyone serve themselves from the sheet pan, scooping on tomato sauce and grabbing garlic bread slices. Grate on lots of Parm.

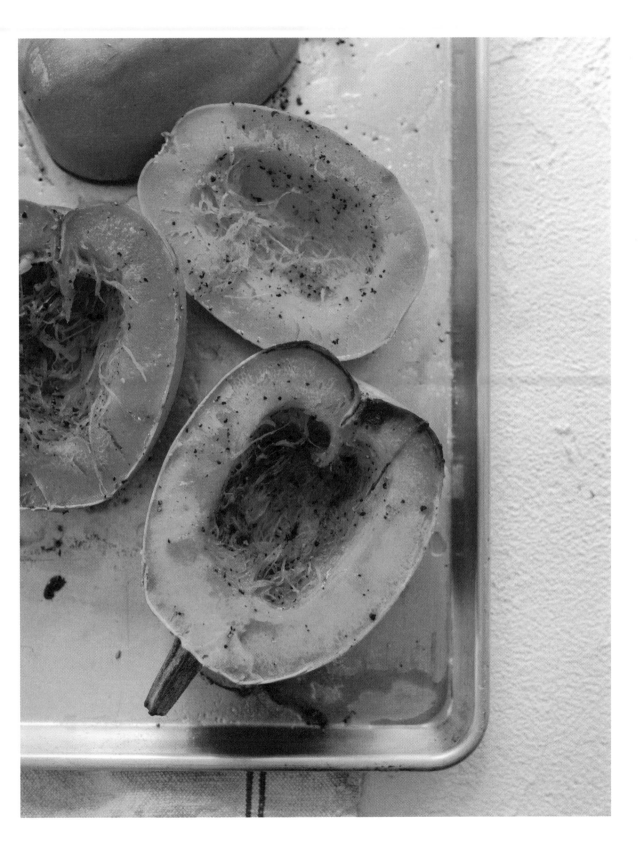

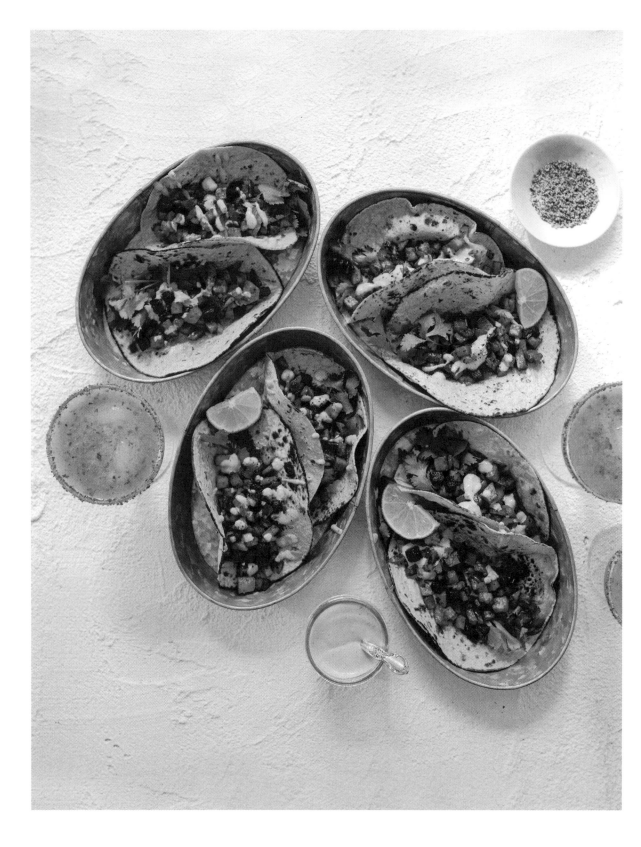

Flannel Root Veggie Tacos with Chipotle Crema & Cilantro

Serves: 4

_____

Vegetables

2 pounds mixed root vegetables–multicolored beets and sweet potatoes, plus parsnips, carrots, turnips, celeriac, chopped into ¼-inch cubes

1 red onion, chopped into ½-inch pieces

2 tablespoons grapeseed oil

2 teaspoons chili powder

½ teaspoon ground cumin

½ teaspoon ground coriander

½ teaspoon smoked paprika

Salt

Pepper

Crema

½ cup sour cream

1 canned chipotle pepper, plus a teaspoon of adobo sauce

2 cloves garlic, minced

1 lime, half juiced, the other half sliced for garnish

Serving

12 soft corn tortillas or 1 package of street-taco size if you can find them

½ bunch fresh cilantro, leaves and tender stems

Tiny Cubes are back for a Mexican-spiced autumn taco! The spicy, smoky sauce and vibrant cilantro make this a roast-whatever's-in-your-CSA-box dinner that you'll crave on fall and winter nights. For a taco party, blend up a pitcher of Pear Pitcher Margaritas (page 257) and create a spread by adding warm pinto beans, avocado, and pickled onions.

1.   Preheat oven to 425°F.

2.   Spread root vegetables and onion onto a baking sheet. Toss with oil, spices, and ¾ teaspoon each salt and pepper.

3.   Roast for 35–40 minutes or until soft and slightly crispy around the edges, tossing halfway through.

4.   Place crema ingredients in a blender with ¼ teaspoon salt and puree until smooth. Add a bit more lime juice or water if it's too thick.

5.   Char the tortillas on both sides over an open flame, using tongs to flip. Spoon veggies down the middle of each taco, and serve with a drizzle of sauce, sprigs of cilantro, and limes for squeezing.

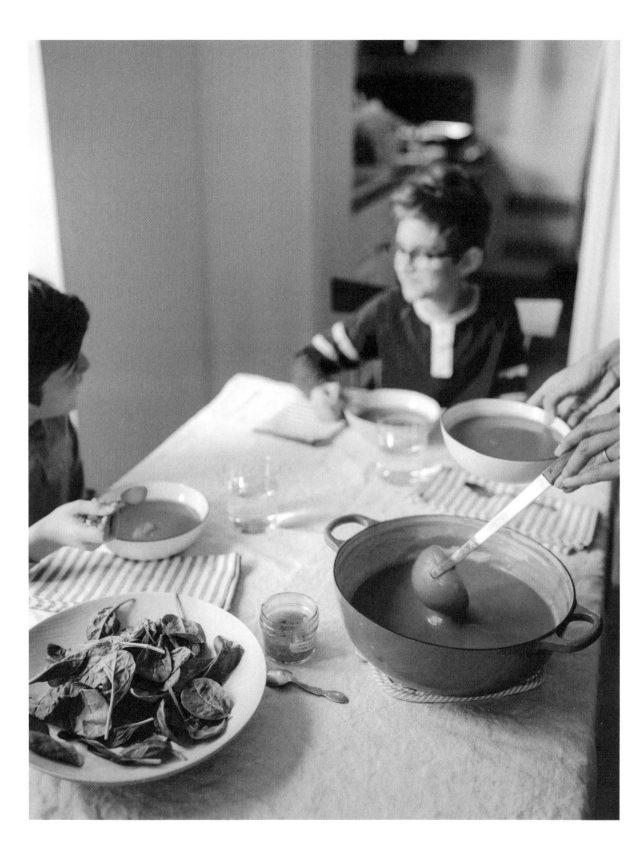

First Squash Soup

Serves: 6

---

2 tablespoons extra-virgin
olive oil

1 large yellow onion,
chopped

2 carrots, peeled and diced

3 stalks celery, diced

5 cloves garlic, minced

¼ teaspoon ground nutmeg

⅛ teaspoon cayenne pepper,
optional

2 teaspoons paprika

½ teaspoon curry powder

1 bay leaf

4 cups low-sodium chicken
or vegetable stock

1 medium butternut squash,
peeled and cut into cubes

1 teaspoon salt

1 teaspoon pepper

½ cup half-and-half or
coconut milk, up to 1 cup,
depending on taste

Optional, for serving:
¼ pound salad greens with
Amazing Apple Cider
Vinaigrette or crusty bread

This is autumn in a bowl. You make it with whatever squash calls your name at the market, when the air says it's officially fall.

1. Heat a Dutch oven or soup pot over medium heat and pour in olive oil.

2. Stir in onion, carrots, and celery. Sauté until veggies begin to soften, about 5 minutes. Add garlic, spices, and bay leaf; cook an additional minute.

3. Pour in the broth along with squash, salt, and pepper. Bring to a boil, then partially cover and reduce heat. Simmer until squash is fork-tender, 20–25 minutes.

4. Remove bay leaf and, using an immersion blender, puree the soup until completely smooth. Stir in half-and-half or coconut milk; taste for seasoning. If the soup is too thick, add a little water.

5. Serve hot with crusty bread, a simple salad, or grilled cheese and repeat all season long.

Amazing Apple Cider Vinaigrette

⅓ cup extra-virgin
olive oil

3 tablespoons apple cider
vinegar

1 tablespoon maple syrup

1 teaspoon Dijon mustard

½ shallot, minced

½ teaspoon salt

½ teaspoon pepper

Place all the ingredients in a jar, cover with the lid, and shake until emulsified. Refrigerate for up to a week.

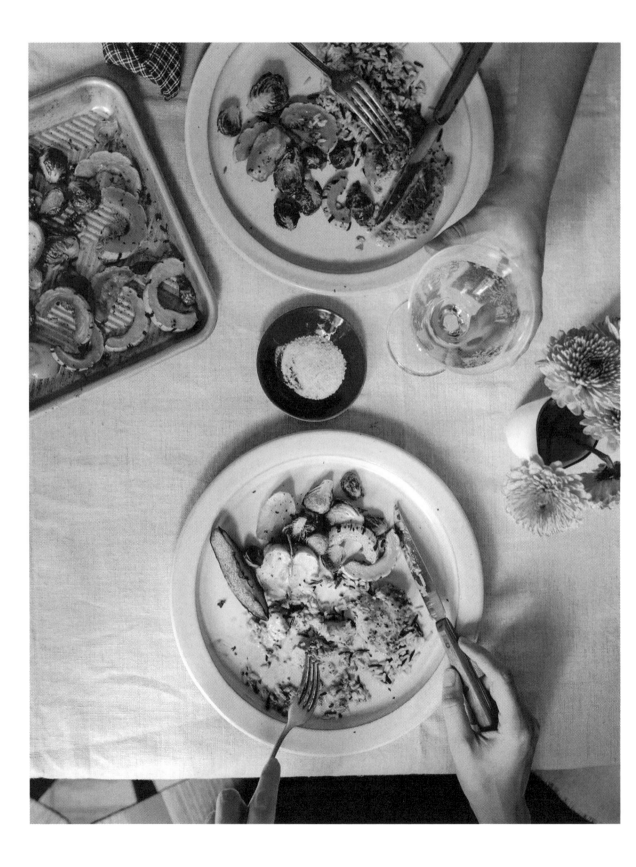

Pork Medallions with Creamy Rosemary Pan Sauce & Roasted Fall Veggies

Serves: 4

―――――――――

Roasted fall veggies & rice

1 delicata squash, cut in half lengthwise, seeds scooped, and sliced into ½-inch moons

1 small acorn squash, cut in half, seeds scooped, and sliced into ½-inch wedges

1-2 apples, ½-inch slices (keep seeds for prettier presentation)

½ pound Brussels sprouts, trimmed and halved

1 cup wild rice

Pork and pan sauce

1-2 tablespoons extra-virgin olive oil

1 pork tenderloin, cut into 8 medallions and pounded to flatten a bit

1 tablespoon butter

1 large shallot, finely chopped

½ cup dry white wine

1 tablespoon Dijon mustard

½ cup heavy cream

3 sprigs rosemary, leaves removed from stems and minced

1 teaspoon maple syrup

Salt

Pepper

Let's talk pan sauce. After you remove any seared meat from a pan, you're left with bits of browned goodness. Concentrated flavor waiting to be released, it just needs a little coaxing with a splash of wine and butter. Stir in any herbs you may have in the fridge, and voilà— you're basically a chef without the months of training.

1. Preheat oven to 400°F.

2. On a sheet pan, toss the squash, apples, and Brussels sprouts with oil and ½ teaspoon each salt and pepper. Transfer to oven and roast for 30 minutes or until squash is tender, flipping halfway through.

3. Cook wild rice according to package directions. Set aside.

4. Season each pork medallion with salt and pepper on both sides. Heat a sauté pan over medium-high heat and, when hot, add 2 tablespoons oil. Sear pork in batches, 2–3 minutes per side, until nicely browned. Transfer to a large plate and keep warm.

5. In the same pan, melt 1 tablespoon butter. Stir in shallot and cook until soft, 2 minutes. Deglaze with wine and let it reduce, another 2–3 minutes.

6. Whisk in mustard, cream, rosemary, and maple syrup with a pinch of salt; reduce heat to low.

7. After 1–2 minutes, place pork back in the pan to heat through. Serve immediately with the roasted vegetables and rice.

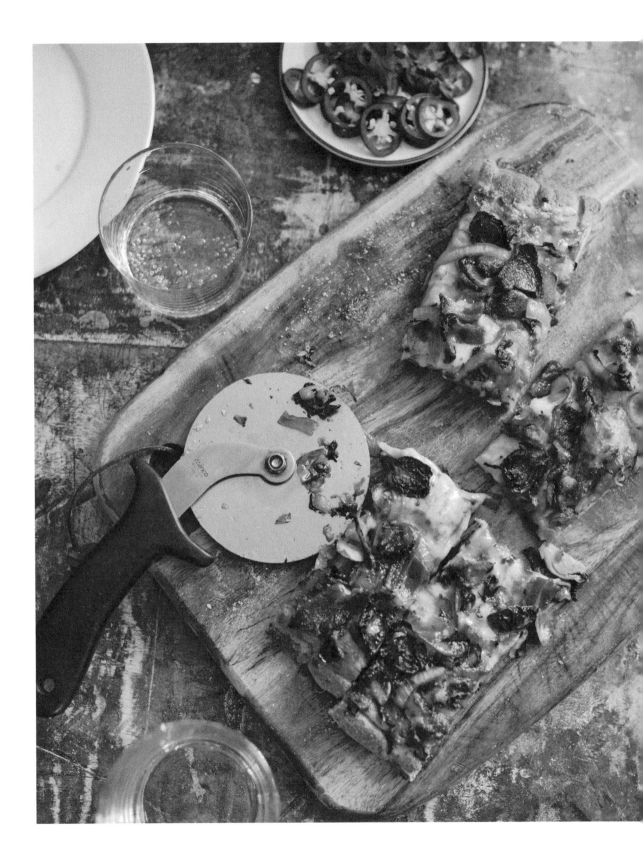

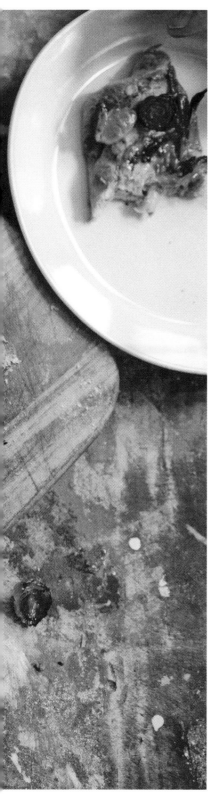

The Lumberjack Pizza with Brussels Sprouts & Bacon

Once upon a time in late November, a lumberjack walked into a Brooklyn pizza joint. All the hipsters thought he was from the neighborhood because of his beard and rugged boots, so they gave him a slice of their Brussels-sprout-and-bacon pizza. He was not a fan of green stuff, but to his surprise, his taste buds were very happy when he took a bite. He now has a garden full of green stuff and makes all kinds of things with them, but his favorite is this pizza. (After all, he is a lumberjack, and bacon reigns supreme.)

When you set this on the table, tell your kids Lumberjack Pizza is for dinner. And when they ask why it's called that, tell them, "Take a bite and I'll tell you a little story."

Giving recipes fun names to entice kids really works, and it's even successful with grown-ups. Stories aren't just for bedtime.

Serves: 4

---

5 slices bacon, cut into ½-inch pieces

1 large yellow or red onion, sliced

2 cloves garlic, minced

½ pound Brussels sprouts (outer leaves removed), sliced

2–3 sprigs fresh thyme, leaves removed from stems

16-ounce ball of homemade or store-bought pizza dough

2 tablespoons cornmeal

1 cup shredded mozzarella cheese

⅓ cup grated Parmesan cheese

Salt

Pepper

1.   Preheat oven to 500°F and move an oven rack to just below the broiler. Put a baking steel on the rack and let it get hot for 45–60 minutes. If you don't want to use the broiler during the last minute of baking, put the steel anywhere in your oven.

2.   Place bacon into a large sauté pan set over medium-low heat. Cook for about 5 minutes (once it's rendered some of its fat)—you don't want it too crispy because it will finish in the oven. Remove bacon with a slotted spoon and set aside.

3. Increase heat to medium-high and add onion, garlic, and Brussels sprouts to the bacon fat. Season with ¼ teaspoon salt and ½ teaspoon pepper. Sauté for 7–8 minutes, stirring occasionally, until veggies are fully cooked. Remove from heat and stir in thyme. Set aside.

4. Divide the pizza dough in half to make two pizzas. Holding the first piece in your hands, begin to gently stretch it into a round or oval shape. Stretching instead of rolling allows those delicious bubbles to form.

5. Spread 1 tablespoon cornmeal onto a pizza peel, then place the stretched pizza dough on top; continue stretching until it's very thin. Throughout the topping process, make sure the dough can move around on the peel. Lift and add more cornmeal wherever it's sticking.

6. Top with half the mozzarella cheese, leaving a border around the edges, followed by half the Brussels sprouts and bacon. Sprinkle with half the Parmesan cheese.

7. Working quickly (but carefully), slide the pizza onto the baking steel. Bake for 5–7 minutes or until crust is golden brown and cooked through and cheese is bubbly. Then turn the broiler on for another minute. Make sure to check after 30 seconds, because things go from charred to completely burnt in a matter of seconds.

8. Prepare the second pizza while the first one is baking. Cut and serve immediately.

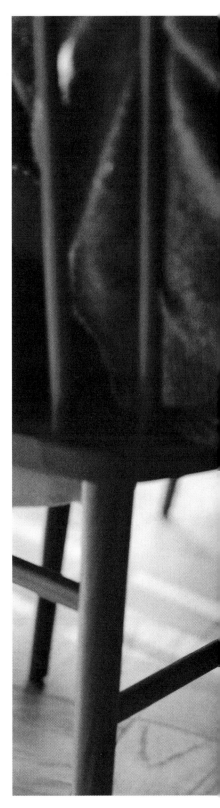

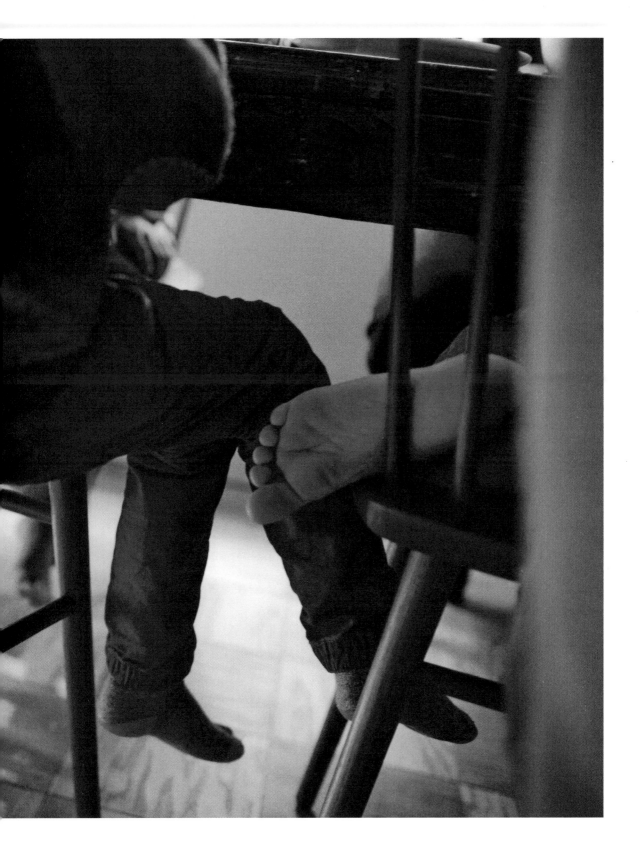

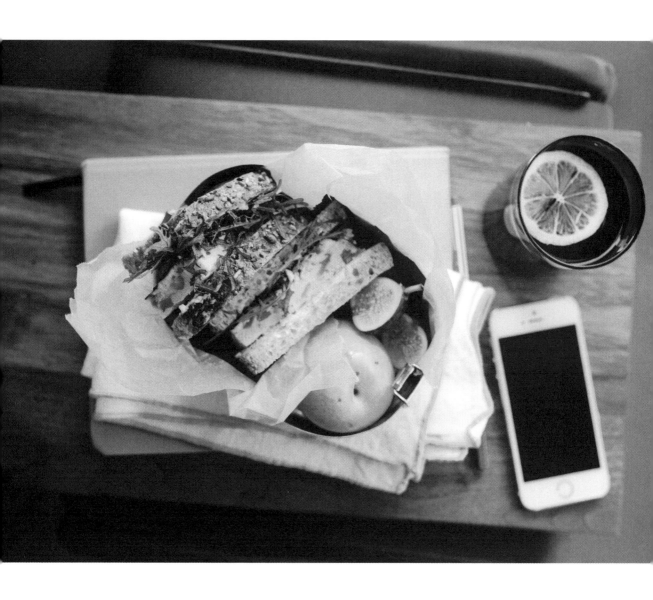

Neighborhood Café Frittata Sandwich with Early-Autumn Fruit

Serves: 4

Frittata

7 large eggs

I tablespoon extra-virgin olive oil, for the skillet

I medium yellow onion, finely diced

I large red sweet pepper, finely diced

3 cloves garlic, minced

I tablespoon unsalted butter, for the pan

3 ounces chèvre

2 tablespoons mixed herbs: parsley, dill, and/or chives

Salt

Pepper

Sandwich

8 slices good, grainy bread that's really soft on the inside and crusty on the outside

⅓ cup mayonnaise

I small bunch delicate greens

Wrapped in parchment or tucked into a steel lunch box, this is the ultimate way to create inspiring café vibes for a portable breakfast or lunch. It's also just the thing for feeding a crowd. Pack with fleeting late-summer or early-autumn fruits like market grapes, fresh figs, husk cherries, or pluots.

1. Preheat oven to 375°F.

2. Crack the eggs into a medium bowl and whisk well with ½ teaspoon each salt and pepper. Set aside.

3. Heat oil in a skillet set over medium heat. Once it's hot, add onion and pepper with a pinch of salt, stirring occasionally for 5–7 minutes, until soft. Add the garlic during the last 30 seconds; turn off the heat.

4. Butter an 8-by-8-inch baking pan; scrape in the vegetables and spread evenly.

5. Pour eggs carefully over vegetables. Dollop spoonfuls of chèvre throughout, then scatter herbs over the top, pushing them into the mixture a little.

6. Bake for about 15 minutes or until eggs just slightly quiver. Set aside to cool. You can make this a day ahead, too, so you can wake up and pack your sandwich in less than 5 minutes.

7. Slice frittata into 4 squares. Spread mayo (add grated garlic for a slight kick) on bread slices and sandwich in frittata squares with a handful of greens.

Seasonal frittata variations

Spring: asparagus, feta, dill-chive mayo
Summer: poblano and corn, cheddar, chipotle mayo
Autumn: squash and leeks, asiago, rosemary mayo
Winter: shredded kale and carrots, Gruyère, garlic mayo

One-Bowl Banana Pumpkin Pancakes

Serves: 4

(makes about 16 pancakes)

————————

1 ripe banana, about
¹/₃ cup mashed

¹/₃ cup pumpkin puree

¼ cup coconut sugar

1 cup oat milk

1 tablespoon coconut oil,
melted, plus extra for pan

2 teaspoons vanilla extract

1 cup oat bran

2 tablespoons wheat germ

2 tablespoons ground
flaxseed

2 teaspoons baking powder

¹/₈ teaspoon salt

Maple syrup, whipped cream,
and/or pats of butter
for serving

There's something incredibly satisfying about making these pancakes on a fall morning. Mixing the pumpkin with so many harvesty grains feels like stirring up the season in a bowl.

1. Grab a large bowl and mash in the banana, then add pumpkin, sugar, milk, coconut oil, and vanilla. Mix well.

2. Add the oat bran, wheat germ, flaxseed, baking powder, and salt; stir to combine. Let the batter sit for 5–10 minutes to thicken.

3. Set a nonstick griddle over medium-low heat and brush with coconut oil.

4. Once it's hot, add 2 tablespoons batter for each pancake, leaving a few inches between them. Nudge batter just a tiny bit into a circle.

5. Cook for 2–3 minutes, until speckled and browned underneath; flip and cook for another 2 minutes.

6. Transfer to a plate and keep warm. Serve with toppings.

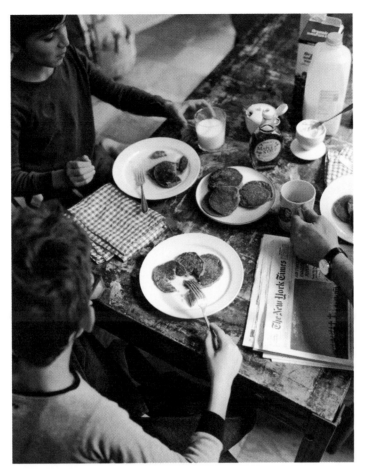

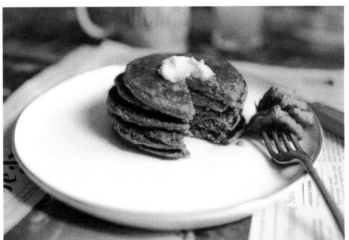

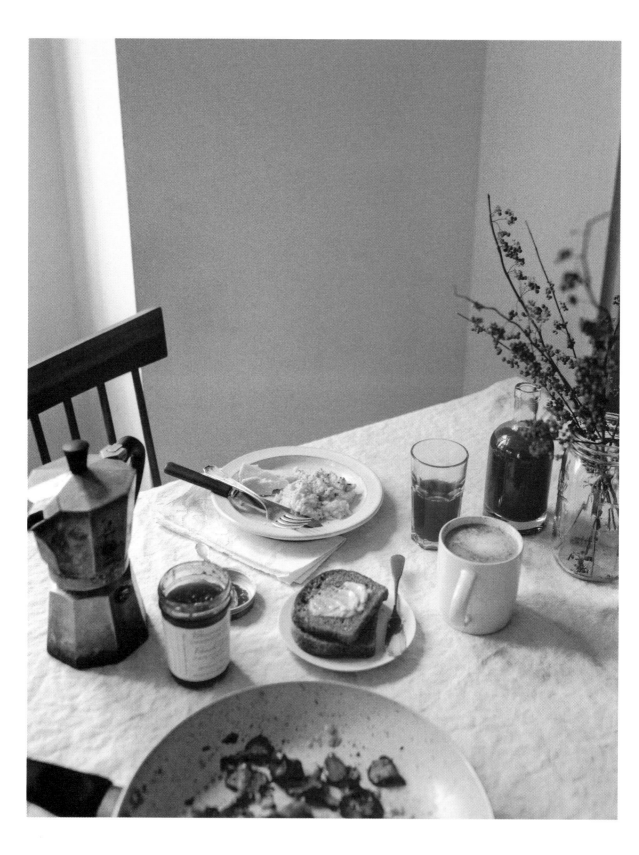

Fall Scramble with Market Mushrooms & Aged Cheese

Serves: 2

_____

3 tablespoons unsalted butter, divided

10 ounces mixed mushrooms, large ones sliced in half or quartered

2 tablespoons fresh herbs: a mix of parsley, thyme, and/or basil, chopped

5 large eggs

Salt

Pepper

1 ounce aged cheddar, sliced, for serving

4 slices hearty bread, toasted, for serving

Rethink mushrooms—have them for breakfast. And when we say "mushrooms," we mean delicately flavored, buttery market ones, not the bland, grayish sponge-like ones usually found at the grocery store. They're the reason people say, "I hate mushrooms."

1. Heat a large sauté pan over medium-high heat. Once hot, swirl in 2 tablespoons butter and add mushrooms in an even layer. Don't stir too often or you'll have gray, soggy mushrooms instead of slightly brown, caramelized ones. Just shake the pan occasionally; they take 5–7 minutes to cook. Add a mix of any leftover herbs you have. Parsley really shines here.

2. In a medium bowl, beat the eggs until really frothy. The more air you incorporate into them, the more fluffy they'll be when you cook them. Add a little water (about 1 tablespoon) and ¼ teaspoon each salt and pepper.

3. Melt the remaining tablespoon of butter in a nonstick pan over medium-low heat. Add the eggs. Stir continuously in swiping motions, keeping the eggs from the edge of the pan. Cook until not quite fully set (about 3–4 minutes); they will continue cooking in the pan off the heat. This prevents overcooked, rubbery eggs.

4. Serve immediately with the mushrooms, cheese, and good toast.

Huckle's Multigrain Harvest Muffins

Makes 12 muffins

―――――――――

½ cup oats

1 cup walnuts, chopped

8 tablespoons unsalted butter, divided
(2 tablespoons cut into small pieces, 6 tablespoons melted)

1 cup whole wheat flour

½ cup cornmeal

½ cup ground flaxseed

½ cup wheat germ

½ cup oat bran

¾ cup sugar

½ teaspoon salt

2 teaspoons baking powder

½ teaspoon baking soda

¾ cup buttermilk,
at room temperature

2 large eggs,
at room temperature

2 teaspoons vanilla extract

2 apples, peeled and grated

Most "muffins" are really cupcakes in disguise. A breakfast muffin should (1) be dense and moist, (2) use nutty, whole-grain flours, and (3) not be ridiculously sweet. A real muffin tides you over until lunch.

1.   Preheat oven to 350°F. On a small sheet pan, mix oats and walnuts together and add butter pieces on top. Transfer to the oven for 10–12 minutes, until everything gets a little color and smells toasty.

2.   Meanwhile, in a large bowl, whisk all the dry ingredients together.

3.   In a measuring cup, combine buttermilk, eggs, melted butter, and vanilla. Mix well with a fork.

4.   Pour the wet ingredients into the dry using a spatula.

5.   Fold in grated apples.

6.   Grease a 12-cup muffin tray or use liners, and fill each to the top with batter (these are mega muffins). Top with the oat-walnut mix and bake for 25 minutes or until a toothpick comes out clean.

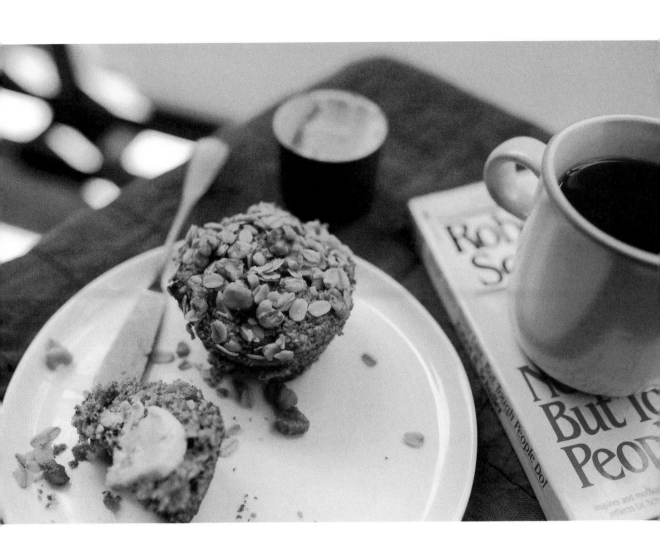

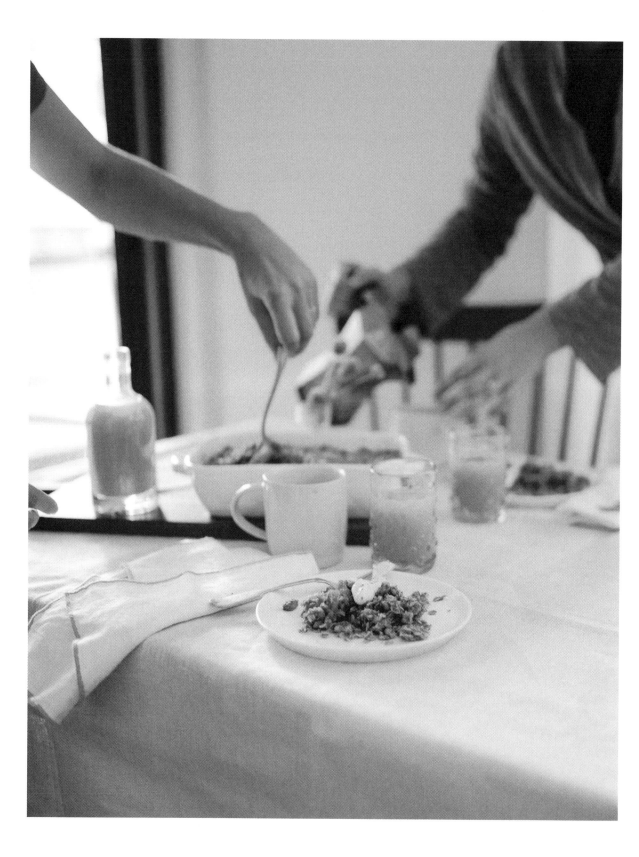

Apple-Walnut Breakfast Crisp

Serves: 6

_____

5 baking apples–Granny Smith, Braeburn, Jonagold, or Winesap–peeled, cored, and cut into chunks

Juice of ½ lemon, about 2 teaspoons

1½ teaspoons ground cinnamon, divided

¼ teaspoon ground nutmeg

1½ cups rolled oats

¼ teaspoon salt

¾ cup walnuts, chopped

½ cup almond or cashew meal

½ cup maple syrup

½ cup coconut oil, melted

Yogurt, ice cream, or coconut whipped cream, for serving

One autumn morning you'll wake up and see nature's cue that the seasons are changing: a blanket of white frost. This is what farmers wait and plan for. It's when growing season officially ends and all of nature shifts gears to signal hibernation prep. Which, in turn, is our cue to bake, bake, bake. On cold mornings, slide this crisp in the oven and wake everyone up with wafts of warm spices and baking apples.

1. Preheat oven to 350°F.

2. In a 9-by-13-inch baking dish, toss the apples with lemon juice, ½ teaspoon cinnamon, and the nutmeg.

3. In a bowl, mix the oats, 1 teaspoon cinnamon, salt, walnuts, and nut meal.

4. In a liquid measuring cup, measure the maple syrup and coconut oil and whisk to combine. Pour over oat mix and stir to coat well.

5. Spoon oat mixture evenly over the apples, transfer the baking dish to the oven, and bake for 35 minutes or until apples are bubbling and topping is golden brown.

6. If you'd like, serve with yogurt for breakfast (or ice cream for dessert).

Apple-Picking Shrub (and a Cocktail)

Serves: 2

_____

Shrub

I pound really good apples, any sweet-tart varieties

I cup apple cider vinegar

½ cup sugar

¼ teaspoon vanilla extract

⅛ teaspoon ground cinnamon

⅛ teaspoon ground cardamom

⅛ teaspoon ground nutmeg or mace

Cocktail

I tablespoon sugar

½ teaspoon pumpkin spice mix

Crushed ice

2 sprigs fresh rosemary, divided

Juice of ½ lemon

3 ounces vodka

1½ ounces Apple-Picking Shrub (recipe above)

Shrubs might sound complicated and kombucha-ish, but the process couldn't be easier. Use any mix of sweet-tart varieties to add complexity to the flavor—Crispin, Gala, Granny Smith, Honeycrisp, Fuji, Braeburn, Pink Lady, Jonagold, Winesap, or Gravenstein. This is perfect for when your apple-picking apples don't look like they'll last much longer.

1. Shrub: Chop the apples and place in a high-speed blender along with the vinegar; puree well.

2. Pour into a mason jar, using a spatula to scrape out everything; stir in sugar and spices.

3. Cover and let this sit out at room temperature for 6–8 hours, then refrigerate for 2–3 days.

4. Strain into another jar, pressing down well on the solids to extract every last bit of syrup. Keep in the fridge for up to 3 weeks, and pour yourself a drink whenever the mood strikes.

5. Ways to serve: (1) Fill a glass a quarter of the way with shrub, then top with sparkling water. (2) Make a cocktail, like this:

6. Cocktail: To make the spiced sugar mixture for the rim, combine sugar and spices on a small, flat plate.

7. Prep two coupes or small glasses. Rub around the rims with the juiced lemon half. Dip rims in sugar-spice mixture. Fill both glasses halfway with crushed ice.

8. In a cocktail shaker, muddle one of the rosemary sprigs; toss in a handful of ice.

9. Pour in lemon juice, vodka, and shrub. Shake for 10 seconds.

10. Divide between glasses and garnish each with ½ sprig rosemary. Cheers!

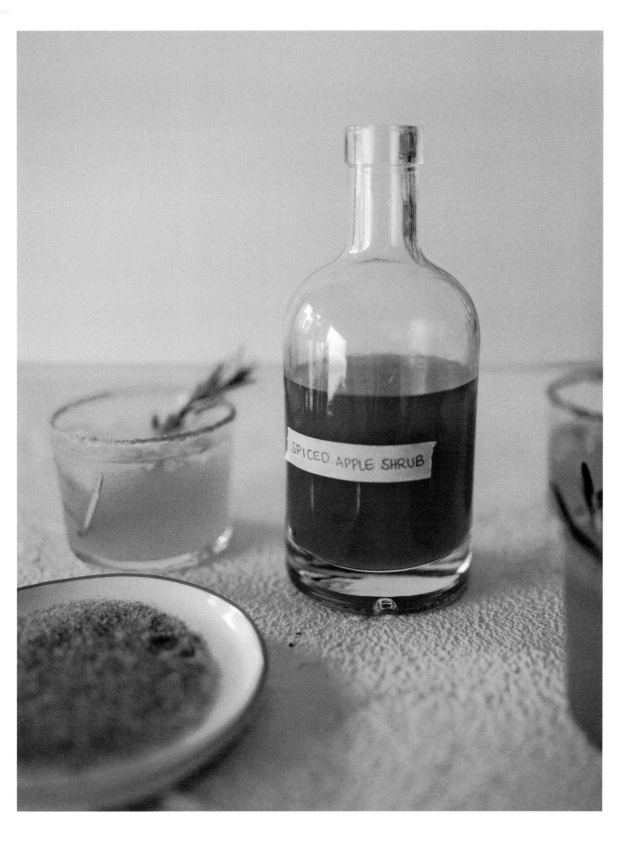

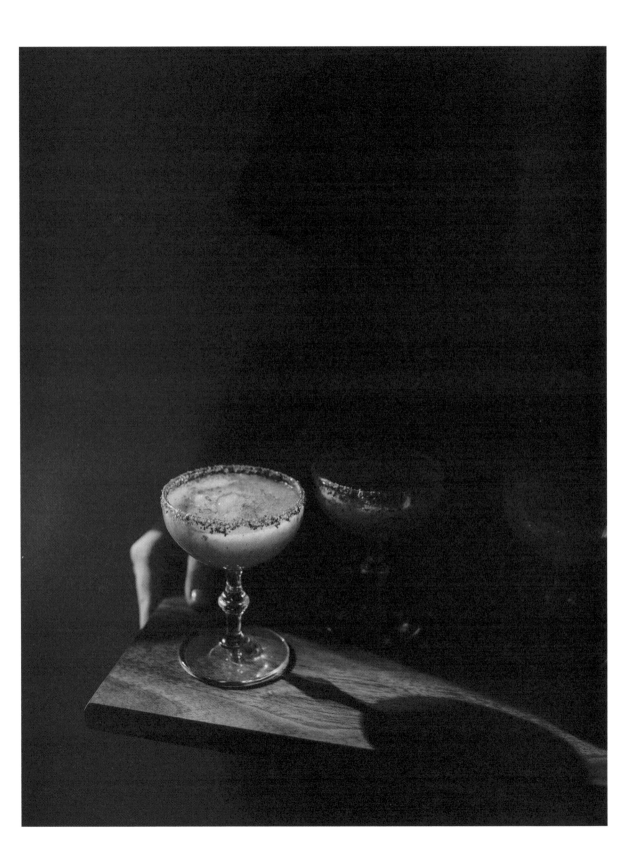

Pear Pitcher Margaritas with Chile-Lime Rims

Serves: 4

_____

Margarita

2 ripe Bosc or Bartlett pears

$1/3$ cup lime juice, from about 3 limes

$2/3$ cup tequila blanco

2 tablespoons maple syrup

Ice cubes, for the blender and each glass

A small handful fresh cilantro, leaves and tender stems

Cardamom bitters, optional

Rim salt

2 teaspoons chile powder

2 teaspoons fine salt

1 teaspoon lime zest, from one of the above limes pre-juicing

Fuel an entire fall fiesta with the push of a blender button. There are no bottled pear concentrates or simple syrups to simmer, and the result is a refreshing burst of spicy, crisp autumn flavors. It's something you'd imagine sipping at the bar of a trendy modern taqueria, except you pulled it off at home, without any of the individual cocktail shaking. For a larger crowd, make extra pitchers a few hours before to have in the fridge and just keep 'em coming.

1. Peel pears and scoop out just the seeds; the slightly harder parts of the flesh will puree well. Chop into large chunks and place in the blender.

2. Add lime juice, tequila, maple syrup, and ¾ cup ice. Give everything a long whir until you have a smoothie-like consistency. Add the cilantro and pulse a few more times for green, herby flecks.

3. Now let the flavors mingle in the blender while you prepare the rims.

4. On a small plate, mix the chile powder, salt, and lime zest.

5. Grab 4 glasses—about 6-ish ounces each. Run one of the spent lime wedges along each rim, then dip in the salt mixture, evenly coating the rim.

6. Fill glasses halfway with ice, add 1–2 dashes of optional bitters, then pour 4 margaritas for 4 lucky people.

Pear Galette with So Much Hazelnut Crumble

Serves: 4

Dough

1½ cups all-purpose flour

¼ teaspoon salt

2 tablespoons sugar

8 tablespoons unsalted butter, really cold and cut into ½-inch pieces

⅓ cup ice water

I large egg, beaten (with a splash of water), for egg wash

Hazelnut crumble

½ cup hazelnut meal (you can do this in a food processor)

3 tablespoons sugar

Pear filling

3 pears, ripe but firm

½ teaspoon ground cinnamon

I teaspoon vanilla extract

I teaspoon lemon juice

2 tablespoons sugar

3 tablespoons unsalted butter, cut into small pieces

Vanilla ice cream, for serving

Kinda like a pie, but half the work and twice the fancy.

1. Whisk flour, salt, and 2 tablespoons sugar in a large bowl.

2. Toss cold cubed butter into the flour mix and, using a pastry cutter, cut the butter into tiny pieces until it looks like crumbled dough.

3. Add half the ice water and use a rubber spatula to fold the flour over, pressing down. You're not stirring, but rather lifting and pressing down, adding more water as you go. Test the dough by squeezing lightly with your hand. If it doesn't hold together, add another tablespoon of ice water. Shape the dough into a flat disk and cover with plastic wrap. Refrigerate for at least 1 hour, up to 3 days.

4. In a small bowl, mix the hazelnut meal and 3 tablespoons sugar.

5. Thinly slice pears on a mandoline. In a bowl, gently toss with cinnamon, vanilla, lemon juice, and 2 tablespoons sugar.

6. Take the dough out of the fridge and roll it out into a 12-inch circle on a lightly floured surface. If it's too cold and hard to roll, wait 5 minutes. Don't worry about the perfect circle—the beauty of a galette is its rustic appearance.

7. Fold dough in half and then in half again and transfer to a sheet pan. Unfold and spread the hazelnut mix on top, leaving a 2-inch border.

8. Add ⅓ of the sliced pears, keeping that 2-inch border, and dot with 1 tablespoon of butter pieces. Repeat two more times until you have a beautiful butter-topped mound of pears in the middle. Fold the dough edges up over the pears, to make a 2-inch rim.

9. Transfer galette to the fridge for 30 minutes to chill (flaky crust).

10. Preheat oven to 375°F.

11. Brush galette with egg wash and transfer to the oven for 45 minutes or until crust is golden brown and a knife cuts through the pears easily. Allow to cool slightly. Get that vanilla ice cream out and serve. Or pack it and take it to a friend's house.

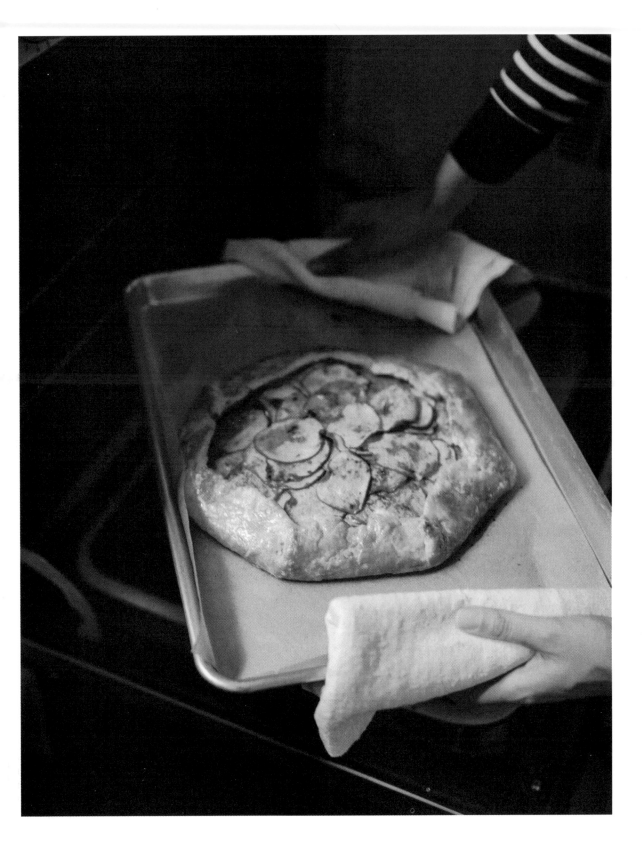

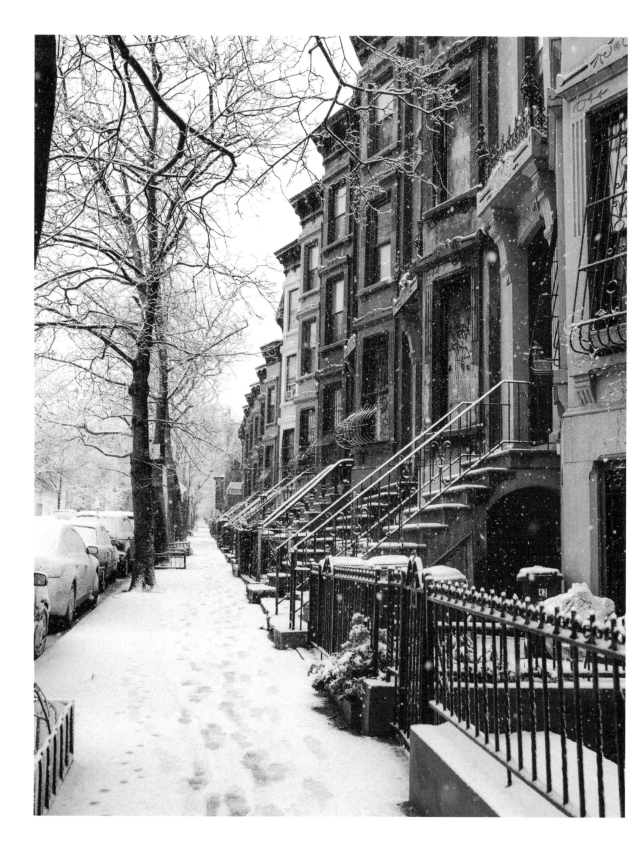

Winter

NOTICE WHAT'S HAPPENING OUTSIDE (NATURE) . . .

More than any other season, we want to hurry winter along, fast-forward to the next season. But the bareness, deadness, cold—it's all necessary. Animals hibernate; plants transition to a state of dormancy, holding their energy in reserve, building up for new growth later. There's a pause. Because, come springtime, growth won't be as abundant without it.

. . . AND INSIDE (HUMAN NATURE)

Instead of wishing winter away, embrace her wisdom and use it for reflection, self-acceptance, and waiting with peace. She's a tough grandma who wants us to rest well and make quality time for others. Transformation begins in the pause. So get cozy. When you feel your coziest, you'll want to share that feeling with others. The best traditions and holidays happen in winter—memories shared around the fire and in the kitchen are often the ones that get passed down from generation to generation. Cherish them and start new ones to pass along.

HERE'S WHAT TO LOOK FORWARD TO:

Catching snowflakes on your tongue, hot toddies, candles and evening tea, building a snowman, snowball fights, hot chocolate with massive marshmallows, night sledding on the steepest hill you can find, baking cookies, a really good blanket, flannel pj's, caroling on Christmas Eve, skiing, trimming the tree, holiday parties.

Your Winter Kitchen Plan

COOK 3X A WEEK:

Choose three dinners.

Add on breakfasts, something

sweet, and a drink, too, if you'd

like. Make a grocery list.

Remember to think in

cooking categories (page 34)

and add a new kitchen habit that

will help you stick to your

plan (pages 31-51).

After 4 weeks, mix and match

favorite recipes to cook the rest

of the season.

Week 1

Monday	Charred Brussels Sprouts Carbonara
Tuesday	Tacos Americano
Wednesday	The Chicken Caesar Salad
Thursday	Seared Fish with Sage Caper Pan Sauce Skillet Carrots & Parsnips
Friday	Friday Night Baked Potato Bar

Week 2

Monday	Don't-Get-Takeout Takeout
Tuesday	Game Night Nachos with Homemade Queso & Charred Cauliflower
Wednesday	Repeat Red Lentil Soup
Thursday	Extra-Crispy Pork Schnitzel with Leek & Cabbage Sauté
Friday	Beef Braise (to Spoon over Rutabaga Mash)

Week 3

Monday	Bolognese with Broken Lasagna & Broken Rules
Tuesday	Easiest Chicken Taqueria Tacos
Wednesday	Persian Winter Vegetable Stew with a Lot of Herbs
Thursday	Sticky Korean Ribs with Creamy Savoy Slaw
Friday	Zuppa Toscana

Week 4

Monday	Roasted Romanesco & Toasted Farro with Warm Cherry Pepper Vinaigrette
Tuesday	The Best Crispy Fish Tacos I Had in Tulum
Wednesday	Bistro Celery Root & Leek Soup with Pumpernickel Croutons
Thursday	You Can Roast a Whole Chicken (with Rosemary Roasted Potatoes)
Friday	Famous BBQ Chicken Pizza with Extra Cilantro

Breakfasts, Drinks, Something Sweet

Breakfast	PaperGal Breakfast Sandwich
Breakfast	Very Vanilla Steel-Cut Oats with Baked Pears
Breakfast	Huevos Hacedores
Breakfast	Lemon-Poppy Pancakes with Warm Berry Compote
Happy Hour	Grapefruit-Fennel & Allspice Gimlet
Happy Hour	Apricot Bourbon Smash
Drink	Miracle Elixir
Sweet	Coconut Lime Loaf
Sweet	Say-Anything Cake

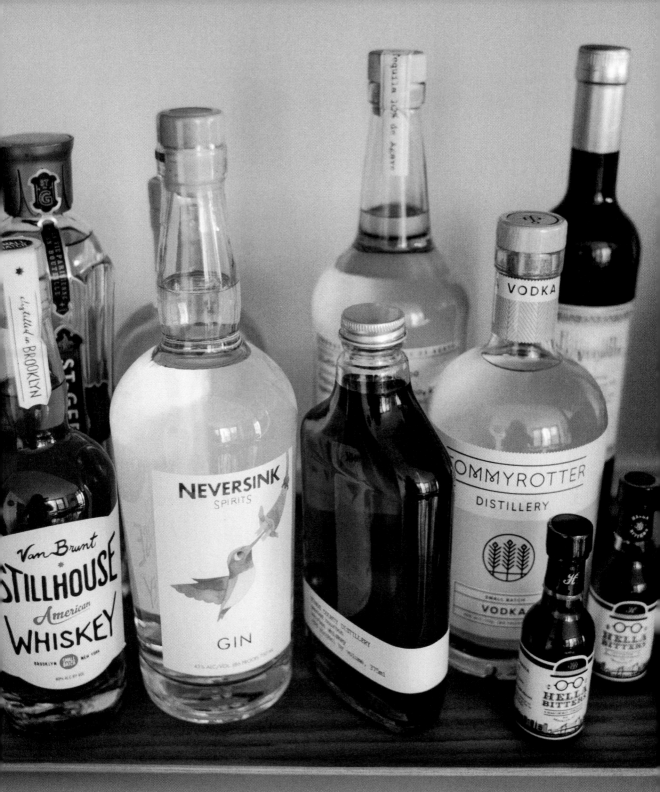

Charred Brussels Sprouts Carbonara

Serves: 4

½ pound Brussels sprouts, large ones if possible

½ pound short ruffled pasta, like reginetti or campanelle

4 ounces pancetta or bacon, finely diced

2 large eggs, super fresh and the best you can find, beaten

½ cup freshly grated Parmesan or Pecorino Romano cheese, or a combination of both

2 tablespoons unsalted butter

Extra-virgin olive oil

Salt

Pepper

This is a humble and filling snowed-in kind of dinner. Pasta water is used to make the sauce, and there's just a handful of other ingredients you probably already have.

1. Preheat oven to 375°F. Remove leaves from Brussels sprouts; slice the stems so you can easily separate into leaves. When you're down to the hearts and can't remove any more leaves, keep them—you'll roast those, too.

2. Drizzle the sprouts with a tablespoon or so of oil on a sheet pan, sprinkle generously with salt and pepper, and toss to coat well. Keep the hearts and leaves separated on the sheet pan. Slide into the oven for 10–15 minutes or until leaves are browned in some spots and crispy; transfer leaves to a plate and continue roasting the hearts for 5–10 more minutes, until browned and tender. Transfer hearts to the plate, too.

3. Meanwhile, bring a large pot of well-salted water to a rolling boil. Cook pasta just 1 minute shy of package directions, right before it's al dente. Reserve a cup of salty, starchy pasta water and drain pasta. Or time it well and use a spider strainer to transfer pasta directly to the pan (in step 6) and leave water in the pot.

4. Set a large sauté pan over medium-high heat and cook pancetta, stirring often, for 5–8 minutes, until browned and just slightly crisp. Transfer to Brussels sprout plate.

5. Meanwhile, in a measuring cup, beat eggs with the cheese, a pinch of salt, and a few cracks of pepper, and gradually stream in ½ cup hot pasta water while continuing to beat. This tempers the eggs without turning them to scrambled eggs.

6. Turn heat down to low under the pan with pancetta fat. Working quickly, pour in egg mix and butter. Whisk to form a silky sauce. Add pasta, tossing to coat well. Use more pasta water if needed to thin the sauce. Taste for seasoning.

7. Add in reserved Brussels sprouts and pancetta. Grate extra cheese on top, then dig in!

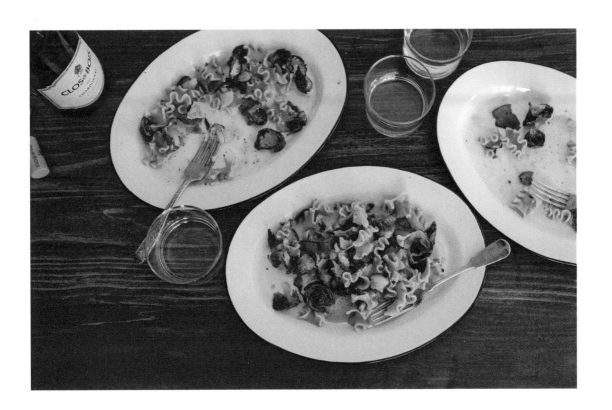

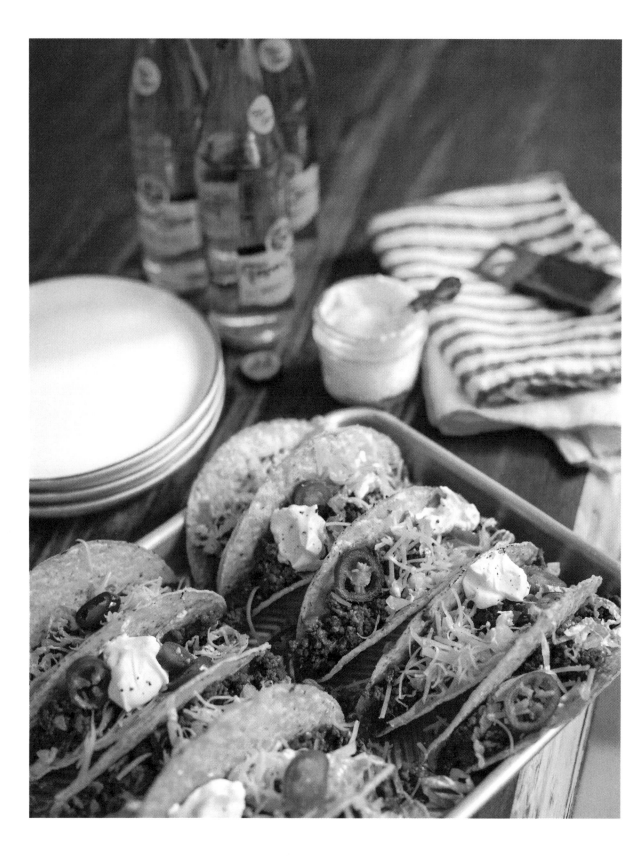

Tacos Americano

Serves: 4

_____

1 tablespoon extra-virgin olive oil

1 yellow onion, diced

3 cloves garlic, minced

2 teaspoons chili powder

1 teaspoon ground cumin

1 teaspoon dried oregano

1 teaspoon ground coriander

1 teaspoon paprika

3 tablespoons tomato paste

1 pound ground beef

1 cup water

1 teaspoon coconut sugar

1 teaspoon salt

½ teaspoon pepper

8–12 hard taco shells

½ head romaine lettuce, finely chopped

4 ounces sharp cheddar cheese, shredded

Sour cream, for serving

Pickled jalapeños, for serving

That quintessential, inauthentic taco from our childhoods, all grown up. This is one of our ultimate go-to dinners, which is on the table in no time. Since everyone asks for seconds, sometimes we add a can of beans to stretch it out.

1. Heat oil in a sauté pan over medium heat.

2. Add onion and cook until soft, about 2 minutes. Stir in garlic and spices for 1 minute. Add tomato paste, stirring occasionally for 2 more minutes.

3. Add the ground beef, breaking it up into tiny bits with a wooden spoon; cook until no longer pink, about 5 minutes.

4. Pour in water with coconut sugar, salt, and pepper. Stir well, cover, and simmer for 15 minutes.

5. Serve in hard taco shells with romaine, cheese, sour cream, and pickled jalapeños.

The Chicken Caesar Salad

Serves: 4

Croutons

½ loaf good bread,
cut into cubes

3 tablespoons extra-virgin
olive oil, more if needed

½ teaspoon turmeric

1 teaspoon dried thyme

½ teaspoon paprika

Dressing

1 egg yolk

1 clove garlic (2 if you're like
us and love things garlicky)

1 teaspoon anchovy paste

2 teaspoons Dijon mustard

1 teaspoon Worcestershire
sauce

2 teaspoons red wine vinegar

Juice of ½ lemon
(about 1 tablespoon needed)

2 tablespoons Parmesan
cheese, grated

½ cup grapeseed oil,
or any neutral oil

Chicken

3 boneless, skinless chicken
breasts, about 1¼ pounds,
pounded to an even thickness

1 tablespoon lemon pepper
seasoning

1½ teaspoons paprika

Extra-virgin olive oil

We haven't met anyone who doesn't love a good Caesar salad. Even kids. Yet most of us think icky thoughts when we learn there are *anchovies* in the dressing. Ironically, they're the whole reason we love this salad so much. That's why restaurant dishes taste so complex and multidimensional—they layer the stinky, intense, and exotic. Push the boundaries in your kitchen, too.

1. Preheat oven to 350°F.

2. On a sheet pan, toss the bread with oil, spices, and ¼ teaspoon each salt and pepper. Spread in one even layer and transfer to the oven for 15 minutes or until lightly browned. Let cool. If not using immediately, store in an airtight container for up to 3 days.

3. In a medium bowl, whisk together all the dressing ingredients (except oil) with ½ teaspoon each salt and pepper.

4. In a slow, steady stream, drizzle in oil, whisking constantly (it helps to put the bowl on a kitchen towel to keep it steady) to get a thick dressing. Add a tablespoon of water and whisk to thin the consistency, adding more if you'd like. Taste for salt and pepper. Refrigerate for up to 3 days.

5. Season both sides of chicken with lemon pepper, paprika, and ½ teaspoon each salt and pepper.

6. In a skillet, drizzle 1–2 tablespoons oil and set over medium-high heat.

7. Once pan is hot, sear the chicken for 3–4 minutes, until slightly crispy on edges. Turn over and cook for another 2–3 minutes or until chicken feels firm to the touch. Transfer to a plate and keep warm.

8. Toss romaine with a couple of tablespoons of dressing to lightly coat. Serve with sliced chicken, plenty of Parmesan, croutons, and extra dressing on the side.

Salad

2 heads romaine, chopped

Parmesan cheese, shaved or grated

Salt

Pepper

To make into wraps for lunch: Warm large flour tortillas in microwave or hold over an open flame for a few seconds. Spread Caesar dressing to your heart's content and add a handful of romaine, sliced chicken, and some Parmesan cheese. Then roll snugly and slice in half.

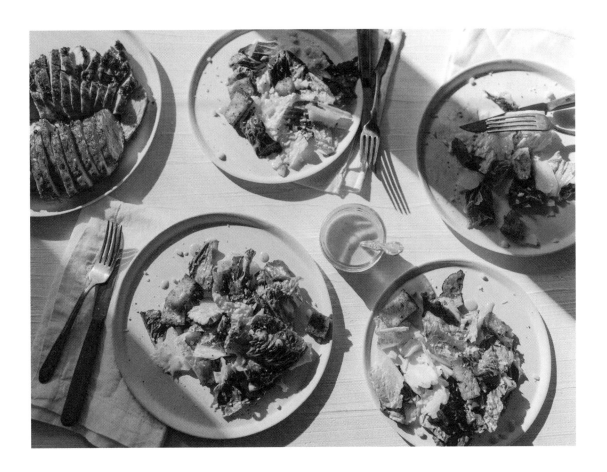

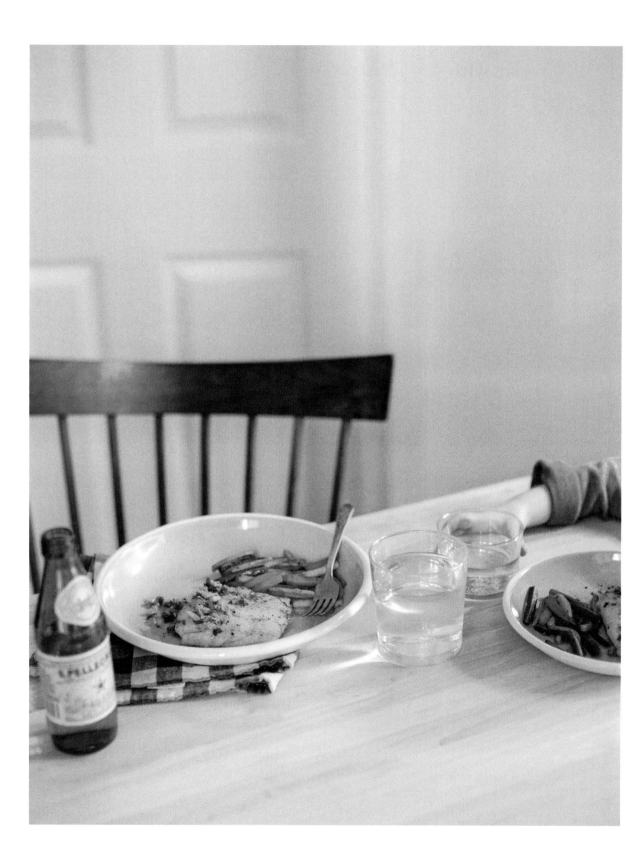

Seared Fish with Sage Caper Pan Sauce

Serves: 4

———————

4 haddock fillets, or any white fish, 1¼ pounds

2 tablespoons all-purpose flour

1 tablespoon extra-virgin olive oil

4 tablespoons unsalted butter, divided

1 small shallot, minced

2 cloves garlic, minced

¼ teaspoon crushed red pepper

⅓ cup dry white wine

½ cup low-sodium vegetable stock

1 lemon, half thinly sliced, the other half zested and juiced

3 tablespoons capers, drained

2 tablespoons fresh sage, minced

2 tablespoons fresh Italian parsley, minced

Salt

Pepper

This is the antidote to any gray winter day and also the answer to getting out of your stretchy pants after all the holiday baking. Light, briny, bright, herby, with just a *liiittle* butter.

1.   Season the fish generously with salt and pepper. Put the flour in a shallow bowl and dredge the fillets on both sides, shaking off the excess.

2.   Heat a large sauté pan over medium-high heat. Add olive oil and 1 tablespoon butter. Once the butter foams, cook fish for 2–3 minutes on each side until nicely browned and fish is no longer translucent. Total time will depend on the thickness of fish. Transfer to a warm plate. Do this in 2 batches if the pan isn't big enough.

3.   In the same pan, melt another tablespoon of butter, add shallot, and sauté, stirring occasionally, for 2–3 minutes. Stir in garlic and crushed red pepper. After 30 seconds, whisk in the wine and vegetable stock, getting all the brown bits.

4.   When the wine and stock reduce a bit (about 5 minutes), add the lemon juice, zest, capers, the remaining 2 tablespoons of butter, and ¼ teaspoon each salt and pepper. Simmer a couple more minutes, until the sauce thickens, then add in lemon slices and fresh herbs.

5.   Gently lay the fish back in to warm through; then serve with Skillet Carrots & Parsnips.

Skillet Carrots & Parsnips

1 tablespoon unsalted butter

1 tablespoon extra-virgin olive oil

3 carrots, peeled and sliced into matchsticks

2 parsnips, peeled and sliced into matchsticks

½ teaspoon all-purpose seasoning

Salt

Pepper

This is root veggies proving they can be a quick, weeknight side—glazed in butter, with a pinch of seasoning, and no sheet pan to wash.

1. Set a skillet over medium heat and swirl in the butter and oil.

2. Once hot, add the carrot and parsnip matchsticks. Sprinkle with a really big pinch of salt. Crack in some pepper and add the all-purpose seasoning. Stir occasionally for 3–4 minutes to get a little color, then cover for another 3–4 minutes to steam through, until vegetables are tender. Serve right away.

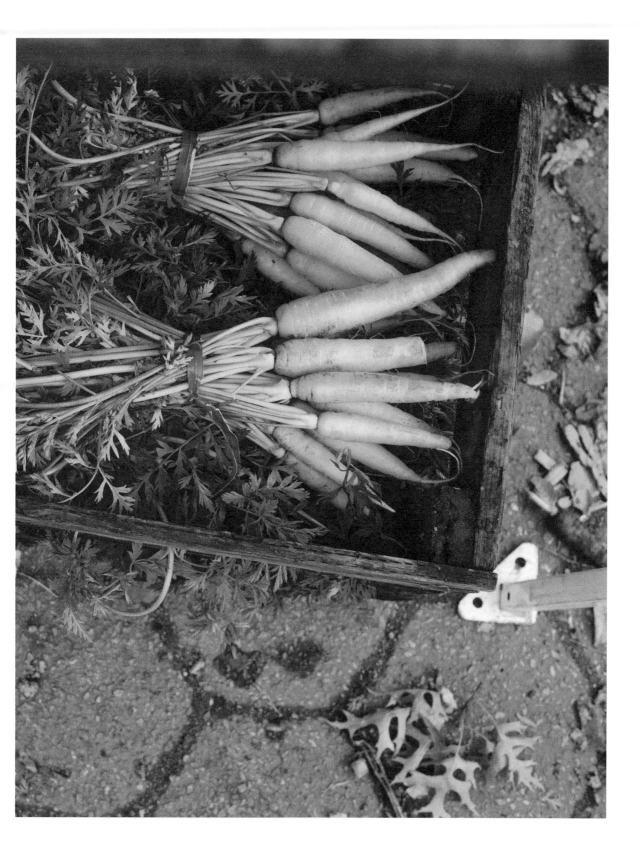

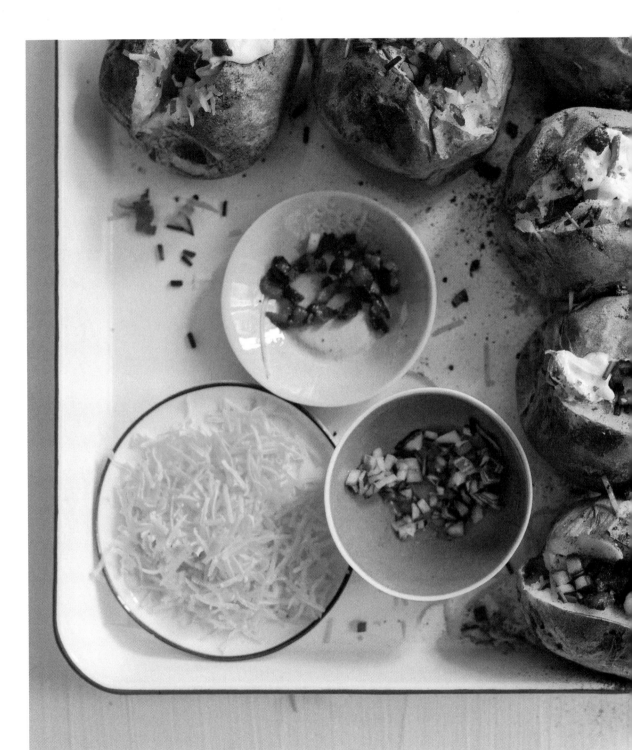

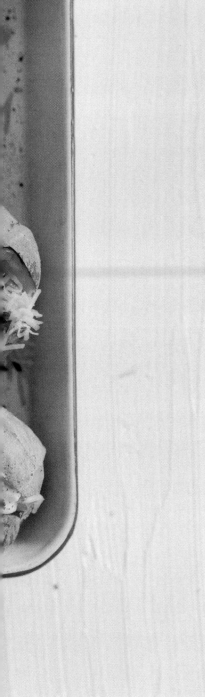

Friday Night Baked Potato Bar

You may already know how to save dinner by piercing some potatoes, tossing them in the oven, and smothering them in butter and bacon. So this is basically just a reminder that it doesn't have to feel like a budget, afterthought meal. Presentation is everything, and people freak out when they get to choose their own toppings. You can impressively feed a massive crowd this way, too, and maybe even serve with a big, crunchy salad.

Serves: 4

½ pound bacon

4 russet potatoes, scrubbed and dried, or more if smaller

1 tablespoon extra-virgin olive oil

3 tablespoons unsalted butter, sliced

½ red onion or ½ bunch chives or scallions, finely chopped

4 ounces cheddar cheese, shredded

Sour cream, for dolloping

Paprika, for dusting

Salt

Pepper

1. Preheat oven to 375°F.

2. Place bacon on a sheet pan in a single layer.

3. Pierce the potatoes all over with a fork. Rub each with a little olive oil and season with salt. Transfer to the oven, placing them directly on the oven rack, and slide the sheet pan with bacon on the rack below to catch any drippings. Roast for about an hour, depending on size. Remove the bacon after 20–25 minutes, depending on how crispy you like your bacon (then crumble it up). Put another pan in the oven to catch any potato drippings.

4. Cut the potatoes in half lengthwise, add some butter on top, season with more salt and some pepper, and start loading them up with fixins. Serve immediately.

Don't-Get-Takeout Takeout

Serves: 4

Sauce

½ cup low-sodium
chicken stock

6 cloves garlic, grated
or finely minced

1 tablespoon fish sauce

1 tablespoon oyster sauce

1 tablespoon roasted red
chile paste

1 teaspoon soy sauce

1 teaspoon cornstarch

½ teaspoon coconut sugar

½ teaspoon dried basil

Crushed red pepper
or Sriracha, to taste

Meat and vegetables

1½ pounds meat: top sirloin
steak; boneless, skinless chicken
thighs or breasts; pork loin

1½ pounds seasonal vegetables:
onions, broccoli, peppers,
asparagus, snap or snow peas,
peas, green beans, zucchini,
eggplant, carrots, spicy peppers

1½ cups jasmine rice,
for serving

Salt

Pepper

Grapeseed oil, for pan

We all know the regret of spending $67 on takeout when we could've made something at home for $50 less. All because of failing to plan. Make a jar of this legit stir-fry sauce ahead and you'll be able to fight the takeout urge when you're in a bind.

1. In a small jar with a lid, combine all the sauce ingredients and shake really well for 10–20 seconds. Use immediately or refrigerate in a jar for up to a week.

2. Slice meat into thin slices or bite-size pieces. Set aside for 15 minutes to come to room temperature.

3. Slice vegetables into bite-size pieces.

4. Cook rice according to package directions.

5. Set a large skillet over medium-high heat and drizzle in a tablespoon of oil. Put in half the vegetables and season with salt and pepper. Sauté until just tender (but not overcooked), about 5–7 minutes for most. Add a splash of water or stock for thicker vegetables to steam and cook through faster. You can also cover with a lid if you'd like to speed up the process. Repeat for remaining half. Transfer to a bowl or plate.

6. In the now empty skillet, drizzle in 2 tablespoons oil to completely coat the bottom. Using tongs, set in half the meat in one layer; season lightly with salt and pepper. Wait about 3 minutes, until browned underneath, then flip for another couple of minutes. Stir around, then transfer to a bowl or plate and repeat with remaining meat.

7. Scrape all the meat back into the skillet along with any accumulated juices. Pour in all the sauce and simmer for 2 minutes.

8. Serve right away with rice and vegetables.

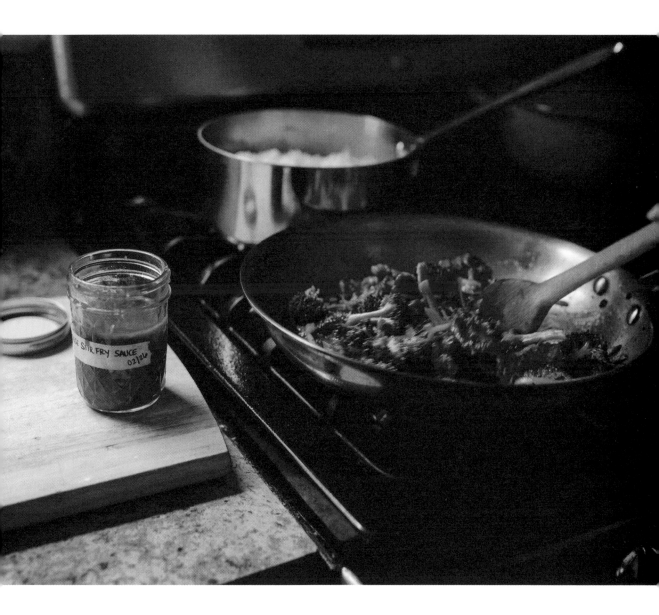

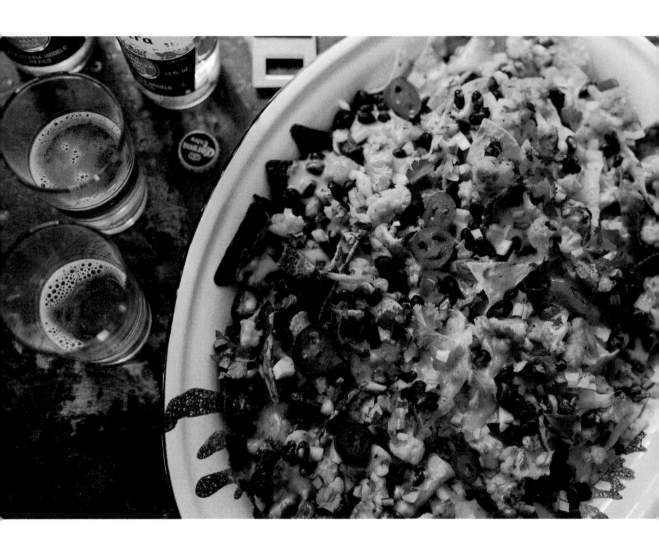

Game Night Nachos with Homemade Queso & Charred Cauliflower

Serves: 6

Charred cauliflower

I small head cauliflower, cut into tiny, ½-inch florets

Grapeseed oil

Salt

Pepper

Queso

2 tablespoons unsalted butter

2 cloves garlic, minced

1½ teaspoons chili powder

2 tablespoons all-purpose flour

1½ cups whole milk

4 ounces Monterey Jack cheese, shredded

4 ounces cheddar cheese, shredded

Assembly

2 bags yellow and blue tortilla chips

I 15-ounce can black beans

Garnishes

Sour cream

Pickled jalapeños

½ red onion, finely chopped

½ bunch cilantro, finely chopped

I lime, cut into wedges

We've developed a few nacho rules to avoid anyone pulling out that dreaded, sad, no-topping nacho from the nacho pile. Here goes: chip layer, toppings, cheese, chip layer, toppings, cheese. And toppings should be cut into tiny cubes or small bite-size pieces so that there's a chip for every topping and a topping for every chip.

1. Preheat oven to 400°F.

2. Toss cauliflower with a couple of tablespoons of oil and ½ teaspoon each salt and pepper. Transfer to the oven for 20–25 minutes or until cauliflower is tender with nice crispy bits. Shake the pan halfway through roasting to ensure even cooking. Remove from oven and set aside.

3. To make queso, melt butter in a small pot; stir in garlic and chili powder. Cook for 1 minute, making sure the mixture doesn't burn.

4. Whisk in flour, stirring continuously, until a thick paste forms.

5. Whisk in milk and, once it's simmering, add the cheese as well with ¼ teaspoon each salt and pepper.

6. Keep whisking until the cheese is completely melted and gooey. You can turn off the heat and reheat if needed.

7. On a large rimmed baking sheet, spread half the tortilla chips in an even layer. Top with half the cauliflower and half the black beans, anywhere your heart desires, then drizzle half the cheese sauce over the top. Repeat with the remaining chips, cauliflower, beans, and cheese sauce. Place the nachos in the oven and bake for 10–15 minutes or until everything is looking bubbly and delicious.

8. Serve immediately with all the garnishes you desire: sour cream, pickled jalapeños, red onion, cilantro, lime wedges.

Repeat Red Lentil Soup

Serves: 4

————————

1 tablespoon extra-virgin olive oil

1 red or yellow onion, finely diced

2 stalks celery, diced

2 carrots, diced

5 cloves garlic, minced

1 bay leaf

½ teaspoon turmeric

½ teaspoon curry powder

1 teaspoon paprika

4 cups low-sodium vegetable or chicken stock

1 cup red lentils

1 teaspoon salt

½ teaspoon pepper

1 cup coconut milk

Warm flatbread or naan, for serving

This is the weekly soup that will keep you from ordering takeout (again) during a hectic Wednesday. It's on repeat during the colder months for a reason. It's really fast, it's cheap to make, and the kids love it.

1. Heat oil in a soup pot or Dutch oven over medium heat.

2. Add onion, celery, and carrots; sauté for 5–7 minutes or until the veggies soften.

3. Stir in garlic, bay leaf, turmeric, curry powder, and paprika; cook for 1 minute.

4. Pour in the stock and lentils. Season with salt and pepper and bring to a boil. Reduce heat and simmer, partially covered, for 15 minutes or until lentils are cooked.

5. Taste for seasoning and pour in the coconut milk. Serve with warm flatbread or naan (smothered with butter).

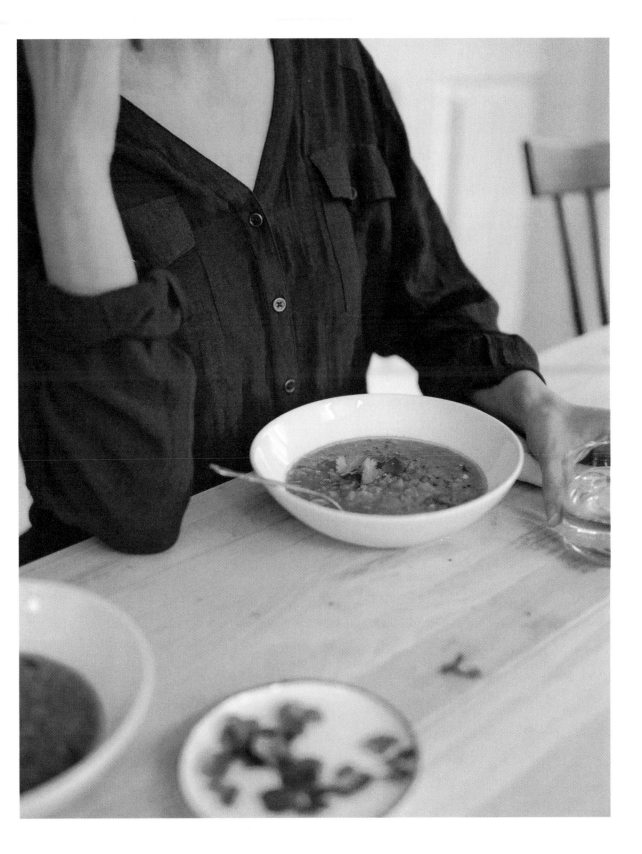

Extra-Crispy Pork Schnitzel with Leek & Cabbage Sauté

Serves: 4

Schnitzel

1 pork tenderloin, 1–1¼ pounds, sliced into ½-inch-thick rounds

⅓ cup all-purpose flour

2 large eggs

1½ cups panko breadcrumbs

3 tablespoons fresh Italian parsley, finely chopped

6 tablespoons extra-virgin olive oil

Salt

Pepper

Really good mustard, for serving

Extra crispy, that's how we like our schnitzel. If you're going to go through all the work of pounding meat, busting out three dredging dishes, and dipping the meat in flour, egg, and breadcrumbs, the result better be crispy schnitzel, not soggy schnitzel. Enter panko. Also, in case you're thinking of forgoing the cabbage sauté, because cabbage . . . One of our teenagers who said sautéed cabbage is gross, upon watching the rest of us scarf it down, decided to try it. You know the rest of this story. She ate more than any of us and even asked if there was extra. Make the cabbage: you'll love it.

1. With a meat mallet, pound the pork between two pieces of plastic wrap sprinkled with a bit of water (this prevents them from sticking) until the cutlets are super thin but not tearing apart. Season them with a total of ½ teaspoon each salt and pepper.

2. Prepare your dredging station by setting up 3 shallow dishes. Place flour in the first, crack eggs into the second, and mix panko and parsley in the third. Divide 1 teaspoon each salt and pepper among all 3 dishes. Using a fork, whisk the contents of each dish, leaving the eggs for last.

3. Coat the pork in flour, dip it in the egg (allowing the excess to drip off), then dredge in panko, covering completely. Press down lightly if needed. You can sauté the pieces immediately or put the cutlets on a sheet pan to rest in the fridge for up to an hour.

4. Heat a ⅛-inch layer of olive oil in a large sauté pan over medium-high heat. When hot, add as many pork cutlets as you can without touching. Cook them for 3–4 minutes on each side, or until crispy, deep golden brown, and opaque inside. Transfer to a paper-towel-lined plate.

Leeks and cabbage

2 leeks (white and light green parts), thinly sliced

1 small green cabbage, halved, core removed, and sliced into ¼-inch-thick pieces

2 tablespoons unsalted butter or extra-virgin olive oil

5.   Place leek slices into a bowl with cold water. Rub them all well to remove the grit, allowing dirt to fall to the bottom of the bowl. Scoop leeks out and set aside.

6.   Pour oil or butter into a large skillet or braiser over medium heat. When hot, add leeks and cabbage with ½ teaspoon each salt and pepper. Partially cover and cook, stirring occasionally until soft, wilted, and golden, about 15 minutes.

7.   Serve cabbage and schnitzel with really good mustard (it's like the ketchup of Germany, Austria, and Belgium).

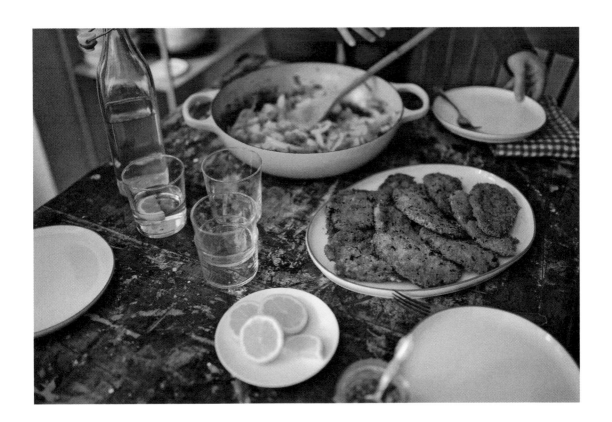

Beef Braise (to Spoon over Rutabaga Mash)

Serves: 6

_____

Beef braise

2 tablespoons bacon fat

2 pounds chuck roast,
cut into 2-inch pieces

1 large white onion, diced

3 stalks celery, diced

5 cloves garlic, minced

2 tablespoons tomato paste

2 tablespoons all-purpose flour

1½ cups red wine

2 cups low-sodium
chicken stock

5 fresh thyme sprigs

1 bay leaf

1 teaspoon fish sauce

2 teaspoons soy sauce

3 carrots, cut into large chunks

½ pound pearl onions, peeled

Rutabaga mash

3 pounds rutabaga, peeled
and cut into ½-inch pieces

6 tablespoons unsalted butter,
chopped into a few pieces

Salt

Pepper

It ain't winter until you braise something. Invite some people over and, when they walk in from the cold, they'll immediately smell *home*.

1. Preheat oven to 350°F.

2. Heat the bacon fat in a Dutch oven over medium-high heat.

3. Season the meat with salt and pepper. When the bacon fat has melted, add the meat in batches. Do not overcrowd. Sear on all sides; this will take 7 minutes. Transfer to a bowl or large plate and continue with remaining meat.

4. Add the onion and celery to pot. Sauté until the veggies begin to brown, 7–10 minutes. Add the garlic and tomato paste and cook an additional minute. Sprinkle flour over top and cook for 1 minute.

5. Pour in the wine and stock. Add thyme, bay leaf, fish sauce, soy sauce, and ½ teaspoon each salt and pepper and stir well.

6. Return the meat and its juices to the pot and bring to a boil. Cover and place in the oven for 1 hour. Then, stir in the carrots (you're adding them here so they don't get mushy). Return to the oven for 30 more minutes.

7. Remove the pot from the oven and add pearl onions, cover again, and return to the oven for 30 minutes. The meat should be fork-tender and the onions fully cooked. Remove the thyme sprigs, taste for seasoning, and keep warm.

8. Meanwhile, make the rutabaga mash. Place rutabaga cubes into a medium pot, cover with well-salted water, and bring to a boil. Turn the heat down and simmer, partially covered, until rutabaga is very soft and crumbles when pierced with a fork, about 30 minutes. If it's not soft enough, it won't puree well.

9. Drain, reserving 1 cup of cooking water. Return rutabaga to pot, scatter butter pieces on top, stir, and cover until butter melts and coats all the cubes. Season with ½ teaspoon each salt and pepper and puree with an immersion blender, adding cooking water a few splashes at a

Butter-basted mushrooms

2 tablespoons unsalted butter

10 ounces mixed wild mushrooms

time until creamy, super smooth, and thick. Taste for salt and keep warm.

10. In a large sauté pan, melt 2 tablespoons butter over medium-high heat. When the foam subsides, add the mushrooms and sauté until browned. The trick is to not constantly stir. If you allow them to sear a little, they develop a beautiful color. Set aside.

11. When ready to serve, spoon the beef braise and mushrooms over the rutabaga mash. Garnish with parsley if you have it on hand.

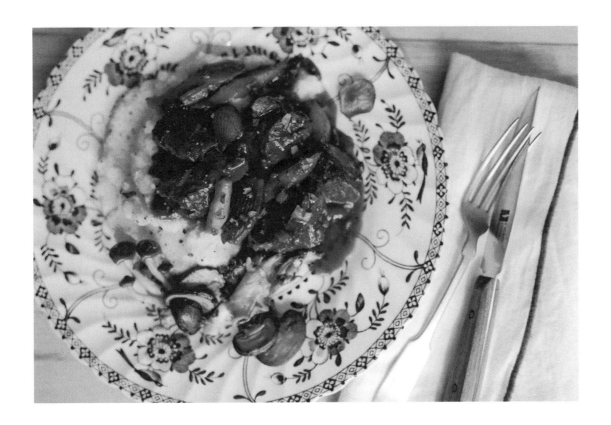

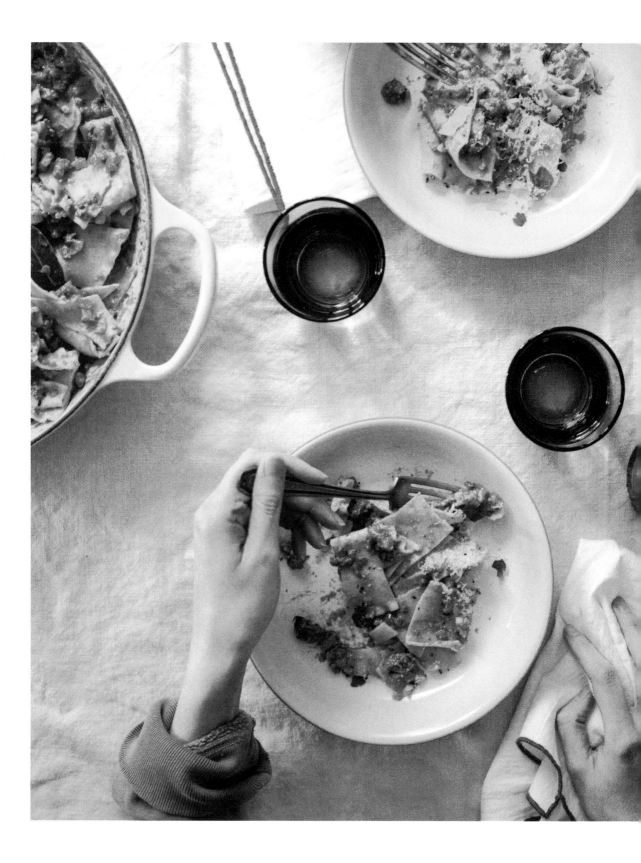

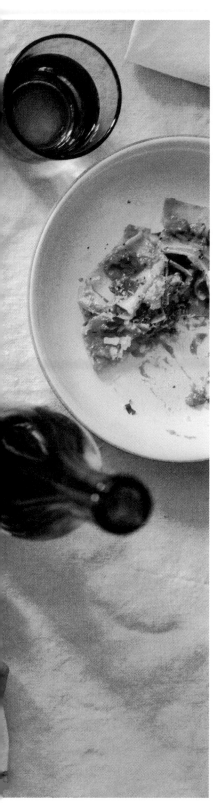

Bolognese with Broken Lasagna & Broken Rules

A lot of Bolognese recipes out there, at some point in the text, will say something about the traditional way of doing things. But there are ways to personalize within the parameters of honoring tradition. This is a crowd-pleasing, comforting pasta to make again and again. Each time, try it out with slight tweaks to develop your secret recipe. It's a good thing to ask—*How can I break the rules and make it better?*

Serves: 6

---

2 tablespoons extra-virgin olive oil

I tablespoon unsalted butter

I yellow onion, finely diced

2 stalks celery, finely diced

2 carrots, peeled and finely diced

5 cloves garlic, minced

2½ teaspoons mixed dried herbs: oregano, basil, thyme

⅛ teaspoon freshly ground nutmeg

I pound ground beef

I cup dry white wine

3 ounces tomato paste

I 28-ounce can crushed tomatoes

I bay leaf

½ cup half-and-half or heavy cream

I pound lasagna noodles, broken into short I-inch strips

¼ bunch fresh Italian parsley, chopped

Parmesan cheese, grated

Salt

Pepper

Make It Yours:

Pasta: We love thin, wide noodles for this—like pappardelle, rombi, or broken-up lasagna pieces. But you could use whatever you like!

Fat: All oil, all butter, combination, a little bit of bacon fat, or super-tiny cubes of pancetta.

Meat: Go with more if you want more, up to 1½ pounds—beef, turkey, pork.

Wine: White or red.

Herbs and spices: Fresh or dried herbs, paprika.

Tomatoes: Tomato paste, crushed, diced, whole that you crush yourself.

Dairy: Half-and-half, heavy cream, just a few pats of butter. Parmigiano, Romano, or pecorino.

Secret ingredients: 1–2 teaspoons of soy sauce, anchovies, fish sauce, ketchup, Worcestershire sauce.

1. Heat a deep sauté pan over medium-high heat.

2. Add oil and butter to the pan. When butter is melted, add onion, celery, and carrots. Season with ½ teaspoon salt and cook for about 4 minutes or until the vegetables are soft.

3. Add garlic, herbs, and nutmeg, and continue to cook for 1 more minute.

4. Add beef and cook until no longer pink, breaking it up with your spoon into smaller bits. Pour in the wine and cook until reduced.

5. Stir in tomato paste and cook for a minute. Add the crushed tomatoes, bay leaf, ½ teaspoon salt, and ¾ teaspoon pepper. Simmer for at least 30–35 minutes, but you could go up to 2 hours for max flavor.

6. Pour in dairy and simmer for 2 more minutes. Taste for seasoning.

7. Bring a large pot of salted water to boil. Once boiling, add pasta and cook according to package instructions. Drain and combine with Bolognese sauce and parsley. Serve right away with grated Parmesan and more pepper.

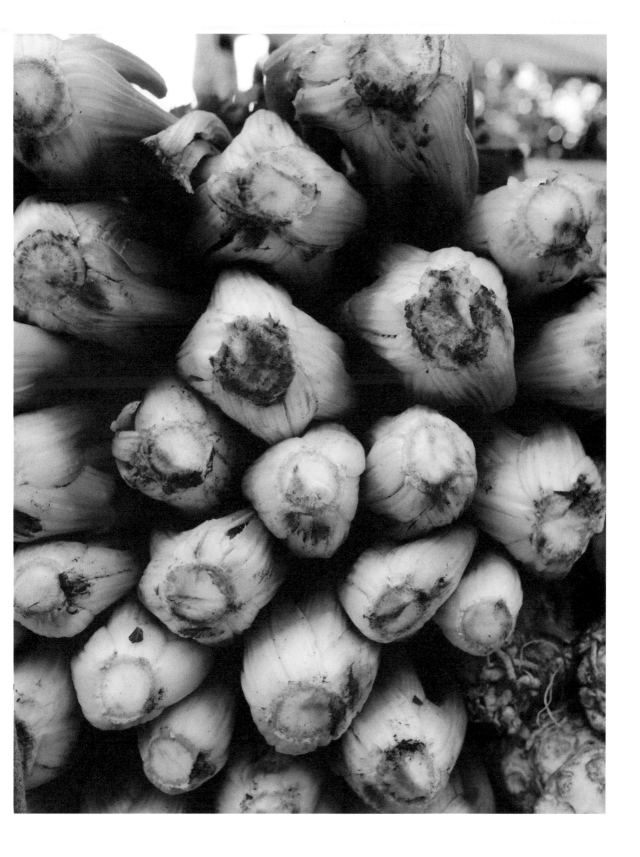

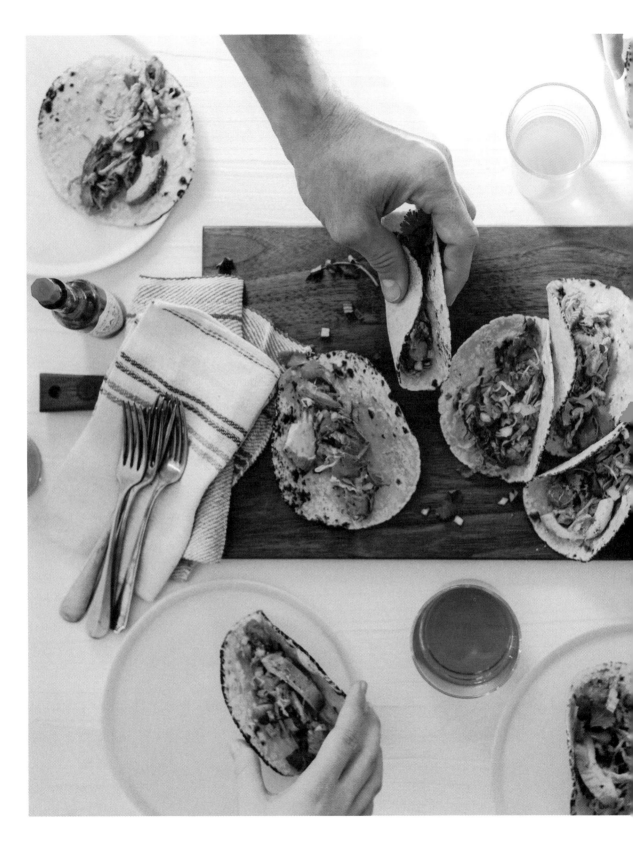

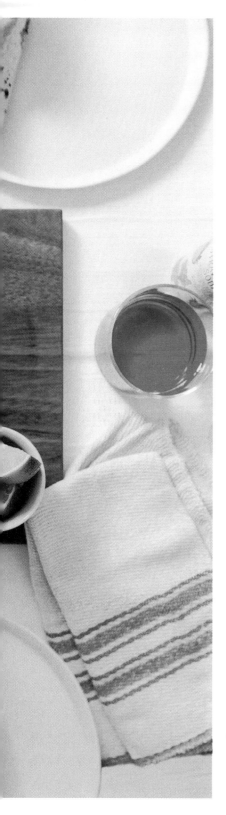

Easiest Chicken Taqueria Tacos

This was previously a slow-cooker recipe. But one day we tried it in a Dutch oven and the results were drastically different. We love the idea of a hands-off meal that cooks itself on the countertop, but the truth is, depth and good texture are always lacking. We're going to include directions for both methods so you can compare, too.

Serves: 8

2½ pounds boneless, skinless chicken thighs, at room temperature

Salt

Pepper

1 tablespoon grapeseed oil, or more if needed

2 tablespoons fajita seasoning or taco seasoning

8 ounces salsa verde, your favorite jarred brand (keep in mind that some are spicier than others)

2 packages soft corn tortillas

Serve with your favorite Taco Tuesday fixings: guac or sliced avocados, salsa, hot sauce, chopped cilantro, chopped red onion, sour cream, shredded lettuce, shredded cheese

1. Preheat oven to 325°F and position a rack in the center.

2. Set a Dutch oven over medium-high heat and drizzle in oil. Season chicken generously with salt and pepper (hold back a little if the fajita or taco seasoning has salt), then brown in batches once the oil is hot, about 2 minutes per side, making sure not to cook through. Add more oil if needed.

3. Nestle all the browned chicken back in the pot (or in the slow cooker), sprinkling the top evenly with fajita seasoning, then pour in the salsa verde. The chicken shouldn't be fully submerged. Cover and slide in the oven for 1½–2 hours or set the slow cooker to 4–5 hours on low.

4. Once chicken is cooked to fall-apart tender, using forks or your hands, pull it apart, discarding any bits of fat. If the chicken seems cooked but too tough, and it isn't coming apart into chunks easily, it just needs 30 minutes more.

5. Serve with warmed corn tortillas and your favorite fixings.

Persian Winter Vegetable Stew with a Lot of Herbs

Serves: 4

2 tablespoons extra-virgin olive oil

1 yellow onion, diced

2 carrots, peeled and diced

5 cloves garlic, minced

1 tablespoon tomato paste

½ teaspoon turmeric

½ teaspoon ground coriander

½ teaspoon ground cumin

1 teaspoon paprika

1 teaspoon salt

1 teaspoon pepper

1 quart vegetable or chicken stock

1 cup water

⅓ cup dried basmati or jasmine rice

1½ cups cooked or canned chickpeas

⅔ cup Swiss chard stems, chopped

2 cups diced turnips

1 cup Swiss chard leaves, chopped

½ cup fresh cilantro, chopped

½ cup fresh Italian parsley, chopped

1-2 tablespoons fresh mint, chopped

Juice of 1 lime

A winter stew with a hint of Persian spices, greens, legumes, grains, herbs, veggies, and broth to warm every inch of you, with plenty left over for the next day.

1. Heat the oil in a soup pot over medium heat. Add onion and carrots; cook, stirring occasionally, until soft, about 4 minutes.

2. Add the garlic, tomato paste, turmeric, coriander, cumin, paprika, half the salt, and pepper and cook another minute.

3. Pour in stock and water with remaining salt, rice, chickpeas, chard stems, and turnips. Simmer for 15 minutes, until the rice is just cooked.

4. Stir in the chard leaves and simmer another 2 minutes. Turn off the heat and stir in cilantro, parsley, mint, and 2 teaspoons lime juice. Taste and add more lime juice, salt, and pepper if needed.

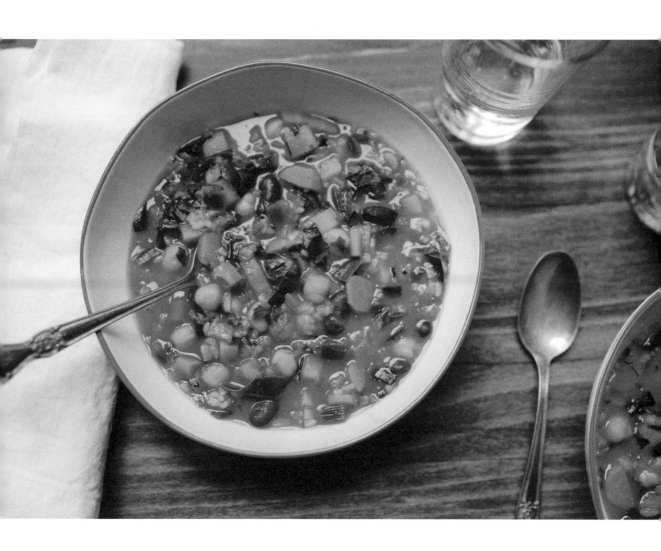

Sticky Korean Ribs with Creamy Savoy Slaw

Serves: 4

_____

Ribs

1 rack baby back ribs

1 tablespoon grapeseed oil

2 scallions, trimmed
and chopped

5 cloves garlic, minced

1 tablespoon minced ginger

2 tablespoons soy sauce

¼ cup hoisin sauce

2 tablespoons rice wine
vinegar

2 tablespoons brown sugar

¼ cup gochujang
(Korean red pepper paste)

Salt

Pepper

These taste like they come from a barbecue joint. The meat falls off the bone and inevitably makes any grown person lick their fingers to get every last drop of sauce. They're awesome for a crowd, because multiple racks can cook on a sheet pan at once, low and slow in the oven, not requiring too much of your attention.

_____

Kitchen note: If you choose to use spare ribs instead (they're more meaty and cost less), they'll need an extra hour or so of cooking time.

1. Preheat oven to 300°F.

2. Tear a long piece of aluminum foil and put it on a sheet pan. Lay the ribs on top and season with salt and pepper. Fold the foil around the ribs, making a packet. Be sure it's completely sealed: you need the ribs to steam inside.

3. Transfer the sheet pan to the oven and cook ribs for 2½ hours. They should be fully cooked and almost falling off the bone. If they're tough, put them back in the oven for another 20–30 minutes.

4. In a small saucepan, heat oil over medium-low heat. Add scallions, garlic, and ginger and cook until soft, about 5 minutes, stirring often so garlic doesn't burn.

5. Add remaining ingredients, whisking to combine. Cook sauce until it reduces slightly, about 5–10 minutes. Taste; if it's not sweet enough, add more sugar. Set aside.

6. Remove ribs from the oven, carefully opening the foil. Pour out any drippings and discard, if needed. Turn the oven up to 425°F and brush a layer of the sauce over the ribs.

7. Return to the oven and roast for 30 minutes, basting the ribs in more sauce every 10 minutes or so. If you like your ribs more charred, place them under the broiler for 1–2 minutes. Serve extra sauce on the side.

Savoy slaw

I egg yolk

I teaspoon Dijon mustard

½ teaspoon sesame oil

I clove garlic, minced

½ cup grapeseed oil, plus more if needed

3 tablespoons rice wine vinegar

I savoy cabbage, finely sliced

8. In a small bowl, whisk the egg yolk, mustard, sesame oil, and garlic.

9. Stream in grapeseed oil very slowly, drop by drop, making sure you are stirring constantly. When it's combined, add another little drizzle. Continue this long and mundane (but 100 percent worth the effort) process until all the oil is used. Stir in the rice wine vinegar and season to taste with salt and pepper. If it's too thick, add a teaspoon or so of water just to loosen the dressing. Set aside.

10. In a salad bowl, toss the savoy cabbage with half the dressing to coat and top with a tablespoon of black sesame seeds if you happen to have them. Serve immediately with the remaining dressing on the side.

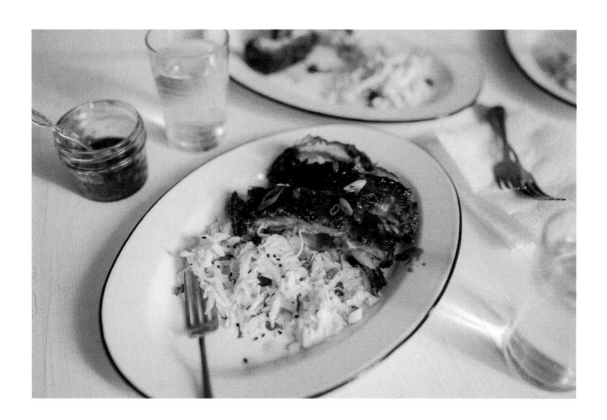

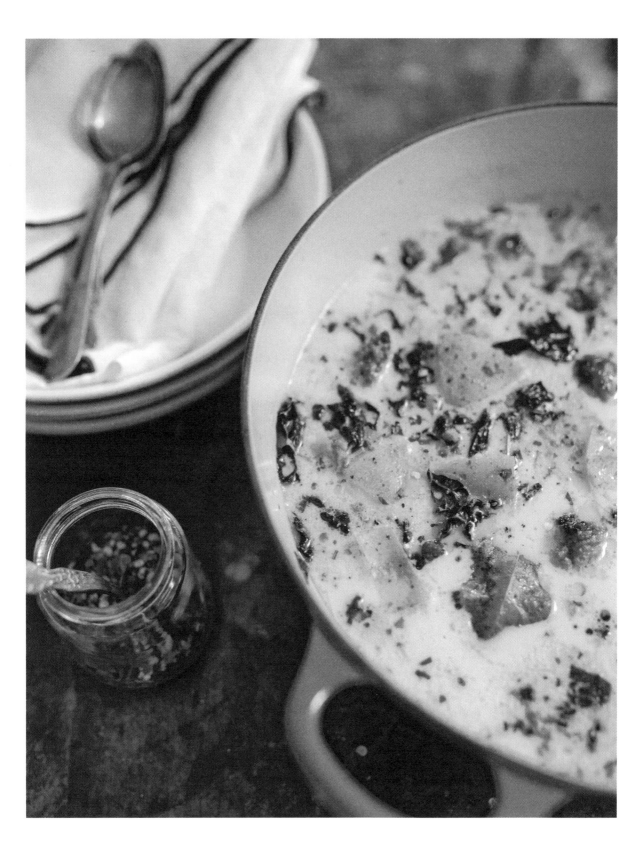

Zuppa Toscana

Serves: 6

2 tablespoons extra-virgin olive oil

I pound sweet Italian sausage

I yellow onion, chopped

4 cloves garlic, minced

¼ teaspoon crushed red pepper, optional

½ cup dry white wine

2 tablespoons fresh Italian parsley, chopped

I bay leaf

4 cups low-sodium chicken stock

I cup water

2 russet potatoes, scrubbed, peel left on, cut into ½-inch chunks

½ bunch lacinato kale, stems discarded and leaves chopped

I cup half-and-half

Salt

Pepper

Optional, for serving: crusty bread

You know this soup. It's a special recipe from Il Giardino d'Oliva (okay, Olive Garden) and an ode to Sunday lunches in the 'burbs. For the full effect, serve with a bottomless breadstick basket. *Mangia.*

1. Set a Dutch oven or stock pot over medium-high heat. Add oil and crumble in the sausage. Let it brown a bit before stirring; you want the sausage to get some color with crunchy bits here and there. When the sausage is no longer pink, 5–6 minutes, transfer to a small bowl with a slotted spoon.

2. Remove excess oil from the pot, leaving about a tablespoon in there. Add onion, sprinkle with a little salt, and sauté for 5 minutes or until soft. Add garlic and red pepper flakes and cook an additional minute.

3. Pour in wine, and scrape up any brown bits on the bottom of the pot. Let the wine reduce by half, then stir in parsley, bay leaf, stock, water, sausage, potatoes, and ¾ teaspoon each salt and pepper. Bring the soup to a boil, then reduce to a simmer for 15 minutes or until the potatoes are fork-tender.

4. Add in kale and cook until it just wilts, about 3 minutes. Turn off heat and stir in the half-and-half. Taste for seasoning and serve in bowls with crusty bread.

Roasted Romanesco & Toasted Farro with Warm Cherry Pepper Vinaigrette

Serves: 4

Romanesco and farro

2 heads romanesco or small cauliflower, broken into 1-inch florets

1 tablespoon grapeseed oil

1 cup farro

Breadcrumbs

2 tablespoons unsalted butter

½ cup breadcrumbs

Vinaigrette

½ cup extra-virgin olive oil

2 small shallots, minced

6 cloves garlic, minced

½ teaspoon crushed red pepper

4 teaspoons anchovy paste or about 6 fillets, minced

1 tablespoon red wine vinegar

12 jarred hot and sweet cherry peppers, thinly sliced

¼ cup Parmigiano-Reggiano, grated, plus extra for serving

¼ cup fresh Italian parsley, chopped

Salt

Pepper

Have you had romanesco? It looks like broccoli and cauliflower's relative from outer space. And this is one of our favorite ways to eat it—mixed with chewy grains, crunchy breadcrumbs, and a sweet-and-spicy skillet dressing.

1. Preheat oven to 400°F. Toss romanesco with grapeseed oil, ½ teaspoon of salt, and a few cracks of pepper. Spread out on a sheet pan and roast for about 30–35 minutes or until tender and browned in a few spots. Toss halfway through roasting. Transfer to a bowl and keep warm.

2. Place farro in a small pot and cover with water by a couple of inches. Add ½ teaspoon salt. Bring to a low boil, then simmer for about 30 minutes, until al dente. Drain well, then spread on the same sheet pan from before. Slide under the broiler for 8–10 minutes, tossing halfway through, or until lightly toasted.

3. Grab a sauté pan and melt the butter over medium heat. Throw in the breadcrumbs with a huge pinch of salt. Stir often, for about 5 minutes, until golden brown and toasty smelling. Transfer to a plate.

4. In the same sauté pan, pour in the olive oil over medium heat. Add the shallots and let them sizzle in the oil for 4–5 minutes. Then in go the garlic, crushed red pepper, anchovy paste or minced anchovies, vinegar, sliced cherry peppers, and half the Parmesan for just another minute. Season with a few cracks of pepper and ½ teaspoon salt. Turn off the heat.

5. Dump all the toasted farro into the sauté pan with the warm vinaigrette and toss well with the parsley. Divide onto plates; top with romanesco, breadcrumbs, and extra grated Parmesan.

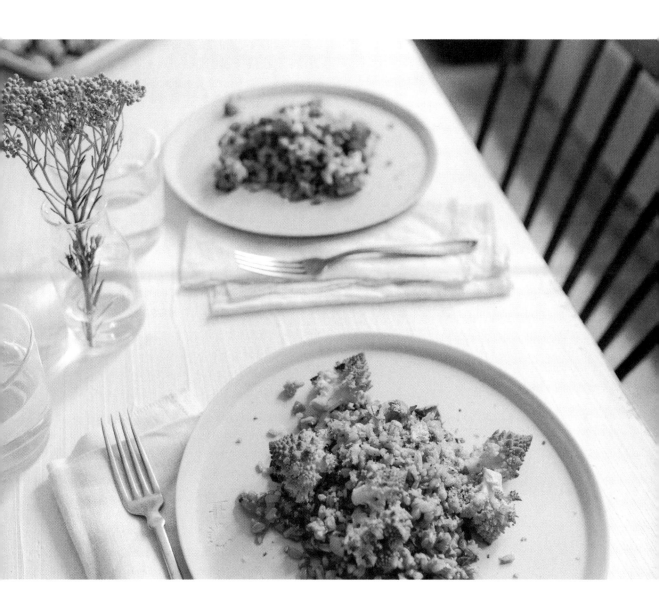

The Best Crispy Fish Tacos I Had in Tulum

Serves: 4

_____

Yucatán sauce

½ cup sour cream

¼ cup mayonnaise

2 cloves garlic, minced

I lime, half juiced for sauce and the other half cut into wedges for garnish

2 tablespoons fresh cilantro, chopped

Salt

Pepper

Tacos

I cup all-purpose flour

I teaspoon paprika

I teaspoon ground coriander

½ teaspoon chili powder

2 large eggs

I pound cod or halibut fillets

½ cup grapeseed oil

I package corn or flour tortillas

½ small green cabbage, finely shredded

Fresh cilantro, for garnish

Optional, for serving: avocado, thinly sliced; radishes, thinly sliced; red onion

Tacos in Tulum. Sandy beaches, straw hats, and a cold beer in hand is the only way to enjoy them. Or at least that's what we're imagining, since we've never actually been to Tulum. One day we'll go and see if their fish tacos are as good as we dream them to be.

_____

Kitchen note: We've tried the beer batter recipes before, but they get soggy fast. The key to extra-crispy fish is to dip it in an egg wash, dredge in seasoned flour, then pan-fry or deep-fry until golden and crispy.

1. In a small bowl, whisk the sauce ingredients with ½ teaspoon each salt and pepper. Refrigerate for up to 3 days, adding a splash of water to loosen consistency if needed.

2. In a shallow baking dish, mix the flour, paprika, coriander, chili powder, 1 teaspoon salt, and ½ teaspoon black pepper. Set aside.

3. In another shallow baking dish, whisk the eggs with ¼ teaspoon each salt and pepper. Set aside.

4. Cut the fish into ½-inch-thick strips. Sink fish into the egg mixture. Let the excess drip off, then dredge it in the flour mixture so that all sides are nicely coated. Set aside on a large plate or sheet pan while oil heats up. In a medium pan with deep sides, heat oil to 375°F. If you don't have a thermometer, you can test the oil by cooking one piece of fish: if it starts to sizzle right away, you know the oil is hot enough.

5. When oil is ready, add fish in a single layer, but do not overcrowd the pan (you don't want sad and soggy fish). You'll need to do this in at least 2 batches. Cook for about 2 minutes and turn onto the other side for another minute. The fish should look nice and golden brown, with a crispy outside. Transfer to a paper-towel-lined plate and continue cooking the rest of the fish.

6. Char tortillas on an open flame. Nestle 2 pieces of fish in each, then some cabbage (plus any other optional toppings) and a good drizzle of the sauce. Garnish with extra cilantro and lime.

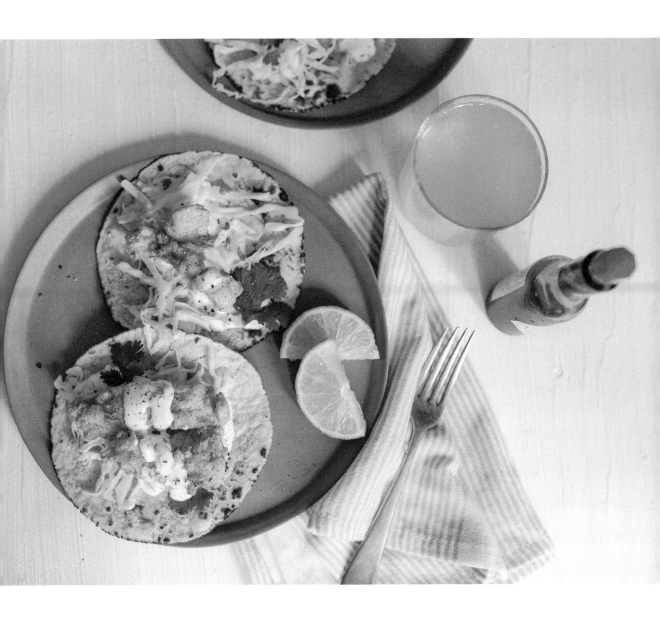

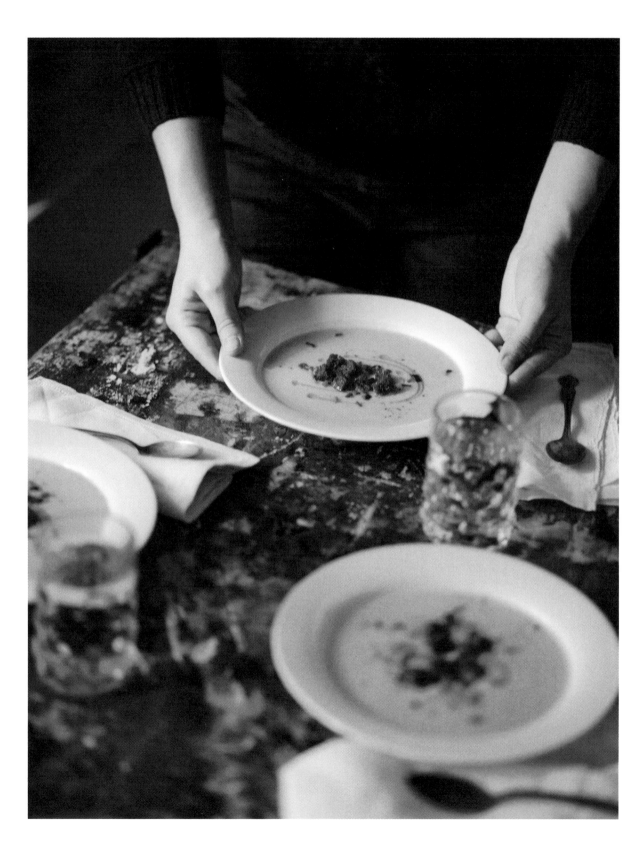

Bistro Celery Root & Leek Soup with Pumpernickel Croutons

Serves: 6

Soup

3 slices thick-cut bacon, finely chopped

2 leeks, white and light green parts, thinly sliced and rinsed well

6 cloves garlic, minced

2 stalks celery, diced

½ teaspoon crushed red pepper

1 russet potato, peeled and chopped into ½-inch chunks

1½ pounds celery root (also called celeriac), peeled and chopped into ½-inch chunks

6 cups low-sodium chicken stock or swap out 2 of those cups with water

1 teaspoon apple cider vinegar

½ cup heavy cream

Extra-virgin olive oil, for drizzling

¼ cup fresh chives, chopped

Croutons

6 slices pumpernickel bread, cut into tiny ¼-inch cubes

2 tablespoons unsalted butter, melted

3 tablespoons extra-virgin olive oil

3 tablespoons fresh rosemary, very finely minced

Salt

Pepper

Without its toppings, this is a very good but very bare soup. All dressed up with a sprinkle of chives, bits of bacon, a drizzle of oil, and buttery herbed croutons, it's another soup entirely. Make this for wintry date nights at home. And imagine you're at a Paris bistro in January, next to a window, watching it snow.

1. Heat a soup pot or Dutch oven over medium heat. When hot, add bacon, stirring a few times until browned and crisped, 7–10 minutes. Transfer bacon to a paper-towel-lined plate with a slotted spoon. Set aside.

2. You should be left with about a tablespoon of bacon fat in the pot; if not, toss in a pat of butter or a drizzle of olive oil. Add leeks, garlic, celery, and crushed red pepper and give everything a few stirs. Sauté for about 5 minutes, until softened, then add the potato and celery root along with 1½ teaspoons salt and ¾ teaspoon pepper; stir.

3. Pour in the chicken stock and bring to a low boil, then let the soup simmer, partially covered, for 30–40 minutes or until the celery root can be very easily pierced with a fork.

4. While soup is simmering, preheat oven to 450°F. Toss bread really well with the remaining crouton ingredients, ½ teaspoon salt, and ¼ teaspoon pepper in a shallow dish. Spread out on a sheet pan and toast for 7–10 minutes, until bread is crisp.

5. Puree the soup in a blender until silky. Pour in the vinegar and heavy cream. Stir well, then taste for salt and pepper.

6. Ladle into shallow bowls and top with a drizzle of good olive oil, reserved bacon, chives, and rosemary croutons.

You Can Roast a Whole Chicken (with Rosemary Roasted Potatoes)

Serves: 4–6

Chicken

2 tablespoons dried herbs: oregano, thyme, marjoram, rosemary, basil; any combination or single herb

8–10 cloves garlic, minced into a paste

2 tablespoons red wine vinegar

3 tablespoons unsalted butter, melted

4–5-pound whole chicken, patted dry, no need to rinse, let it come to room temperature while you prep everything else

1 onion, cut into quarters (no need to peel)

½ lemon

Extra-virgin olive oil

Salt

Pepper

Okay, people, listen: the whole roast-chicken thing is something you can do! You're just going to slather the bird in a wet rub and stuff it with onion and lemon. The result is crispy skin and juicy meat. No special Boy Scout knots for trussing; no basting multiple times. Plop it in a cast-iron skillet (or whatever baking dish you have on hand), wash your hands, and then transfer it to the oven. Roast it, rest it, eat it.

1. Preheat oven to 400°F.

2. In a small bowl, combine the herbs, garlic, vinegar, melted butter, 2 teaspoons salt, and 1 teaspoon pepper. Using a fork, mix vigorously to get a whipped paste consistency.

3. Set the chicken, breast side up, into a cast-iron skillet (or baking dish). Gently loosen the chicken skin with your fingers, starting at the bottom of the breasts and, working your way up, get about half the paste under there. The skin releases pretty easily. Smear the remaining herb paste on the chicken on/in every possible space; don't forget about the legs, either.

4. Stuff chicken with the onion and lemon and transfer to the oven for 1 hour.

5. There are a few ways to be sure about doneness. (1) It's super crispy everywhere and firm to the touch, not rubbery. (2) Make a little incision in the thickest part of the thigh and take a peek. The juices should run clear (not pink), the meat should be fully opaque (nothing translucent), and you can see the cooked fibers of the meat if you poke around with the knife. (3) The drumstick detaches from the chicken almost effortlessly. (4) A meat thermometer in the thickest part of the thigh (not touching the bone) should register 165°F. If it's not done, slide in the oven for another 15–20 minutes. Let it rest for 10 minutes so that juices settle. Get ready for some crispy skin.

Rosemary potatoes

2 pounds red or gold potatoes, skins left on and scrubbed, halved or quartered if large

2 tablespoons fresh rosemary, minced

6. After you get the chicken in the oven, toss the potatoes on a large sheet pan with 2 tablespoons oil, rosemary, and a few generous pinches of salt and pepper.

7. Place in the oven, on a rack below the chicken, and roast for 35–45 minutes, depending on the size of the potatoes. (Start them after the chicken has been in for 20 minutes so they finish at the same time.) Toss them halfway through cooking. Remove from the oven and serve immediately.

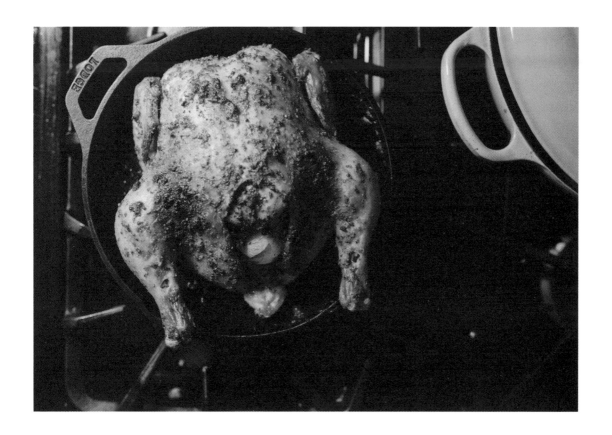

Winter

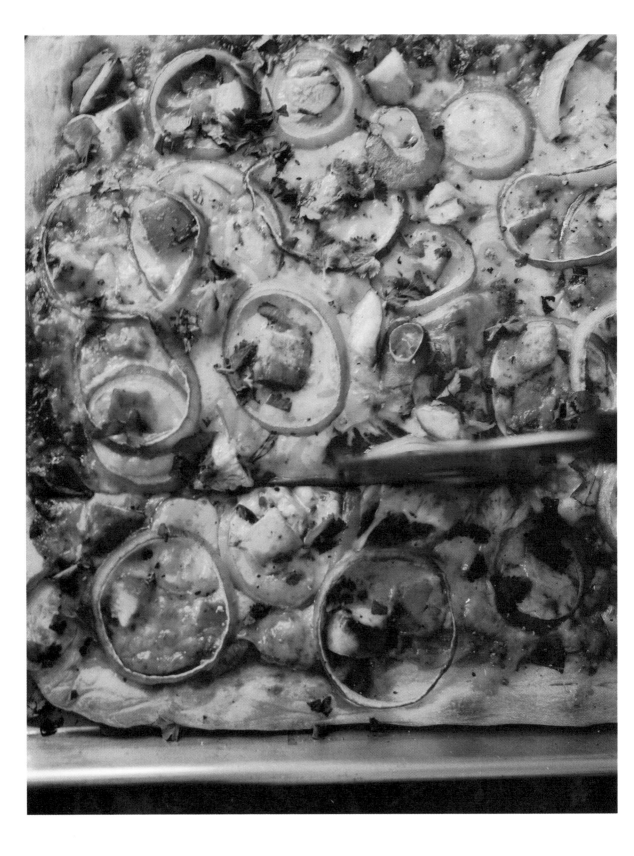

Famous BBQ Chicken Pizza
with Extra Cilantro

Serves: 4-6

---

2 small boneless, skinless chicken breasts, ½–¾ pound

¾ cup barbecue sauce, divided

Extra-virgin olive oil, for pan

1 16-ounce ball of homemade or store-bought pizza dough

6 ounces shredded cheddar cheese

4 ounces shredded Monterey Jack cheese

1 small red onion, sliced

2-3 tablespoons fresh cilantro, chopped

Salt

Pepper

Never a leftover slice when we make this. We've had people politely say, "Maybe just a slice" and then scarf down three more slices right after. The point is, for the purists, this seems like an odd combination and possibly too sweet. But the chicken, red onion, and cilantro are such a perfect combination. And the extra cilantro means "extra." It's not a garnish; it's an ingredient.

1.   Preheat oven to 400°F.

2.   On a small baking dish or sheet pan, brush the chicken breasts generously with ¼ cup of the barbecue sauce and season with salt and pepper. Transfer to the oven for 15 minutes. Remove from oven, cut into bite-size pieces, and set aside.

3.   Raise temperature to 450°F.

4.   Grease a large sheet pan with a little drizzle of oil. Hold the dough in your hands and begin to gently stretch it, which allows for those delicious bubbles. Set the dough on the pan and continue stretching to fill the sheet pan.

5.   Brush dough with ½ cup barbecue sauce, leaving a border around the edges. Top with the cheese, diced chicken, onion, and a sprinkle of salt and pepper. Transfer to the oven for 10–15 minutes or until cheese is completely melted and the crust is golden brown. Garnish with chopped cilantro and serve immediately.

PaperGal Breakfast Sandwich

Serves: 4

Cherry pepper–cheddar spread

1 cup shredded cheddar cheese

3 tablespoons pickled cherry peppers, finely chopped

2 tablespoons grated onion

¼ cup mayonnaise

Sandwich

6-8 strips really good thick-cut bacon

4 brioche buns

2 tablespoons unsalted butter, at room temperature

2 tablespoons grapeseed oil

4 large eggs, from a good farm, with really orangey-yellow yolks

1 small bunch mâche, or your favorite market greens

Your favorite hot sauce, for serving

Salt

Pepper

Inspired by our favorite Austin breakfast food truck, this is *the best* breakfast sandwich ever. It comes with a sunny side of Texas patio vibes.

Kitchen note: You're using up the jar of cherry peppers you got for the romanesco grain bowl (page 298).

1. Mix all the spread ingredients in a bowl, along with ½ teaspoon each salt and pepper. Refrigerate up to 1 day and bring to room temperature before serving.

2. Place bacon in a single layer on a sheet pan; slide into a 375°F oven for 15–20 minutes, until browned. Break strips in half and set aside.

3. Heat a skillet, preferably nonstick, over medium heat. Slather butter on the insides of all 8 bun halves. Once pan is hot, working in batches, set buns in, cut side down, to toast for 2–3 minutes, taking care not to burn. Set buns aside and keep warm.

4. Wipe out the skillet and pour in oil, enough to coat the bottom well.

5. Crack in eggs, leaving an inch in between (do this in 2 batches if needed). Fry for about 5 minutes, until whites and yolks are set. To accomplish this without the bottom getting too crispy before the yolk is cooked, spoon hot oil from the pan over the egg fairly often. Give them a good sprinkle of salt and pepper. Set aside.

6. Spread 3 tablespoons of cherry pepper–cheddar mix on each bottom bun. Make a bed of bacon with 3–4 bacon halves, then add an egg and greens. Add dashes of hot sauce if you'd like, then top with bun. This is a pick-it-up-with-both-hands or a knife-and-fork kind of sandwich.

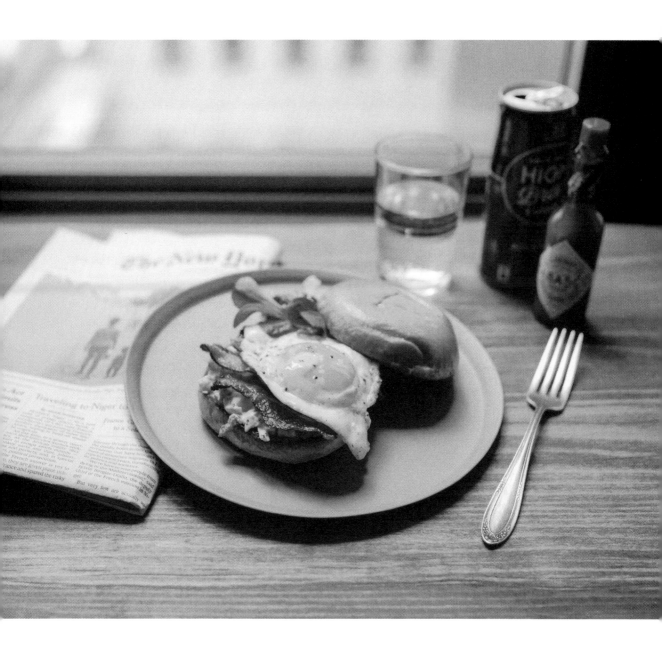

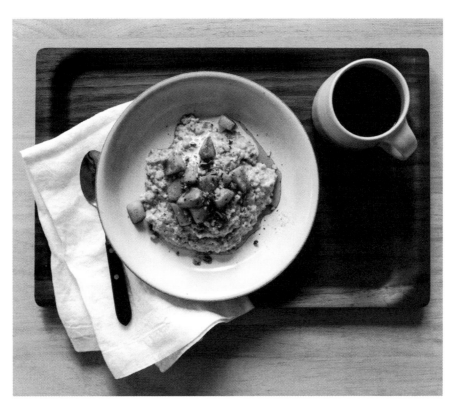

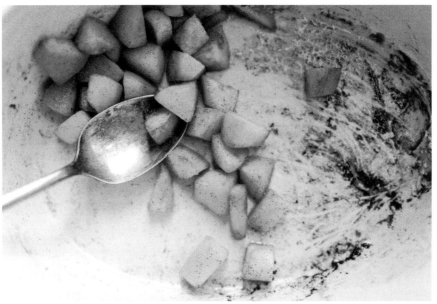

Very Vanilla Steel-Cut Oats
with Baked Pears

Serves: 2–3

Pears

3 ripe Bosc, Anjou, or Bartlett pears, chopped into small cubes

1 tablespoon vanilla bean paste

1 tablespoon unsalted butter

2 tablespoons coconut sugar

Juice of ¼ lemon

Oatmeal

1 cup steel-cut oats

3½ cups water

¼ cup full-fat coconut milk

2 tablespoons coconut sugar

2 teaspoons vanilla extract

Salt

Other topping options

Chocolate shavings, hemp hearts, dusting of cinnamon, toasted walnut pieces, drizzle of maple syrup, drizzle of coconut cream or heavy cream

Morning oatmeal doesn't have to be boring, and it can be a regular thing. Keep the baked pears refrigerated in a jar; reheat in a super-small pot. Keep the rest of your favorite toppings corralled in your cupboard within easy reach.

1. Preheat oven to 375°F. In a small baking dish, toss pear cubes with remaining ingredients and a pinch of salt. Bake for 30 minutes or until soft, basting with the sweet, buttery syrup twice throughout baking. Set aside to cool, then refrigerate in a jar for up to a week. Reheat to serve.

2. Add oats, ¼ teaspoon salt, and water to a medium pot. Bring to a low boil, then turn the heat down to a simmer. Add coconut milk, sugar, and vanilla extract. Simmer, uncovered, for 20–30 minutes, until oatmeal is tender and liquid is absorbed. Scoop into shallow bowls and top with warm pears (plus juices) and extra toppings.

Huevos Hacedores

Serves: 4

Cilantro sauce

½ bunch fresh cilantro,
leaves and tender stems

5 slices pickled jalapeño

I clove garlic

⅓ cup yogurt or mayonnaise

⅓ cup sour cream

A squeeze of lime

Fritters

½ pound sweet potato
(I medium-large), shredded
lengthwise on the large holes
of a box grater

½ bunch lacinato kale,
sliced into very thin ribbons

½ yellow onion, finely minced

I teaspoon paprika

2 tablespoons all-purpose flour,
or a gluten-free blend

Grapeseed oil, for skillet

Eggs

Extra-virgin olive oil, for skillet

4 large eggs, or more to order

Salt

Pepper

Red pepper flakes

Optional, for serving: sliced
avocado and cilantro sprigs

Hacedores means "doers and makers," and you may remember from Spanish class that *huevos* = eggs. Which together translates to: eggs for people like you, who need to recharge from all the doing and making. This is the Dilly Dally's cooler-weather cousin.

1.   Place all the cilantro sauce ingredients in a blender with ½ teaspoon salt; pulse until completely smooth with a few herb specks. Refrigerate for up to 3 days.

2.   Toss all the fritter ingredients except oil in a bowl with ½ teaspoon each salt and pepper.

3.   Heat a large skillet over medium-high heat and drizzle in 3 tablespoons oil, enough to coat the bottom.

4.   Once oil is hot, take about ¼ cup of the fritter mixture between your hands, pressing together so it adheres (doesn't have to be flat, you'll shape in the pan). Carefully place it in the skillet and flatten with a fish spatula. Working quickly, make 3 more and add them to the skillet, leaving about an inch in between.

5.   Cook for 3–4 minutes on each side (flipping gently), until golden brown and crisp. No peeking, let them do their thing, otherwise they'll fall apart. Transfer to a warm platter in a 200°F oven. Repeat for remaining fritters.

6.   Set a nonstick skillet over medium heat and add 2 tablespoons oil, enough to coat the bottom well.

7.   Crack in eggs, leaving an inch in between (do this in 2 batches if needed). Fry them for about 5 minutes, until the whites and yolks are set. To accomplish this without the bottom getting too crispy before the yolk is cooked, spoon hot oil from the pan over the eggs fairly often. Sprinkle with salt, pepper, and red pepper flakes for some heat.

8.   To serve, overlap 2–3 fritters per plate, add avocado slices, top with an egg, and drizzle generously with cilantro sauce.

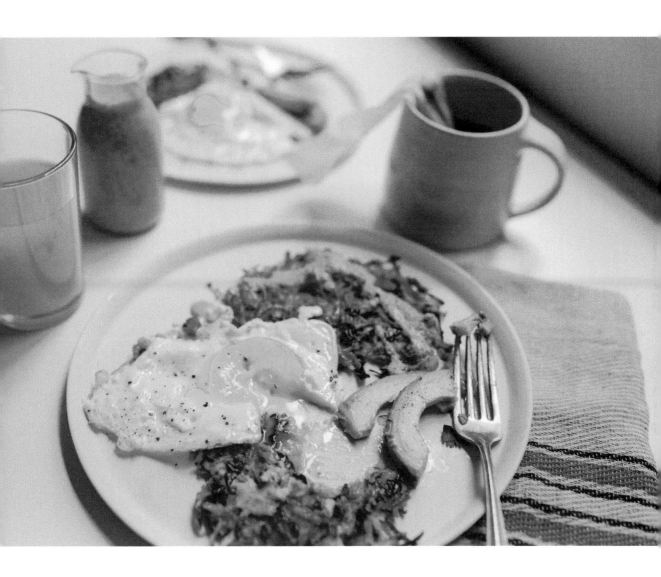

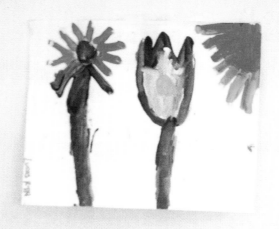
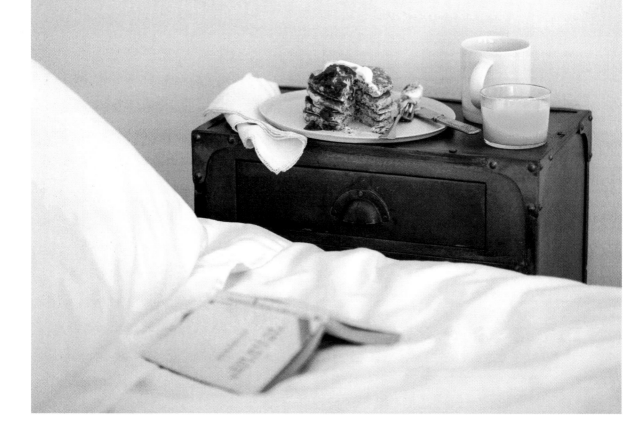

Lemon-Poppy Pancakes with Warm Berry Compote

Serves: 4

_____

Berry compote

1½ cups frozen mixed berries or just raspberries

1 teaspoon vanilla extract (or 2 teaspoons vanilla bean paste)

1 teaspoon lemon juice

¼ cup sugar or maple syrup

¼ cup water

Pancakes

1½ cups all-purpose flour

2 tablespoons sugar

2 teaspoons baking powder

½ teaspoon baking soda

¼ cup poppy seeds

¼ teaspoon salt

1 cup ricotta cheese, room temperature

1 large egg, room temperature

1 cup buttermilk, room temperature

1 teaspoon vanilla extract

Zest of 1 lemon, plus 2 teaspoons juice

2 tablespoons unsalted butter, melted, plus extra for brushing pan

Whipped cream or crème fraîche, for serving

This is one recipe in the book that you're *not* going to make. Bookmark this page and hand it over to someone else. This weekend you feast in bed, so grab a pile of magazines or the book you've been wanting to finish. You'll be getting room service. They say you teach people how to treat you, and we like to teach people to feed us.

1. Place all the compote ingredients in a small saucepan set over medium heat. Simmer for 10–15 minutes, stirring occasionally until thickened and coats the back of a spoon. Set aside and keep warm.

2. In a large bowl, whisk flour, sugar, baking powder, baking soda, poppy seeds, and salt.

3. In a smaller bowl, whisk together the ricotta, egg, buttermilk, vanilla, lemon juice, zest, and melted butter.

4. Pour the wet ingredients into the dry and mix until just combined. The batter will be thick and fluffy.

5. Heat a griddle or nonstick pan over medium heat. Brush on a little butter, then add ¼ cup batter for each pancake, leaving an inch in between. Nudge the batter a bit with a spatula to create an even round.

6. Cook for 2–3 minutes on each side until deeply golden and set, flipping gently. Transfer to a warm platter in the oven and continue until you've used up all the batter. Serve immediately with plenty of berry compote and dollops of whipped cream or crème fraîche.

_____

Kitchen note: In the spring and summer, top with ripe berries or peaches.

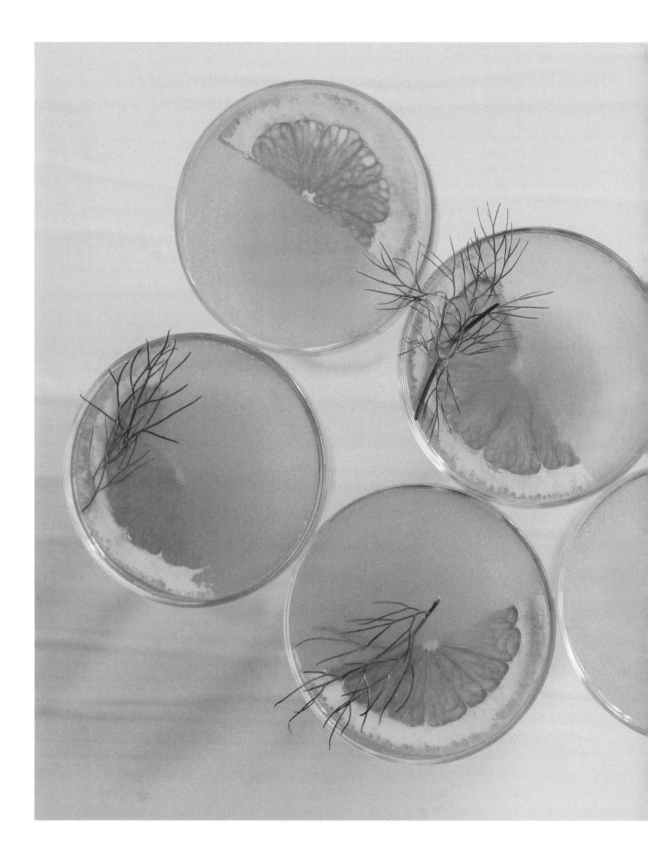

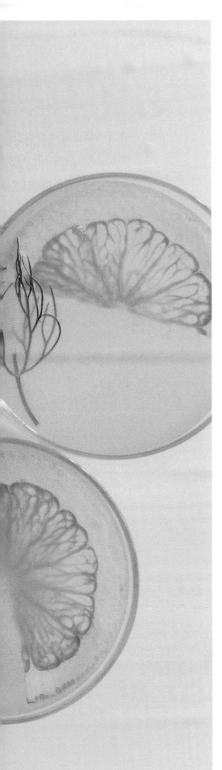

Grapefruit-Fennel & Allspice Gimlet

A pretty coral-colored cocktail that smells so good it could be a perfume, but it's also strong, spiced, complex, herbal, tart, and sweet. All good qualities to liven up a midwinter get-together.

Serves: 2

I small fennel bulb;
save the fronds for garnish

Juice of I grapefruit,
plus slices for garnish

Juice of I lime

I ounce St. Elizabeth
Allspice Dram

1½ teaspoons raw honey

3 ounces gin

Ice cubes

Cardamom bitters or
grapefruit bitters, optional

1. Using a box grater, finely grate the fennel. You'll need 4 tablespoons for every 2 cocktails. In the bottom of a cocktail shaker, muddle the fennel really well.

2. Add in a handful of ice and pour in 3 ounces grapefruit juice, 1 ounce lime juice, allspice dram, honey, and gin.

3. Shake, shake, shake, then strain into 2 ice-filled glasses. Add 1 or 2 dashes of optional bitters. Garnish with thinly sliced grapefruit and a fennel frond.

Apricot Bourbon Smash

Serves: 2

4 ounces bourbon

1-2 tablespoons apricot preserves, depending on how sweet you'd like it

Juice of 1 lemon
(2 ounces needed)

Ice cubes

2 cinnamon sticks

A cocktail for *once upon a midnight dreary, in the bleak December* (or never-ending January). When you're *pondering, wondering, fearing, doubting, dreaming dreams no mortals ever dared to dream before.* And *suddenly there came a tapping, as of someone gently rapping, rapping at your chamber door.* 'Twas just your offspring parched and weary . . .

1. In a cocktail shaker, combine the bourbon, apricot preserves, and lemon juice and shake for 10 seconds, until there are no clumps of apricot preserves.

2. Fill two glasses with ice and pour in the drink.

3. Using metal tongs, hold the cinnamon sticks over an open flame. Turn them so they don't burn too much on any side. You'll start to smell the cinnamon after about 10 seconds. Garnish each drink with a smoky cinnamon stick.

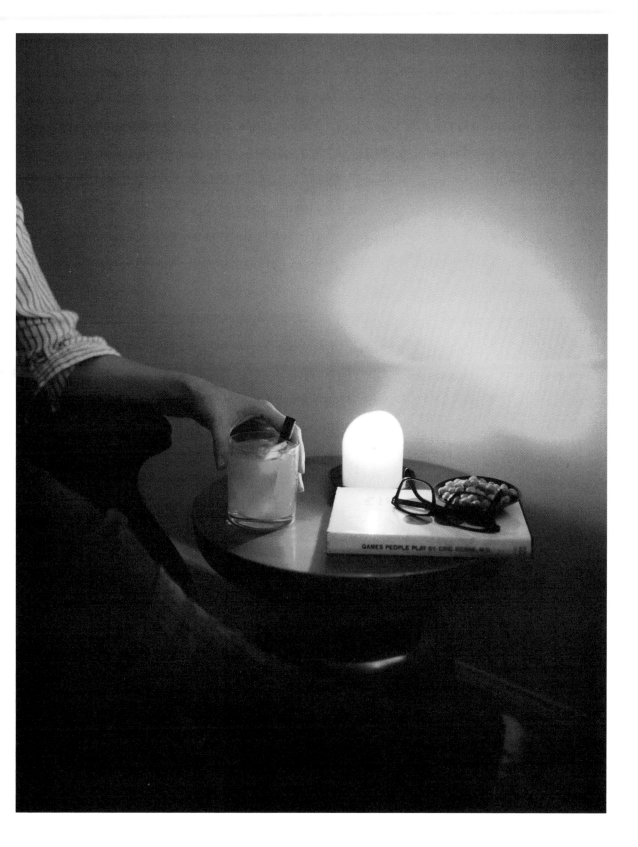

Miracle Elixir

Make this the minute you feel an ever so faint scratchy throat. You know, the kind that could turn into something more but you can't tell if it's a cold coming or if you just haven't been drinking enough water (again). Drink when almost sick, full-blown sick, or just because it's really good.

———————

Note: You could double or triple the recipe to keep a big batch in the fridge for up to a week. Reheat cups as needed.

Serves: 2

———————

2-3-inch piece fresh ginger; you can reuse for another batch

3 cups water

I small lemon, halved

2 tablespoons raw honey, or to taste

1. Wash ginger and thinly slice. No need to peel it.

2. In a small saucepan, bring the water and ginger to a boil. Cover with a lid and reduce heat to simmer for 15 minutes. Turn off heat and steep for longer if you want. The longer it steeps, the stronger the ginger flavor.

3. Pour the tea through a fine mesh strainer into two mugs. Into each mug stir the juice of ½ lemon and a tablespoon of honey (or both to taste).

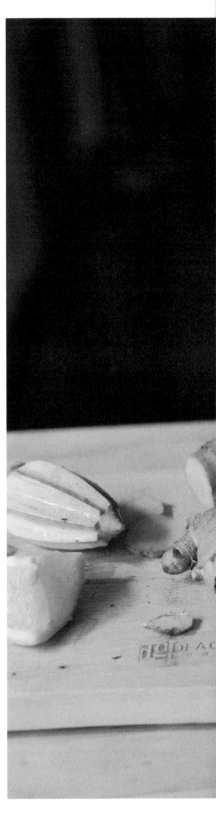

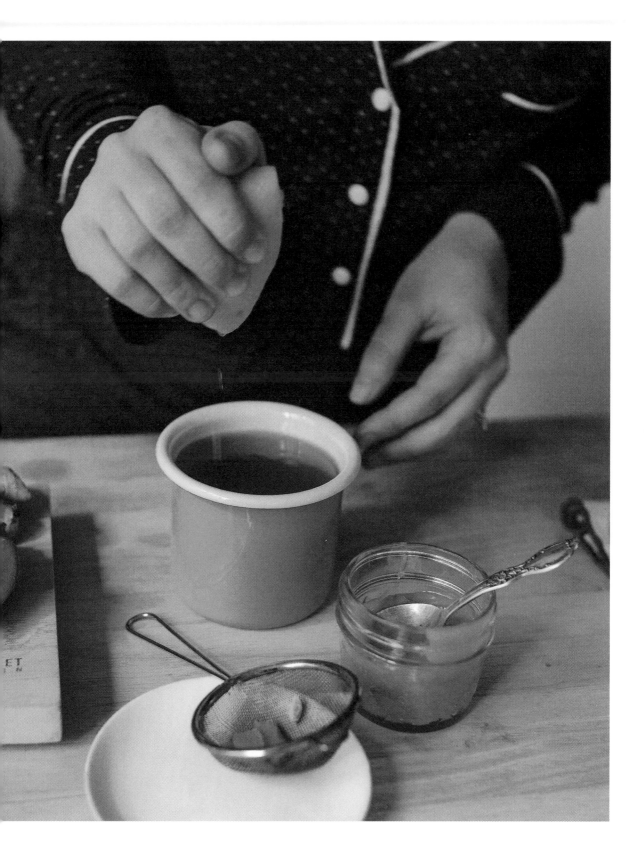

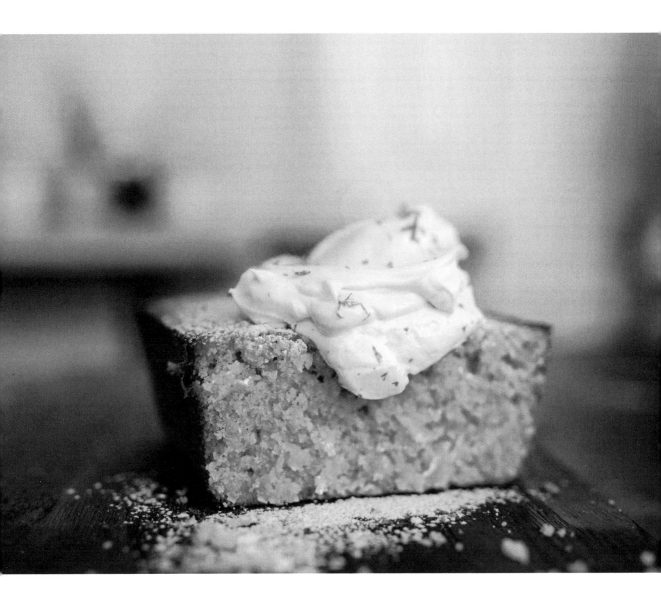

Coconut Lime Loaf

Serves: 8

---

1 cup almond meal

1 cup cornmeal, fine
or medium ground

1 cup unsweetened
shredded coconut

1½ teaspoons baking powder

¼ teaspoon salt

8 tablespoons unsalted butter,
softened

¾ cup sugar

2 large eggs,
at room temperature

¾ cup full-fat coconut milk

2 limes, both zested and 1 juiced

2 teaspoons vanilla extract

Whipped cream, for serving

There comes a time in February when your sanity basically hinges on boarding a plane to Very Far Away. The next best thing is a warm slice of this tropical-esque loaf.

1. Preheat oven to 350°F.

2. In a medium bowl, whisk together the almond meal, cornmeal, coconut, baking powder, and salt. Set aside.

3. Beat the butter and sugar in the bowl of a stand mixer fitted with a paddle attachment, or use a handheld mixer.

4. After about a minute, add the eggs one at a time, making sure to mix well after each. Follow with the coconut milk, lime zest, lime juice, and vanilla.

5. Fold the dry ingredients into the wet ingredients with a spatula, taking care not to overmix. Pour into a buttered 9-inch loaf pan and transfer to the oven for 40–45 minutes, baking until cake is golden brown and a toothpick comes out mostly clean. It won't rise very much.

6. Cool cake slightly for 15 minutes, then take it out of the pan. Serve slices with a dollop of whipped cream and extra lime zest.

Say-Anything Cake

Serves: 6

Vanilla cake

½ cup unsalted butter,
at room temperature

I cup brown sugar

½ cup sugar

2 cups all-purpose flour

½ teaspoon salt

1½ teaspoons baking powder

½ teaspoon baking soda

2 large eggs,
at room temperature

½ cup sour cream, at room
temperature

I tablespoon vanilla extract

I cup whole milk,
at room temperature

Chocolate frosting

½ cup unsalted butter

²/₃ cup cocoa powder

I cup powdered sugar

²/₃ cup heavy cream

½ teaspoon vanilla extract

Decorating

Sprinkles or white icing

This cake is fuss-free and easy, for any day and any reason—celebrating, appreciating, apologizing, comforting, or just because you need cake.

1. Cake: Preheat oven to 350°F.

2. In a stand mixer fitted with the paddle attachment, beat the butter and sugars until light and fluffy, 5–7 minutes. Scrape the sides occasionally.

3. Mix the dry ingredients together in a bowl and set aside.

4. Add the eggs to the stand mixer bowl and mix for another minute.

5. Then add the sour cream and vanilla; mix well.

6. Turn the mixer to the lowest setting and add half the flour mixture, then half the milk, remaining flour, and remaining milk. Do not overmix.

7. Grease a 9-by-13-inch cake pan, pour the cake batter in, and even out the top with a spatula. Transfer to the oven and bake for 25–30 minutes or until a toothpick comes out clean. Remove from oven and set aside to cool completely.

8. Frosting: Melt butter in a saucepan over medium heat.

9. Whisk in cocoa powder, then turn off heat.

10. Add the powdered sugar (it will get really clumpy). Whisk in heavy cream and vanilla until glossy and super smooth, about 3 minutes. Allow to cool completely.

11. Spread the frosting over the cake. Write what you need to say. Top with sprinkles.

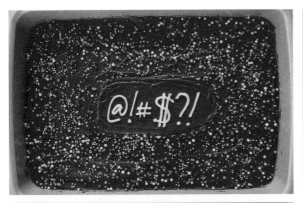

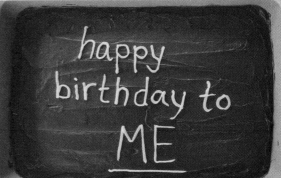

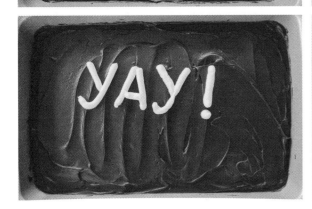

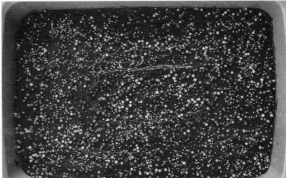

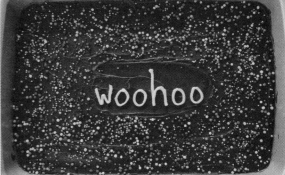

The Whole Point

The last page. You made it.

You're cooking more often in the kitchen and have even added on a few new habits along the way. And there were moments, probably when you least expected them, when you noticed. Those changes you wished so much to make (and some you didn't even know you wanted to make) actually happened. You can't pinpoint when they happened exactly, but they did. That's the Huckle & Goose Effect.

It happens when your kid finally declares broccoli to be the best vegetable, even though it took two years.

It comes in the form of Saturday game nights, with dinner and drinks, now a tradition at your place.

It happens on weekend mornings when you realize you'd rather stay home because you make a mean brunch. You spend less on takeout because of those memorized pantry recipes up your sleeve. That savings account is now growing, slowly but surely.

It's when you completely impress your boss with that afternoon presentation because you actually took a lunch break, saw the sunshine, and sat in the park with your packed lunch.

It strikes in the form of a veggie burger craving even though you went out for burger burgers. You still love them, but you learned to notice when your body's not in the mood for meat.

It's that moment of gratitude that washes over you as you're about to start on dinner. Wait, when did it switch from dread to gratitude? It was almost undetectable, yet here you are. Keep looking for the Huckle & Goose Effect.

Bring your Something Sweet to the new neighbors three houses down. Take a giant bowl of warm Bolognese to friends who just had a baby. When a friend texts about a rough day, say, "Come over," and start simmering the most comforting soup you know how to make in your cheery yellow pot. It's your co-worker's birthday, so you bake a real birthday cake. For the office-wide card signing, everyone had to write *specifically* why work wouldn't be the same without said co-worker. He's smiled a little more ever since.

When you feel the nudge to invite an acquaintance over for dinner, don't dismiss it and give in to the usual *What if it's awkward?* thoughts. Encourage your kids, spouse, roommate to invite someone over a couple of times a month. Make it known that your home is open to all.

If your dinner table is constantly filled with people who look, talk, and think like you, you probably won't really grow in compassion and empathy, or experience the thrill of getting to understand a new perspective. There isn't an equation for this, and don't invite people over *just* because they're different from you. Just be open to it. We're human, and need other humans and each other's stories.

That really is the whole point. In the end, isn't that what we all want? To make our little corner a bit more bright and to invite others into that. There isn't one specific method or way. It's not all about what you cook or eat, the people you surround yourself with, whether you're outside a lot or a little, or how great your routine is. It starts with noticing yourself and layering all these small, everyday things within the context of your personality, time, budget, circumstances, and what's important to you. All these tiny habits, done somewhat consistently, can add up to a pretty great life.

The Whole Point

Acknowledgments

If you're anything like us, this is the page you'll skip. But if you knew us, you'd know there's no way we could've done this by ourselves. Not only that, the amount of time and work that go into a cookbook—geez Louise!

Mandalyn: Our photographer and linen-placement whisperer. It's truly a miracle that we found you. You are a ridiculously talented photographer and human. Thank you for capturing the heart of H&G and jumping into totally unknown creating-a-book-from-scratch territory with us, all while having a thirty-five-pound baby strapped to you during shoots.

Lindsay: Our ever-patient agent. Who saw an ounce of potential in us, refined our vision for this cookbook, and helped make it happen every step of the way.

Julie: Our incredible editor. You're the perfect combination of "run with your vision, I trust you" and "wake up, this sucks, we need to fix it." Our first meeting in the fancy NYC office surrounded by books and lots of people really good at their job felt straight out of a movie, and it hasn't stopped feeling surreal since. We're so profoundly grateful you took a chance on us.

The whole team at Harper: Haley, for keeping us on track. Leah, for designing the book of our dreams. And our copy editor, who kept us PC and saved us from some headnotes that could've upset the Internet trolls.

Cast Iron (Jonny & Richard): You guys have been there since H&G was just a business plan and brought it to life. And then brought our cover to life as well. Please don't become so successful that we can't afford you.

Keri: Thank you for designing a book proposal that made us look legit and got us here in the first place.

Didi: How many pages did you read, and read, and helped us edit and edit and edit. Thank you for saving us from awkward phrasing and sentences that made no sense.

All. Our. Kids. There are seven between us. Thank you for all forcing smiles when we yelled at you to hold spoons "naturally." And for only asking us thirty times a shoot, "Can we eat now?"

And finally our husbands: We had encouraging words from Andrew like "You guys better not suck" and then, when you saw the finished manuscript, you said, "Dude, this could actually sell lots of copies!" Dumitru for always walking in during food styling and stealing food before we got the shot, but also thanks for going to Home Depot with us and making the faux tabletops.

For helping us spruce up the place: Room & Board, Interior Define, Joybird, Minted, Lindsay Letters, Schoolhouse Electric, Yamazaki, Parachute Home, Newgate Clocks, Marshall Speakers, Lostine, Brooklyn Candle Co., Everlane, Rove Concepts, Mifuko, Re-co Bklyn.

For making us love our jobs cooking and styling food even more: Canvas Home, Le Creuset, Santimetre Studio, Baking Steel, R. Murphy Knives, Boo Louis for Ekobo, Aha Life, Crow Canyon, MoccaMaster, The Spice House, Farmhouse Pottery, Blackcreek M&T Co., Kinto, Flotsam & Fork.

Happy hours wouldn't have been happy without: Bittermens, Jack Rudy Co., Casamigos, Barr Hill, Scrappy's Bitters, Kings County Whiskey, Neversink Spirits, Van Brunt Stillhouse.

Authors' Note

One more thing.

Very early on, we decided that if we were going to spend more than two years pitching and brainstorming and writing and shooting and editing a book for home cooks, it needed to be one that would really help you do this in your own home, on a regular basis. No matter your kitchen size, cooking experience, number of pots or kitchen appliances you own.

We quickly found out there's usually a small army behind the scenes of shooting a cookbook. Food stylists, photographers, prop stylists, assistants to the stylists, sometimes rented spaces— and all these food-styling tricks to make the food look extra-perfect and glossy.

But we kept it just us and our photographer. Not just because we couldn't afford the small army, but because it didn't seem fair to celebrate the home cook and then have people trailing behind us making everything prettier.

Almost the entire book was shot in Anca's '70s New York apartment with popcorn ceilings and a meh kitchen. Because that's real life. That's where we eat all the time. We styled the food we cooked so you could do the same. Our photographer helped in every way possible to get that final magic shot. Our kids were in the next room playing with Legos or on their fifteenth episode of something. Our teenagers helped with the dishes when they got home from school. We didn't rent props. We used what we had and were super-selective about buying new things because we'd actually use them long past the shoots.

We really, really want you to know you can cook this way and make things look a little nicer, too. To set out the nice linen and pretty plates, not just when you have people over, and even if it's for Thai takeout. It makes a difference. It's the everyday stuff, just a little happier. That's why we wrote the book.

Index

Page references in *italics* refer to illustrations.

Index

Index

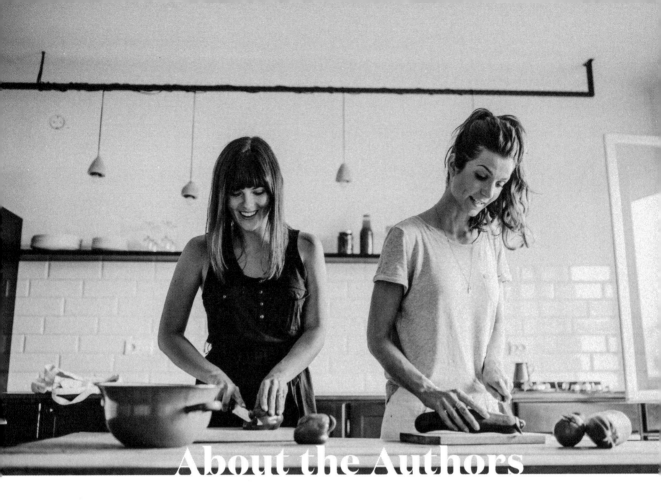

About the Authors

Anca has an affinity for all things spicy and loves to add butter to any recipe she's developing. She has a knack for making people laugh, tends to interrupt people when they talk (she's working on this), and loves to feed as many people as she can. She used to work in PR, was a private chef, and also had a brief stint in TV when she failed to win any money on *Deal or No Deal*. She lives in New York City with her husband, four kids, and one sheepadoodle (who she says is her favorite child).

Christine is equal parts type-A and artistic. She does calligraphy for fun (which landed her in some national publications), has a financial analyst background that kept the company from caving in, and unabashedly sings out loud. It should be noted that, while she's an expert cook, she still gets skeeved at touching a raw chicken. Of all the things she plans and organizes, dinner parties and birthday surprises are her favorites. She lives in Virginia wine country with her husband, three kids, and a potential future kitten (she hasn't decided yet).